Caring for the Heart Failure Patient

Caring for the Heart Failure Patient

A textbook for the health care professional

Edited by

Simon Stewart PhD RN NFESC FAHA
Professor and National Heart Foundation of
Australia Chair of Cardiovascular Nursing
School of Nursing and Midwifery
University of South Australia
Adelaide
Australia

Debra K Moser DNSc RN FAAN
Professor and Gill Chair of Cardiovascular Nursing
University of Kentucky
College of Nursing
Lexington, KY
USA

David R Thompson PhD RN FRCN FESC
Professor of Nursing and Director
Nethersole School of Nursing
Chinese University of Hong Kong
Hong Kong
China

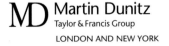
Martin Dunitz
Taylor & Francis Group
LONDON AND NEW YORK

A CIP record for this book is available from the British Library.

ISBN 1 84184 041 6

Distributed in the USA by
Fulfilment Center
Taylor & Francis
10650 Toebben Drive
Independence, KY 41051, USA
Toll Free Tel: +1 800 634 7064
E-mail: taylorandfrancis@thomsonlearning.com

Distributed in Canada by
Taylor & Francis
74 Rolark Drive
Scarborough, Ontario M1R 4G2, Canada
Toll Free Tel: +1 877 226 2237
E-mail: tal_fran@istar.ca

Distributed in the rest of the world by
Thomson Publishing Services
Cheriton House
North Way
Andover, Hampshire SP10 5BE, UK
Tel: +44 (0)1264 332424
E-mail: salesorder.tandf@thomsonpublishingservices.co.uk

Composition by EXPO Holdings, Malaysia
Printed and bound in Spain by Grafos SA Arte Sobre Papel

Contents

Contributors

Cynthia D Adams RN MSN CS
The Care Group, LLC
8333 Naab Road, Suite 400
Indianapolis IN 46260
USA

Linda S Baas PhD RN ACNP
Associate Professor and Director of Acute Care Program
University of Cincinnati College of Nursing
PO Box 210038
Cincinnati OH 45221-0038
USA

John Beltrame BMBS FRACP PhD FESC
Senior Lecturer in Medicine
The University of Adelaide
Northwestern Adelaide Health Service
$c/_o$ The Queen Elizabeth Hospital
Cardiology Unit
28 Woodville Road, Woodville South SA 5011
Adelaide, Australia

Susan J Bennett DNS RN
Professor
Indiana University School of Nursing
1111 Middle Drive, NU 317C
Indianapolis, IN 46202
USA

John Byrne MRCP
Consultant Cardiologist
Department of Cardiology Medical Unit C
Southern General Hospital
1345 Govan Road
Glasgow G51 4TF
UK

Patricia C Clark PhD RN
Emory University
Nell Hodgson Woodruff School of Nursing
531 Asbury Circle NE
Atlanta, GA 30022
USA

Ginger Conway MSN RN CNP
Field Service Instructor and Heart Failure
Nurse Practitioner
University of Cincinnati Medical Center
Internal Medicine – Cardiology Department
PO Box 670542
231 Albert Sabin Way
Cincinnati, OH 45267-0542
USA

Andrew P Davie MD MRCP
Consultant Cardiologist
Department of Cardiology Medical Unit C
Southern General Hospital
1345 Govan Road
Glasgow G51 4TF
UK

Lynn V Doering DNSc RN
Associate Professor
University of California
Los Angeles
School of Nursing
CA, USA

Robert N Doughty
Senior Lecturer in Cardiology
Department of Medicine
University of Auckland
Park Road, Auckland
New Zealand

Sandra B Dunbar DSN RN FAAN
Charles Howard Candler Professor
Emory University
Nell Hodgson Woodruff School of Nursing
1520 Clifton Road NE
Atlanta, GA 30322-4207
USA

Bengt Fridlund PhD RN
Professor of Nursing
Lund University
Lund
Sweden

Marjorie Funk PhD RN FAAN
Professor
Yale University School of Nursing
100 Church Street South
PO Box 9740
New Haven CT 06536-0740
USA

Anna Gawlinski DNSc RN CS ACNP
Clinical Nurse Specialist
Associate Adjunct Professor
Medical Center and School of Nursing
University of California
10775 Wilkins Avenue
Unit 103
Los Angeles CA 90024
USA

Rosemary Gee RN MSN
Emory University
Nell Hodgson Woodruff School of Nursing
531 Asbury Circle NE
Atlanta, GA 30022
USA

John D Horowitz
Professor, Department of Cardiology
University of Adelaide/The Queen Elizabeth
Hospital, 28 Woodville Rd, Woodville
South Australia 5011
Australia

Kimberly Hudson MSN RN
Nurse Practitioner
Middlesex Cardiology Associates
520 Saybrook Road
Middletown, Connecticut
USA

Tiny Jaarsma PhD RN NFESC
Associate Professor
Department of Cardiology
University Hospital Groningen
PO Box 30.001
9700 RB Groningen
The Netherlands

Terry A Lennie PhD RN
Associate Professor
The Ohio State University
College of Nursing
Ohio
USA

Kate MacIntyre
Department of Public Health
Glasgow University
2 Lilybank Gardens
Glasgow G12 8RZ
UK

John JV McMurray MD FRCP FESC FACC
Professor of Medical Cardiology and Honorary
Consultant Cardiologist
Department of Cardiology
Western Infirmary
Glasgow G11 6NT
UK

Jan Mårtensson RN PhD
Assistant Professor
Halmstad University
Halmstad
Sweden

Debra K Moser DNSc RN FAAN
Professor and Gill Chair of Cardiovascular Nursing
University of Kentucky, College of Nursing
527 CON Building
760 Rose Avenue
Lexington, KY 40536-0232
USA

Mark C Petrie
Specialist Registrar in Cardiology
CRI in Heart Failure,
Wolfson Building,
University of Glasgow,
Glasgow G12 8QQ
UK

Mariann R Piano PhD RN
Associate Professor
University of Illinois at Chicago
College of Nursing (MC 802)
845 S. Damen
Chicago, IL 60612
USA

Milton L Pressler MD
Clinical Development
Cardiovascular and Metabolic Diseases
Pfizer Global Research and Development
Ann Arbor
MI 48105
USA

Karen Smith PhD RN NFESC
Clinical Research Fellow in Cardiac Nursing
University of Dundee
Dundee
UK

Simon Stewart PhD RN NFESC
Professor and National Heart Foundation of
Australia Chair of Cardiovascular Nursing
School of Nursing and Midwifery
University of South Australia
4th Floor Centenary Building, City East Campus
Frome Road
Adelaide 5000
Australia

Anna Strömberg RN PhD
Assistant Professor
Department of Medicine and Care
Linköping University
Linköping
Sweden

David R Thompson PhD RN FRCN FESC
Professor of Nursing and Director
Nethersole School of Nursing
Chinese University of Hong Kong
Hong Kong
China

Mary A Woo DNSc RN
UCLA School of Nursing
PO Box 956917
Los Angeles, CA 90095
USA

Preface

There is little doubt that during the past decade heart failure has emerged as a 'growth industry' within the health care systems of developed countries. The reasons for this, of course, are relatively straightforward. The underlying prevalence of heart failure has increased dramatically and we have become much more heart failure 'aware' in terms of screening and detection. As predicted, we now have a situation where greater longevity and survival from previously fatal cardiac events, two key markers of a combination of better public health initiatives, and dramatic changes in medical treatment have left us with a far more vulnerable population in whom heart failure has thrived.

The emergence of an 'epidemic' of heart failure has led to a parallel imperative to limit its impact both on an individual and societal level. Much time and effort has been devoted, therefore, to understanding heart failure and to improving therapeutic options (with the hope of providing a cheap and effective cure). Unfortunately, we rarely see a coordinated and orderly response to health issues and the management of heart failure has suffered accordingly. The likelihood of any one clinician having a complete mastery of the subtleties and nuances of the pathophysiology and treatment of this heterogeneous condition is naturally small – the field is simply too vast. On the other hand, we have seen a dramatic increase in the range and sophistication of therapeutic options for the detection, treatment and overall management of heart failure and, given the right mix of expert opinions, these can be presented and absorbed in a coherent and holistic manner.

It is within this context that we present the first edition of *Caring for the Heart Failure Patient*. This textbook is designed to give the reader an overall view of the most salient and important features of the epidemiology, pathophysiology, treatment and therapeutic management of the patient with heart failure.

We believe *Caring for the Heart Failure Patient* has a number of key features that distinguish it from other textbooks. The first thing you will probably note is that we have assembled a truly international cast of experts to reflect the global nature of heart failure and the similarities in problems and issues that confront those who are forced to deal with this malignant syndrome, irrespective of whether they live in the southern or northern hemisphere and regardless of the type of health care system in which they operate. You may also note that the majority of the contributors are academic cardiovascular nurses. Cardiovascular nurses have effectively filled the 'void' in managing the increasing number of complex cases of heart failure by providing cost-effective care where no other care would have been provided due to the limited capacity of current health care systems. This book is a reflection of the increasing sophistication in cardiovascular nursing and the type of contribution it can make to better outcomes. Finally, you may also note that the title of this book is different. The real emphasis of this textbook is on 'caring' for heart failure rather than just 'treating' heart failure. In addition to being a reflection of the nursing orientation of our international contributors, it also represents an explicit acknowledgement that our ability to effectively manage and ultimately cure heart failure is still suboptimal. In their absence, when our patients (and their carers) are still suffering from the effects of heart failure and are still dying despite our best efforts, there is still scope to offer the therapeutic benefits of individual care and attention to improve the quality of their life and, ultimately, death.

We hope, therefore, that this book will provide a rich resource of information and ideas and equip you to provide quality health care to those affected by heart failure.

Simon Stewart
Debra K Moser
David R Thompson

1 Heart failure: epidemiological considerations for the new millennium

Simon Stewart, Kate MacIntyre and John JV McMurray

Introduction

Epidemiology is not an exact science. This is never more evident than when examining the literature describing the epidemiological features of heart failure. Firstly, heart failure is a complex syndrome with a number of different causes. It is on this basis that the term 'heart failure' is most commonly used to describe a constellation of symptoms. Unfortunately, we do not have a standard definition for heart failure – a fact that may become increasingly obvious to the reader of this textbook.

Given the inherent difficulty in defining and characterizing heart failure, it should come as no surprise that making direct comparisons between those epidemiological studies examining this lethal syndrome is fraught with difficulty. For example, whilst the data derived from the Framingham Heart Study in relation to heart failure remain the gold standard for describing its causes, consequences and overall burden, there are many limitations inherent to this study that should be considered. Whilst these are not unique to Framingham, they are worth mentioning. First and foremost, Framingham represents a relatively small, homogeneous, US-based cohort that largely represents the generation before the heart failure patient of today. Secondly, heart failure in this cohort was originally determined on clinical grounds rather than documented cardiac dysfunction (e.g. left ventricular systolic dysfunction). Although this does not devalue the data relating to this particular cohort, it does provide difficulties in comparing the Framingham cohort with other study cohorts. For example, we know that the risk factor profile for coronary heart disease within the population has changed with changing rates of hypertension, diabetes, smoking and hypercholesterolaemia over time. Modern treatments for many of the precursors of heart failure, including hypertension and heart disease, also differ dramatically than those used previously, as the era of clinical trials has ushered in a whole new armoury of effective pharmacological treatments.

Whilst heart failure is inherently difficult to characterize, it does represent a good example of why we need to undertake epidemiological studies in order to understand how we can prevent debilitating disease states and, often before an effective prevention strategy or cure is introduced, direct health care resources where they are needed most. It is within this context that this chapter summarizes the evidence to suggest that we are experiencing an 'epidemic' of heart failure that is likely to continue without a dramatic victory in our attempts to prevent and treat its most common precursors – hypertension and coronary artery disease.

The paradox of improved treatment of cardiovascular disease states

In recent decades, cardiovascular-related mortality rates have declined appreciably in most industrialized countries.[1] However, coronary heart disease remains a major contributor to morbidity and mortality.[2] Despite effective strategies to curb the incidence of coronary heart disease, the combination of better overall treatment of younger individuals and the trend towards larger and significantly older populations in Western developed countries[3] has resulted in its increased prevalence among older individuals.[2]

A major advance in confronting the impact of heart disease has been the significant reduction in the number of 'premature deaths' (i.e. previously fatal cardiac events in younger individuals).[2] This is not surprising considering the combined impact of more effective primary prevention, acute treatment and secondary prevention strategies designed to reduce the risk of developing coronary heart disease, improve the immediate prognosis for individuals who do experience an acute coronary event and to improve their subsequent prognostic outlook.[4,5]

Paradoxically, however, the initially improved survival prospects of individuals with acute myocardial infarction, for example, have no doubt contributed to an older patient population more susceptible to morbidity associated with advanced coronary heart disease and in particular the development of chronic heart failure.[2] The problems associated with a greater prevalence among older individuals (representing the 'residual' effects of better health care strategies overall), are becoming increasingly apparent. The most obvious example of this phenomenon is the increasing burden of chronic heart failure.[2]

The emergence of a heart failure epidemic

Heart failure, particularly in its chronic form, is now recognized as a major and escalating public health problem among industrialized countries with ageing populations.[6] However, determining its current burden on individual countries remains problematic. This uncertainty is the product of two related problems. In the first instance, heart failure represents a complex pathological process that is the terminal manifestation of a number of diverse cardiac disease states (e.g. ischaemic heart disease, valve disease, endocardial and pericardial problems and idiopathic cardiomyopathy, to list just a few). It is therefore associated with a broad spectrum of clinical presentations and defies simple definition. More importantly, perhaps, to date, there has been no large-scale, systematic investigation of the epidemiological features of chronic heart failure from both a physiological and clinical perspective within the same population.

The majority of epidemiological data relate to the 'symptomatic' syndrome of heart failure. However, there are undoubtedly many asymptomatic patients that might be legitimately labelled with a diagnosis of 'heart failure' (for example, those with asymptomatic left ventricular systolic dysfunction). Alternatively, the large-scale clinical trials largely concentrate on those patients with definitive evidence of left ventricular systolic dysfunction. Data from the Framingham cohort suggest that normal left ventricular systolic function is found in just over half those subjects with symptoms of heart failure.[7] The fact that women are more likely to experience symptoms of heart failure in the absence of systolic dysfunction is clearly one explanation for the gender imbalance inherent to clinical trials.

There are, however, a number of characteristics that are common to those patients who exhibit signs and symptoms of heart failure:

- abnormal neurohormonal regulation;
- unmet metabolic demand;
- breathlessness and associated intolerance to exercise;
- fluid retention

Also, there are typically five types of study used to describe the epidemiological characteristics of heart failure:

- Cross-sectional and longitudinal follow-up surveys of well-defined populations have focused almost exclusively on those individuals with clinical signs and symptoms indicative of chronic congestive heart failure.
- Cross-sectional surveys of individuals who have been medically treated for signs and symptoms of heart failure within a well-defined region.
- Echocardiographic surveys of individuals within a well-defined population to determine the prevalence of left ventricular systolic dysfunction.
- Nation-wide studies of annual trends in heart failure-related hospitalization identified on the basis of diagnostic coding at discharge.
- Comprehensive clinical trial and trial registry data sets. These include a large proportion of individuals who were identified on the basis of having both impaired left ventricular systolic dysfunction and signs and symptoms of heart failure.

Prevalence

Table 1.1[8–21] summarizes the reported prevalence of heart failure according to whether this was estimated from a survey of individuals requiring medical treatment in a primary care setting (receiving treatment from a general practitioner/primary care physician) or from population screening. Despite the wide variation in the reported overall prevalence of heart failure (largely reflecting different research methodologies and study cohorts), these data demonstrate that its prevalence increases markedly with age and that it has become more common over the past few decades.

Studies of patients within a primary care setting

In the UK there have been a number of large studies examining the prevalence of patients being treated for heart failure by a general practitioner. For example, in 1992, Parameshwar et al[11] examined the clinical records of diuretic-treated patients in three general practices in north-west London. From a total of 30 204 patients, a clinical diagnosis of heart failure was made in 117 cases (46 men and 71 women). The overall prevalence rate in this cohort was 3.9 cases/1000. Prevalence increased markedly with age. In those aged under 65 years the prevalence rate was 0.6 cases/1000 vs 28 cases/1000 in those aged 65 years and over. However, objective investigation of left ventricular function was performed in less than one-third of these patients. In 1995, Clarke et al[15]

Table 1.1. *Prevalence of heart failure*

Location of study	Overall prevalence	Age-specific prevalence
Surveys of community-treated patients		
UK national data (1958)[8]	3/1000	–
Rural cohort, USA (1966)[9]	9–10/1000	65/1000 (> 65 yrs)
UK national data (1988)[10]	11/1000	–
London, UK (1992)[11]	4/1000	28/1000 (> 65 yrs)
Rochester, UK (1993)[12]	3/1000 (< 75 yrs)	–
Liverpool, UK (1994)[13]	15/1000	80/1000 (> 65 yrs)
UK national data (1995)[14]	9/1000	74/1000 (65–74 yrs)
Nottinghamshire, UK (1995)[15]	8–16/1000	40–60/1000 (> 70 yrs)
Population cohorts		
Sheffield, UK (1953)[16]	–	30–50/1000 (> 62 yrs)
Georgia, USA (1966)[17]	21/1000 (45–74 yrs)	35/1000 (65–74 yrs)
Framingham, USA (1971)[18]	3/1000 (< 63 yrs)	23/1000 (60–79 yrs)
Sweden (males only) (1984)[19]	3/1000 (< 75 yrs)	80–170/1000 (> 67 yrs)
Gothenburg, Sweden (1989)[20]	–	130/1000 (> 67 yrs)
USA national data[21]	20/1000	80/1000 (> 65 yrs)

reported an even larger survey of chronic heart failure based on similar methods and including analysis of loop diuretic prescriptions for all residents of Nottinghamshire. They estimated that between 13 017 and 26 214 patients had been prescribed frusemide. Case note review of a random sample of those patients receiving such treatment found that 56% were being treated for heart failure. The prevalence rate in this cohort was therefore 8–16/1000. Once again, prevalence increased with advancing age (an estimated 40–60 cases/1000 in those aged > 70 years).

Population studies based on clinical criteria

The National Health and Nutrition Examination Survey (NHANES – 1)[21] reported prevalence of heart failure within the US population. Based on self-reporting, and a clinical scoring system, this study screened 14 407 persons of both sexes, aged 25–47 years, between 1971 and 1975, with detailed evaluation of only 6913 subjects and reported a prevalence rate of 20 cases/1000. The Helsinki Ageing Study in Finland describes clinical and echocardiographic findings in 501 subjects (367 female) aged 75–86 years.[22] Prevalence of heart failure, based on clinical criteria, was 8.2% overall (41 of 501) and 6.8%, 10% and

8.1% in those aged 75, 80 and 85 years, respectively. As might be expected in an elderly population with a clinical diagnosis of heart failure, there was a high prevalence of moderate or severe mitral or aortic valvular disease (51%), ischaemic heart disease (54%) and hypertension (54%). However, of the 41 subjects with 'heart failure', only 11 had significant left ventricular systolic dysfunction (diagnosed by fractional shortening or left ventricular dilation) and in 20 subjects no echocardiographic abnormality was identified. Despite this, the 4-year relative risk of all-cause and cardiovascular mortality associated with chronic heart failure in this population was 2.1 and 4.2, respectively, relative to the overall population.[22] Most recently, using the European Society of Cardiology guidelines for the diagnosis of chronic heart failure the EPICA Study in Portugal identified 551 patients via 365 selected general practitioners (GPs) to estimate the prevalence of heart failure in mainland Portugal in 1998.[23] The overall prevalence in the population aged 25 years or more was 4.4%, with similar prevalence in both men and women. The prevalence of heart failure rose from 1.4% in those aged 25–49 years, 12.7% in those aged 70–79 years and 16.1% in those aged > 80 years.[23]

Prevalence of left ventricular systolic dysfunction

There have been three notable estimates of the population prevalence of left ventricular systolic dysfunction as determined by echocardiography emanating from Scotland,[24] The Netherlands[25] and England.[26] The Scottish study targeted a representative cohort of 2000 persons aged 25–74 years. Of those selected, 1640 (83%) had a detailed assessment of their cardiovascular status and underwent echocardiography. Left ventricular systolic dysfunction was defined as a left ventricular ejection fraction ≤ 30%. The overall prevalence[24] of left ventricular systolic dysfunction using this criterion was 2.9%. Concurrent symptoms of heart failure were found in 1.5% of the cohort, whilst the remaining 1.4% was asymptomatic. Prevalence was greater in men and increased with age (in men aged 65–74 years it was 6.4% and in age-matched women 4.9%).[24] The Rotterdam Study in The Netherlands, although examining individuals aged 55–74 years, reported similar findings. Overall the prevalence of left ventricular systolic dysfunction, defined in this case as fractional shortening of ≤ 25%, was 5.5% in men and 2.2% in women.[25] More recently, Morgan et al[26] studied 817 individuals aged 70–84 years selected from two general practices in Southampton, England. Left ventricular function was assessed qualitatively as normal, mild, moderate or severe dysfunction. The overall prevalence of all grades of dysfunction was 7.5% (95% CI 5.8–9.5%). Prevalence of left ventricular dysfunction doubled between the ages of 70–74 years and > 80 years. A recent study based on patients attending three general practices in Copenhagen, Denmark, and with signs and symptoms indicative of heart failure found similar age- and sex-specific prevalence rates of left ventricular systolic dysfunction as determined by echocardiography – the overall prevalence in those aged ≥ 50 years being 2.9%.[27]

Incidence

It is important to note that there is much less known about the incidence than the prevalence of heart failure. The most detailed incidence data emanate from the Framingham Heart Study.[28] As noted in the introduction to this chapter, this important landmark study is based on the periodic screening of a small, geographically selected semi-urban population in the USA. As with the population-based prevalence studies, heart failure was defined according to a clinical scoring system. The only 'cardiac' investigation was a chest X-ray. After 34 years' follow-up, the incidence rate was approximately 2 cases/1000 in those aged 45–54 years, increasing to 40 cases/1000 in men aged 85–94 years.[18,29] Using similar criteria, Eriksson et al[20] reported incidence rates of 'manifest' heart failure of 1.5, 4.3 and 10.2 cases/1000, in men aged 50–54, 55–60 and 61–67 years, respectively. More recently, Rodeheffer et al[12] also reported the incidence of heart failure in a US population residing in Rochester, during 1981 in persons aged 0–74 years. The annual incidence was 1.1 cases/1000. Once again incidence was higher in men compared with women (1.57 vs 0.71 cases/1000 respectively). It also increased with age – new cases increasing from 0.76 male cases/1000 in those aged 45–49 to 1.6 male cases/1000 in those aged 65–69 years. In a preliminary analysis of the 20-year follow-up of the Renfrew/Paisley cohort in the West of Scotland (comprising 15 406 middle-aged men and women and with the study period ending in 1997), it was found that 4.7% of men and 3.6% of women experienced at least one new hospitalization with heart failure.[30] The Framingham Study reported male and female incidence rates per 100 000 patient-years of follow-up (652 cases detected over 34 years) of 200 and 100 in the age group 45–54 years, and 400 and 300 in those aged 55–64 years.[28] In support of these data, in the Renfrew/Paisley cohort, the equivalent male and female rates in these age groups were 205 and 113 (45–54) and 421 and 314 (55–64) (633 cases detected over 20 years of follow-up).[30]

Cowie et al have reported the most recent incidence study from an area of London with a population of approximately 150 000. In a 20-month period, 220 new cases of heart failure (118 male and 102 females) were identified from referrals to a GP-referred, rapid-access clinic (40 cases) specifically designed to increase detection rates,[31] and continuous surveillance of hospital admissions (180 cases) in the region.[32] Using a broad definition of heart failure, only 26% of those patients referred to the rapid access clinic for confirmation of heart failure were definitively diagnosed as such. Men (33%) were more likely than women (18%) to be found to have heart failure when referred to the clinic. In the male population, the incidence of heart failure was 1.4 per 1000 per year and in women 1.2. The overall incidence rate was 1.3/1000 population per annum. As expected there was a steep gradient in the incidence rate according to age: ranging from 0.02/1000 to 11.6/1000 population per annum in the age groups 25–34 years and 85 years and over, respectively.[32]

Table 1.2. *Incidence of heart failure*

Study	Location	Incidence rate (whole population)	Incidence rate in older age groups
Eriksson et al (1989)[20]	Sweden (men born in 1913)	–	10/1000 (*61–67 yrs*)
Remes et al (1992)[33]	Eastern Finland	1–4/1000 (*45–74 yrs*)	8/1000 (> 65 yrs)
Ho et al (1993)[29]	Framingham, US	2/1000	–
Rodeheffer et al (1993)[12]	Rochester, US	1/1000 (*< 75 yrs*)	16/1000 (*> 65 yrs*)
Stewart et al (2000)[30]	West of Scotland, UK	1–4/1000 (*45–64 yrs*)	
Cowie et al (1999)[32]	London, UK	1/1000	12/1000 (*> 85 yrs*)

Table 1.2[12,20,29,30,32,33] summarizes the data from the major incidence studies.

Hospitalization

Within the context of a number of unavoidable limitations (they are retrospective and cannot account for variations in coding practices and changing admission thresholds), some of the most reliable epidemiological data come from reports of heart failure-related hospital admissions.

Figure 1.1 compares reported hospitalization rates from Scotland,[34,35] the USA,[36,37] Sweden,[38] and The Netherlands on an age-specific basis.[39] It should be noted that these figures are difficult to interpret owing to differences in categorizing these admissions (e.g. whether or not heart failure as a secondary diagnosis is recorded as a heart failure admission) and the limitations of interpreting reported, rather than raw data.

Despite their limitations, these studies reveal three important points in relation to the epidemiology of heart failure. Firstly, all countries report age-adjusted increases

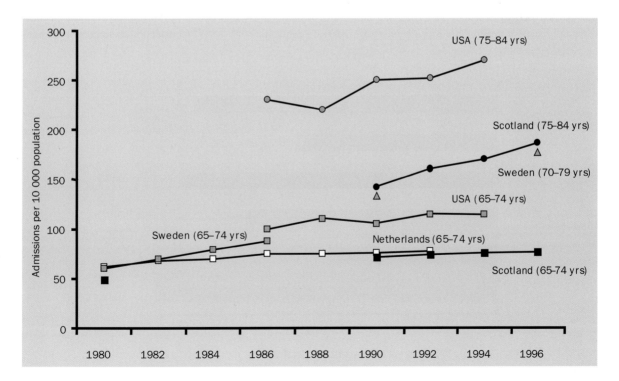

Figure 1.1. *Trends in hospitalization for heart failure.*

in admissions for heart failure during the period 1980–1995; preliminary reports from Scotland[35] and The Netherlands[40] suggest that those admissions associated with a primary diagnosis of heart failure have begun to plateau but there is little doubt that age-adjusted admission rates in older individuals particularly continue to rise. Secondly, in relation to the latter phenomenon, admission rates increase dramatically with age. This has also been shown in Spain[41] and New Zealand.[42] Finally, despite the variance in data collection and reporting, the rates of admission reported in these studies from a range of countries are remarkably similar when age groups are compared directly. In the USA, like many other countries, heart failure has been identified as the most common cause of hospitalization in people over the age of 65 years.[37] An admission for heart failure is frequently prolonged and in many cases followed by readmission within a short period of time.[35] Within the UK about one-third of patients are readmitted within 12 months of discharge,[34,35] whilst the same proportion are reported to be readmitted within 6 months in the USA.[36,37] Such readmission rates are usually higher than the other major causes of hospitalization, including stroke, hip fracture and respiratory disease.[43,44] On a sex-specific basis, men tend to be younger than women when admitted for the first time with heart failure, but because of greater female longevity, the number of male and female admissions are roughly equal. Moreover, the average age of individuals experiencing their first admission for heart failure appears to be increasing.[35,45]

A recent comparison of readmission rates associated with a number of conditions in three states in the USA and three European countries has highlighted the difficulty in comparing different regions owing to confounding variables. As expected, chronic heart failure, along with chronic pulmonary disease was associated with the highest readmission rates in both the USA and Europe. However, there was a clear inverse correlation between index length of stay and readmission rates. In essence, it was found that the shorter the initial length of stay the higher the readmission rate.[46] Although a heart failure-specific study of institutional variations in readmission and mortality rates did not find such an association when adjusting for a limited number of potential confounders,[47] both studies highlight the importance of evaluation of such data on a national and more specifically local level.

Economic burden

The management of heart failure consumes a significant amount of health care expenditure in developed countries. Figure 1.2 shows that heart failure is reported to consume between 1% and 2% of health care expenditure in these countries.[37,38,43–45,48–50] Considering the increasing rates of

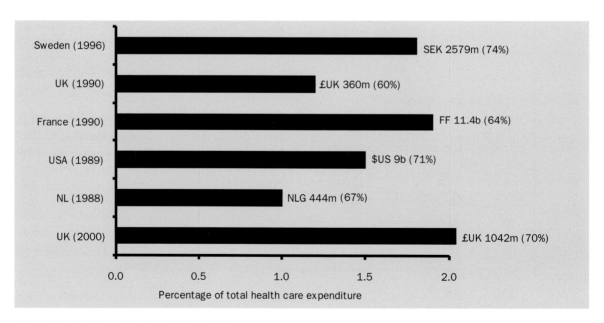

Figure 1.2. *The international cost of heart failure.*

hospitalization in these it is likely that these reported estimates fall short of the current burden of heart failure. Data from the UK best illustrate this. In 1990 heart failure was estimated to cost 1.3% of health care expenditure.[43] A decade later (year 2000 figures) heart failure was estimated to consume approximately 2.1% of expenditure (based 1990 equivalent expenditure levels) and, when the cost of hospitalization associated with a secondary diagnosis of heart failure was also considered, this figure rose markedly to 4%.[44]

Aetiology

Chapters 3 and 4 provide a detailed account of the pathophysiology of acute and chronic heart failure. It is important to note that although our understanding of heart failure in this respect continues to increase, there are still uncertainties about the relative contribution of the disease states commonly associated with this syndrome. For example, coronary heart disease, either alone or in combination with hypertension, *seems* to be the commonest cause of heart failure. It is, however, very difficult to be certain what the primary aetiology of heart failure is in a patient with multiple potential causes. Furthermore, even the absence of overt hypertension in a patient presenting with heart failure does not rule out an important aetiological role in the past with normalization of blood pressure as the patient develops pump failure. Importantly, data from both the Framingham[51,52] and Renfrew/Paisley studies,[30] which represent large-scale population cohorts followed up for a prolonged period, support the crucial role of hypertension in precipitating heart failure before acute manifestations of coronary heart disease emerge.

Some of the more common precursors of chronic heart failure include:

- coronary heart disease (e.g. consequent upon acute myocardial infarction);
- chronic hypertension;
- cardiomyopathy (dilated, hypertrophic, alcoholic and idiopathic);
- valvular dysfunction (diseases of the aortic or mitral valve);
- cardiac arrhythmias/conduction disturbance (heart block and atrial fibrillation);
- pericardial disease (constrictive pericarditis);
- infection (rheumatic fever, Chagas' disease, viral myocarditis and HIV).

Recent data from the Framingham cohort has also confirmed that obesity is likely to fuel more cases of heart failure in the next few decades, most probably due to 'metabolic' cardiovascular disease.[53]

As indicated above, in the initial cohort of the Framingham Heart Study monitored until 1965, hypertension appeared to be the most common cause of heart failure, being identified as the primary cause in 30% of men and 20% of women and a cofactor in a further 33% and 25% cases, respectively.[51] Disturbingly, national data from the USA confirm that hypertension remains largely uncontrolled and a key target for the future 'control' of the heart failure epidemic.[54] Furthermore, ECG evidence of left ventricular hypertrophy in the presence of hypertension carried an approximate 15-fold increased risk of developing heart failure.[51] In the subsequent years of follow-up, however, coronary heart disease became increasingly prevalent prior to the development of heart failure and, as the identified cause of new cases of heart failure, increased from 22% in the 1950s to almost 70% in the 1970s. During this period, the relative contribution of hypertension and valvular heart disease declined dramatically. As such, there was an approximate 5% and 30% decline in the prevalence per decade of hypertension during this period among men and women respectively.[54] The 'apparent' decline in the contribution of hypertension to heart failure most probably reflects the introduction of antihypertensive therapy; the parallel decline in the prevalence of left ventricular hypertrophy supports this supposition. However, as noted above, hypertension, as a major cause of heart failure, remains a major public health concern.[54] It is also probable that during this same period, progressively greater accuracy in determining the presence of coronary heart disease contributed to its increasing importance in this regard.

Any interpretation of the Framingham data also has to consider the fact that heart failure was identified on clinical criteria alone and undoubtedly included individuals without associated left ventricular systolic dysfunction. Conversely, the large-scale clinical trials have largely recruited patients who have reduced left ventricular ejection fractions and applied an extensive list of exclusion criteria. Table 1.3 is a summary of the most common attributed causes and associates of heart failure in a number of clinical trials and registries.[55–61]

In the study of left ventricular function in Western Scotland, 95% vs 71% of symptomatic and asymptomatic individuals with definite left ventricular systolic dysfunction had evidence of coronary heart disease (p = 0.04). Those

Table 1.3. Aetiology of heart failure in clinical trials and registers

	Clinical trials					Registers	
	SOLVD[55]	DIG Study[57]	MERIT-HF[58]	ATLAS[59]	RALES[58]	SOLVD[60]	SPICE[61]
	1991	1997	1999	1999	1999	1993	1999
Size of cohort	2569	6800	3991	3192	1663	6273	9580
Mean age	61	64	64	64	65	62	66
Male	80%	78%	78%	79%	73%	74%	74%
Aetiology of heart failure							
Ischaemic	71%	70%	66%	64%	54%	69%	63%
Non-ischaemic	–	29%	34%	35%	46%	31%	–
Hypertensive	–	9%	–	20%	–	7%	4%
Idiopathic cardiomyopathy	18%	15%	–	28%	–	13%	17%
Valvular	–	–	–	6%	–	–	5%
Other	–	6%	–	–	–	11%	–
Unknown	–	–	–	–	–	–	6%
Comorbidity							
Hypertension	42%	–	44%	46%	–	43%	27%
Diabetes	26%	–	25%	29%	–	23%	–
Atrial fibrillation	10%	–	17%	–	–	14%	–
Current angina	37%	–	–	27%	–		–
Respiratory disease	26%	–	–	–	–	15%	–

individuals with symptomatic heart failure were also more likely to have a past myocardial infarction (50% vs 14%; p = 0.01) and concurrent angina (62% vs 43%; p = 0.02). Hypertension (80%) and valvular heart disease (25%) were also more prevalent in those individuals with both clinical and echocardiographically determined heart failure compared with the remainder of the cohort, including those with asymptomatic left ventricular dysfunction (67% and 0%, respectively).[24] Therefore, the aetiological importance of the many associated causes of heart failure will depend on both the age-cohorts examined, and the type of criteria used to determine the presence of heart failure.

Prognosis

Irrespective of its aetiology or whether it is the subject of aggressive, active treatment (e.g. during acute hospitalization), heart failure is a lethal condition. The reported

prognostic implications of heart failure do vary, however, depending on the type of cohort studied (e.g. population vs clinical trial) the operational definition for heart failure (e.g. clinical vs echocardiographic criteria) and the time-frame in which mortality data is collated (e.g. 1970s vs 1990s). In general, those studies examining subjects selected from the population have far worse outcomes than those patients selected for clinical trials.

Population-based studies

Data from the original and subsequent Framingham cohort suggested the probability of someone dying within 5 years of being diagnosed with heart failure was 62% and 75% in men and 38% and 42% in women, respectively. In comparison, 5-year survival for all cancers in men and women combined within the USA during the same period was approximately 50%.[62]

The Rochester Epidemiology Project has described the prognosis in 107 older patients presenting to associated hospitals with new onset heart failure in 1981, and 141 patients presenting in 1991.[63] The mean age of the 1981 patients was 75 years rising to 77 years in 1991. The 1-year and 5-year mortality rate was 28% and 66% in the 1981 cohort and 23% and 67%, respectively, in the 1991 cohort. In other words, although the same diagnostic criteria used in the Framingham study were used in the Rochester project, the prognosis was somewhat better in the latter.

Another large, representative, epidemiological study reporting long-term outcome in patients with heart failure is the NHANES-I survey.[21] This survey initially evaluated 14 407 adults aged 25–74 years in the USA between 1971 and 75. Follow-up studies were carried out in 1982–1984 and again in 1986 (for those aged ≥ 55 years and alive during the 1982–1984 review). The estimated 10-year mortality rate in subjects aged 25–74 years with self-reported heart failure was 42.8% (49.8% in men and 36% in women). Mortality in those aged 65–74 years was 65.4% (71.8% and 59.5% in men and women, respectively). These mortality rates are considerably lower than those observed in Framingham. However, the patients in NHANES-I were non-institutionalized and their heart failure was self-reported and follow-up was incomplete. It was also carried out in a more recent time period than Framingham and the prognosis for heart failure may have improved (see Scottish data below); although neither study reported an improved prognostic outlook for heart failure over time.

A recent study of a population cohort in west London examined survival in patients with incident heart failure – detected via a screening programme of all GPs and hospitals in the region and diagnosed via a panel of three cardiologists who reviewed all diagnostic data including echocardiography.[64] The survival rate at 1 month in the 220 patients identified in this study was 81%, while 57% survived to 18 months. These rates are not surprisingly higher than that reported above given that a significant proportion of subjects were identified at the point of hospitalization.

Similarly, recent data from the whole Scottish population (approximately 5.1 million), with identification of all patients who experienced their 'first-ever' hospital admission associated with a principal diagnosis of heart failure, has been used to examine two important questions arising from the findings of the above studies:

1) Is the prognosis associated with heart failure improving over time?
2) Is heart failure as malignant as many types of cancer?

Improving prognosis?

Over the period 1986–95 a total of 66 547 patients were admitted to hospital in Scotland for the first time with heart failure. Women (n = 35 507) accounted for more than half (53.4%) of this patient cohort. The median age at admission was 78 years in women and 72 years in men.[45] Just over half (53%) of this cohort was aged over 75 years. Consistent with the Rochester Study,[63] the median age of women (76.0 years in 1986 compared with 79.0 years in 1995) and men (70.7 years in 1986 compared with 73.0 years in 1995) increased significantly over the period of study (p < 0.001).

During the whole period of study the crude case fatality rate at 30 days, 1 year, 5 years and 10 years in men was 19.4%, 44.0%, 75.0% and 87.2%, respectively. The equivalent rates were 20.3%, 44.9%, 76.2% and 89.3% in women, respectively. Not surprisingly, case fatality rates increased markedly with age with 1-month and 1-year case fatality rates increasing from 10.4% and 24.2% in those aged < 55 years to 25.9% and 58.1% in those aged > 84 years. Median survival over the period of study was 1.5 years in men and 1.4 years in women. For those surviving the initial 30-day period, median survival was 2.5 years in men and 2.4 years in women.[45] Figure 1.3 shows the 5-year survival rates in the 1991 cohort of men and women on an age-specific basis, demonstrating decreasing survival rates with age.

Adjusted case-fatality rates

Multivariate analysis confirmed the powerful effect of age on survival. The adjusted risk of death (30-day to end of follow-up) associated with each additional decade of age increased by 1.42-fold in men and 1.38-fold in women. The effect of sex on survival was both modest and complex. There was a highly significant interaction between age and sex, but only for 30-day case fatality. For example, in the short-term, younger women (aged < 65 years) fared worse than younger men, whilst older women (> 65 years) had a better outcome than older men. In the longer term (beyond 30 days), no age–sex interaction was detected and, overall, women had a lower case fatality than men. Greater deprivation was associated with a higher short-term case fatality rate (a 26% and 11% increased risk for those men and women in the lowest deprivation category compared to the highest). The equivalent risk of longer-term case fatality was increased by 10% in men and 6% in women. In general, a prior admission (regardless of the principal cause) increased the risk of death.[45]

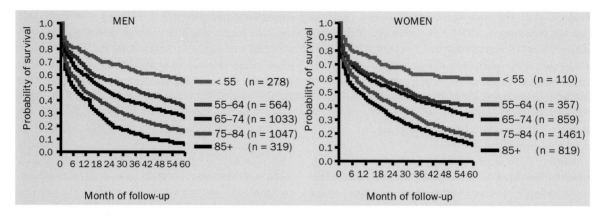

Figure 1.3. *Five-year survival rates following an incident heart failure admission in Scotland (1991).*

After adjustment for age, deprivation and prior admission the risk of 30-day case fatality fell by 26% in men and 17% in women (p < 0.001). Importantly, the adjusted risk of longer-term case fatality for each year of admission also fell by approximately 18% in men and 15% in women (p < 0.001) during this period.[45]

These data, therefore, support the hypothesis that the prognosis in heart failure has improved over time (at least in those hospitalized), although this needs to be confirmed by other studies and in non-institutionalized subjects.

More malignant than cancer?

In a related study, the 5-year survival rates for those patients admitted for the first time with heart failure in 1990 were directly compared with those patients admitted for the first time with the most common types of cancer (specific to men and women) in addition to acute myocardial infarction.[65] Figure 1.4 shows the crude, 5-year sur-

vival rates for each diagnosis, suggesting that heart failure is at least as 'malignant' as cancer and, as expected, has a worse prognosis than a first acute myocardial infarction. Multivariate analysis showed that, with the major exception of lung cancer, heart failure was associated with the poorest longer-term, adjusted survival in men. In women, both cancer of the breast and large bowel were associated with better short-term survival rates in comparison with heart failure. Subsequent long-term survival was more favourable in the former and equivalent in the latter. Alternatively, cancer of the ovary and lung were associated with poorer adjusted survival rates overall in comparison to heart failure.[65]

Consistent with more recent data from the Framingham Study,[66] it was found that heart failure was associated with a significant number of 'premature' life-years lost (on average 9 years per person), being associated with more deaths than the combination of large bowel, prostate and

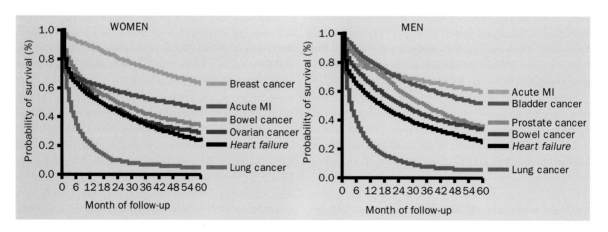

Figure 1.4. *Five-year survival rates: heart failure vs myocardial infarction and cancer (MI, myocardial infarction).*

bladder cancer. In women, despite the fact that proportionately more deaths occurred in those who had already exceeded average life expectancy, heart failure was second only to myocardial infarction in terms of the total number of premature deaths. Both lung and breast cancer, however, by virtue of a greater number of expected life-years lost per person had a greater impact on the population as a whole during this period.

Overall, these Scottish data[65] support those from the US-based Framingham cohort,[62,66] a similar report from Ontario, Canada, that mirrored the approach used in the Scottish study,[67] and the contemporary UK-based population cohort from London,[64] suggesting that heart failure survival rates, in both men and women, are comparable to or even worse than those associated with cancer.

Clinical trial data

Despite careful selection (predominantly younger males with less comorbidity), gold-standard pharmacotherapy and careful management, the mortality rates among participants in clinical trials have also been reportedly high.[68,69] For example, during 10-year follow-up of the original CONSENSUS-1 cohort (n = 253) only five patients were found to be alive.[70] During a mean follow-up of 41 months in the SOLVD study treatment arm, a total of 962 (39.7% in the placebo group vs 35.2% in the enalapril treated group) died.[55] The true contribution of heart failure to overall mortality or coronary heart disease-related mortality is almost certainly underestimated. Although it is highly prevalent among the elderly, is the endproduct of a number of cardiovascular disease states, and has been shown to be associated with extremely poor survival rates, official statistics continue to attribute only a small proportion of deaths to heart failure. A recent study of Scottish death data during the period 1979–92 showed that while heart failure was recorded as the underlying cause of death in only 1.5% of cases, it was found to be a contributory cause in an additional 14.3% of deaths.[71] Importantly, this study demonstrated that one-third of coronary heart disease-related deaths may have been due to heart failure.

Quality of life

Two large studies from the USA have shown that heart failure impairs self-reported quality of life more than any other common chronic medical disorder[72,73] and these data have been confirmed in Europe.[74] Quality of life deteriorates with increasing heart failure severity, and this is associated with increased numbers of physician visits, drug consumption and hospitalization.[75] The prevalence of major depression in a hospitalized cohort of chronically ill patients aged > 60 years was found to be significantly greater in those with chronic heart failure (36.5% vs 25.5% for the remaining cohort). Such depression was both prolonged and largely untreated in the chronic heart failure cohort.[75]

Health-related quality of life is being increasingly recognized as an important endpoint in trials of both pharmacological and nonpharmacological treatment strategies. Rather than solely measuring duration of survival, studies are being designed with a quality of life component in order to determine whether greater longevity equates to poor quality of life before an inevitable death.[76] As the focus on the individual patient becomes more important, quality of life measures are even being incorporated into primary endpoints, rather than being measured as a secondary endpoint, particularly when examining strategies where prolonging survival is not the principal concern. Dyspnoea, confusion and pain are very common during the last few days of life in heart failure, as are anxiety and depression. The majority of patients would prefer 'comfort care' and do not wish active resuscitation. Many would even prefer death.[77,78] It is not surprising, therefore, that there is a growing clamour for more attention to be paid to the end-of-life experience in heart failure and the extension of palliative care services to improve the quality of life for a rising tide of such patients and their carers.[77–82]

Future burden

As noted in the introduction, despite an overall decline in age-adjusted mortality from coronary heart disease in developed countries overall,[1] the number of these patients is increasing.[2,83] This reflects a higher proportion of older individuals in whom the incidence of coronary heart disease and hypertension is highest and the overall ageing of the population. In particular, it has been shown that survival after acute myocardial infarction has increased markedly over the past decade, at least in part because of better medical treatment.[4,5] As coronary heart disease is the most powerful risk factor for heart failure, it is likely that the aforementioned trends will lead to an increase in its prevalence in the future. It will probably become, therefore, a more common manifestation of chronic coronary heart disease as well as contribute to an increasing number

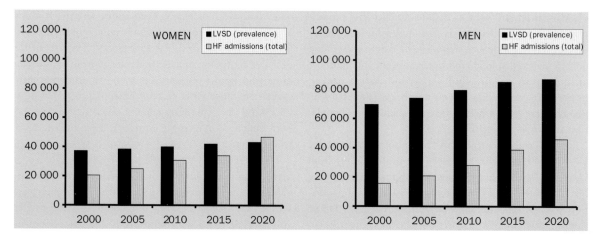

Figure 1.5. Future of heart failure (HF) in Scotland (2000–2020) (LVSD, left ventricular systolic dysfunction).

of deaths.[2,83] Three formal projections of the future burden of heart failure in Australia,[2] The Netherlands[83] and, most recently, Scotland[84] have been undertaken. The projected number of cases of heart failure within the relatively small population of Australia (approximately 18 million people at present) is expected to increase by approximately 70% during the period 1980–2010.[2] Likewise, an analysis of demographic trends in The Netherlands has predicted that the prevalence of heart failure, due to coronary heart disease, will rise by 70% during the period 1985–2010.[83] The most recent analysis of the future burden of heart failure, using Scottish data, suggested that based on population changes alone, the number of men and women with heart failure will rise by 2300 (6%) and 1500 (3%) by the year 2005, and by 12 300 (31%) and 7800 (17%) in the longer term (2020), respectively.[84] On the same basis, the annual number of male and female GP visits is likely to rise by 6% and 2% by year 2005, and by 40% and 16% in the year 2020. It has also been estimated that in the year 2000 about 3500 men and 4300 women in Scotland experienced an incident hospitalization for heart failure. By the year 2020 these figures are likely to increase by 52% (1800 more) and 16% (717 more) in men and women, respectively. Figure 1.5 shows the projected prevalence of left ventricular systolic dysfunction in Scottish men and women during this period in addition to the total number of admissions per annum. It is important to note that systolic dysfunction is much more common in men than women whilst admission rates are more similar – hence the difference in ratios between these two parameters.

Summary

Heart failure represents a growing health problem. Despite some recent evidence of improving morbidity and mortality rates,[35,40,45] currently available pharmacological treatment strategies do not completely ameliorate the high morbidity and mortality rates associated with chronic heart failure – especially in older individuals. As will be discussed in various chapters of this book, there is a clear need, therefore, to develop and implement cost-effective programmes that prevent the development of heart failure (e.g. primary prevention in coronary heart disease). There is also a need for programmes that provide for the early detection and optimal treatment of individuals who develop heart failure despite prevention strategies for example, 'early' screening with brain natriuretic peptide assays[85] and rapid access echocardiography.[86]

Unfortunately, the most urgent need relates to the increasing number of older individuals with chronic heart failure who are hospitalized with an acute episode of heart failure or a related condition. Such individuals have limited survival prospects and are likely to have an extremely poor quality of life and require recurrent hospitalizations before they experience an often traumatic and premature death. Apart from individualized and supportive care, we will need to develop guidelines for applying palliative care in heart failure. To do this will be to acknowledge our therapeutic limitations in prolonging life and the overwhelming nature of the current epidemic of heart failure.

References

1 Tunstall-Pedoe H, Kuulasmaa K, Mahonen M et al. Contribution of trends in survival and coronary-event rates to changes in coronary heart disease mortality: 10 year results from 37 WHO MONICA Project populations. *Lancet* 1999; **353:** 1547–57.

2 Kelly DT. Our future society: a global challenge. *Circulation* 1997; **95:** 2459–64.

3 Caselli G, Lopez AD. Health and mortality among elderly populations. New York: Clarendon Press, 1996.

4 Capewell S, Livingstone BM, MacIntyre K et al. Trends in case-fatality in 117,718 patients admitted with acute myocardial infarction in Scotland. *Eur Heart J* 2001; **21:** 1833–40.

5 Capewell S, MacIntyre K, Stewart S et al. Age, sex and social trends in out-of-hospital cardiac deaths in Scotland 1986–1995: a retrospective cohort study. *Lancet* 2001; **358:** 1213–17.

6 McMurray JJV, Stewart S. Epidemiology, aetiology and prognosis of heart failure. *Heart* 2000; **83:** 596–602.

7 Vasan RS, Larson MG, Benjamin EJ, Evans JC, Reiss CK, Levy D. Congestive heart failure in subjects with normal versus reduced left ventricular ejection fraction: prevalence and mortality in a population-based cohort. *J Am Coll Cardiol* 1999; **33:** 1948–55.

8 Logan WPD, Cushion AA. Morbidity statistics from General Practice. Vol 1. Studies on medical and population subjects (No. 14) London: HSMO, 1958.

9 Gibson TC, White KL, Klainer LM. The prevalence of congestive heart failure in two rural communities. *J Chronic Dis* 1966; **19:** 141–52.

10 Royal College of General Practitioners, Office of Population Census and Survey, and Department of Health and Social Security. Morbidity statistics from general practice: third national study, 1981–82. London: HMSO, 1988.

11 Parameshwar J, Shackell MM, Richardson A, Poole-Wilson PA, Sutton GC. Prevalence of heart failure in three general practices in north west London. *Br J Gen Pract* 1992; **42:** 287–9.

12 Rodeheffer RJ, Jacobsen SJ, Gersh BJ et al. The incidence and prevalence of congestive heart failure in Rochester, Minnesota. *Mayo Clin Proc* 1993; **68:** 1143–50.

13 Mair FS, Crowley TS, Bundred PE. Prevalence, aetiology and management of heart failure in general practice. *Br J General Practice* 1996; **46:** 77–9.

14 Royal College of General Practitioners, Office of Population Census and Survey, and Department of Health and Social Security. Morbidity statistics from general practice: fourth national study, 1991–92. London: HMSO, 1995.

15 Clarke KW, Gray D, Hampton JR. How common is heart failure? Evidence from PACT (Prescribing Analysis and Cost) data in Nottingham. *J Public Health Medicine* 1995; **17:** 459–64.

16 Droller H, Pemberton J. Cardiovascular disease in a random sample of elderly people. *Br Heart J* 1953; **15:** 199–204.

17 Garrison GE, McDonough JR, Hames CG, Stulb SC. Prevalence of chronic congestive heart failure in the population of Evans County, Georgia. *Am J Epidemiol* 1966; **83:** 338–44.

18 McKee PA, Castelli WP, McNamara PM, Kannel WB. The natural history of congestive heart failure: the Framingham study. *N Engl J Med* 1971; **285:** 1441–46.

19 Landahl S, Svanborg A, Astrand K. Heart volume and the prevalence of certain common cardiovascular disorders at 70 and 75 years of age. *Eur Heart J* 1984; **5:** 326–31.

20 Eriksson H, Svardsudd K, Larsson B et al. Risk factors for heart failure in the general population: the Study of Men Born in 1913. *Eur Heart J* 1989; **10:** 647–56.

21 Schocken DD, Arrieta MI, Leaverton PE, Ross EA. Prevalence and mortality rate of congestive heart failure in the United States. *J Am Coll Cardiol* 1992; **20:** 301–6.

22 Kupari M, Lindroos M, Iivanainen AM, Heikkila J, Tilvis R. Congestive heart failure in old age: prevalence, mechanisms and 4-year prognosis in the Helsinki ageing study. *J Int Med* 1997; **241:** 387–94.

23 Ceia F, Fonesca C, Mota T et al, for the EPICA Investigators. Prevalence of chronic heart failure in Southwestern Europe: the EPICA Study. *Eur J Heart Failure* 2002; **4:** 531–9.

24 McDonagh TA, Morrison CE, Lawrence A et al. Symptomatic and asymptomatic left-ventricular systolic dysfunction in an urban population. 1997; **350:** 829–33.

25 Mosterd A, de Bruijne MC, Hoes AW et al. Usefulness of echocardiography in detecting left ventricular dysfunction in population based studies (The Rotterdam Study). *Am J Cardiol* 1997; **79:** 103–4.

26 Morgan S, Smith H, Simpson I et al. Prevalence and clinical characteristics of left ventricular dysfunction among elderly patients in general practice setting: cross-sectional survey. *BMJ* 1999; **318:** 368–72.

27 Schnohr P, Jensen G, Lange P, Appleyard M. The Copenhagen City Heart Study. *Eur Heart J* 2001; **3** (Suppl H).

28 Margolis JR, Gillum RF, Feinleb M, Brasch RC, Fabsitz RR. Community surveillance for coronary heart disease: the Framingham Cardiovascular Disease Study. Methods and preliminary results. *Am J Epidemiol* 1974; **100:** 425–36.

29 Ho KK, Pinsky JL, Kannel WB, Levy D. The epidemiology of heart failure: the Framingham Study. *J Am Coll Cardiol* 1993; **22:** 6A–13A.

30 Stewart S, Hart CL, Hole DJ, McMurray JJ. The incidence and natural history of heart failure in 15,406 men and women over 20 years: the Renfrew/Paisley Study. *Eur Heart J* 2001; **22:** 208.

31 Cowie MR, Struthers AD, Wood DA et al. Value of natriuretic peptides in assessment of patients with possible new heart failure in primary care. *Lancet* 1997; **350:** 1347–51.

32 Cowie MR, Wood DA, Coats JS et al. Incidence and aetiology of heart failure: a population based study. *Eur Heart J* 1999; **20:** 421–8.

33 Remes J, Reunanen A, Aromaa A, Pyorala AK. Incidence of heart failure in eastern Finland: a population-based surveillance study. *Eur Heart J* 1992; **13:** 588–93.

34 McMurray J, McDonagh T, Morrison CE, Dargie HJ. Trends in hospitalization for heart failure in Scotland 1980–1990. *Eur Heart J* 1993; **14:** 1158–62.

35 Stewart S, MacIntyre K, McCleod ME, Bailey AE, Capewell S, McMurray JJ. Trends in heart failure hospitalisations in Scotland, 1990–1996: an epidemic that has reached its peak? *Eur Heart J* 2001; **22:** 209–17.

36 Ghali JK, Cooper R, Ford E. Trends in hospitalisation rates for heart failure in the United States 1973–1986: evidence for screening population prevalence. *Arch Intern Med* 1992; **150:** 769–73.

37 Haldeman GA, Croft JB, Giles WH, Rashidee A. Hospitalization of patients with heart failure: national hospital discharge survey 1985–1995. *Am Heart J* 1999; **137:** 352–60.

38 Eriksson H, Wilhelmsen L, Caidahl K, Svardsudd K. Epidemiology and prognosis of heart failure. *Zeitschrift Fur Kardiologie* 1991; **80:** 1–6.

39 Reitsma JB, Mosterd A, de Craen AJM et al. Increase in hospital admission rates for heart failure in the Netherlands, 1980–1993. *Heart* 1996; **76:** 388–92.

40 Mosterd A, Reitsma JB, Grobbee DE. ACE inhibition and hospitalisation rates for heart failure in The Netherlands, 1980–1998. The end of an epidemic? *Heart* 2002; **87:** 75–6.

41 Rodriguez-Artalejo F, Guallar-Castillon P, Banegas Banegas JR, del Rey Calero J. Trends in hospitalization and mortality for heart failure in Spain, 1980–1993. *Eur Heart J* 1997; **18:** 1771–9.

42 Doughty R, Yee T, Sharpe N et al. Hospital admissions and deaths due to congestive heart failure in New Zealand, 1988–91. *NZ Med J* 1995; **108:** 473–5.

43 McMurray JJV, Hart W, Rhodes G. An evaluation of the cost of heart failure to the National Health Service in the UK. *Br J Med Econ* 1993; **6:** 91–8.

44 Stewart S, Jenkins A, Buchan S, Capewell S, McGuire A, McMurray JJ. The current cost of heart failure in the UK – an economic analysis. *Eur J Heart Fail* 2002; **4:** 361–71.

45 MacIntyre K, Capewell S, Stewart S et al. Evidence of improving prognosis in heart failure: trends in case-fatality in 66,547 patients hospitalised between 1986 and 1995. *Circulation* 2000; **102:** 1126–31.

46 Westert GP, Lagoe RJ, Keskimaki I, Leyland A, Murphy M. An international study of hospital readmissions and related utilization in Europe and the USA. *Health Policy* 2002; **61:** 269–78.

47 Stewart S, Demers C, Murdoch DR et al. Substantial between-hospital variation in outcome following first emergency admission for heart failure. *Eur Heart J* 2002; **23:** 650–7.

48 Launois R, Launois B, Reboul-Marty J et al. Le cout de la severite de la maladie: le cas de l'insuffisance-cardiaque. *J Econ Med* 1990; **8:** 395–412.

49 Van Hout BA, Wielink G, Bonsel GJ et al. Effects of ACE inhibitors on heart failure in The Netherlands: a pharmacoeconomic model. *Pharmacoeconomics* 1993; **3:** 387–97.

50 Konstam M, Dracup K, Baker D et al. Heart failure: evaluation and care of patients with left ventricular systolic dysfunction. Clinical Practice Guideline No 11. AHCPR Publication No 94–0612 Rockville, MD: Agency for Health Care Policy and Research, Public Health Service, US Department of Health and Human Services. June 1994.

51 Levy D, Larson MG, Vasan RS, Kannel WB, Ho KL. The progression from hypertension to congestive heart failure. *JAMA* 1996; **275:** 1557–62.

52 Kannel WB, Ho KK, Thom T. Changing epidemiological features of cardiac failure. *Eur Heart J* 1994; **72:** S3–9.

53 Chobanian AV, Bakris GL, Black HR et al. for the National Heart, Lung, and Blood Institute Joint National Committee on Prevention, Detection, Evaluation, and Treatment of High Blood Pressure; National High Blood Pressure Education Program Coordinating Committee. The Seventh Report of the Joint National Committee on Prevention, Detection, Evaluation, and Treatment of High Blood Pressure: the JNC 7 report. *JAMA* 2003; **289:** 2560–72.

54 Kenchaiah S, Evans JC, Levy D et al. Obesity and the risk of heart failure. *N Engl J Med* 2002; **347:** 305–13.

55 The SOLVD Investigators. Effect of enalapril on survival in patients with reduced left ventricular ejection fractions and congestive heart failure. *N Engl J Med* 1991; **325:** 293–302.

56 Pitt B, Zannad F, Remme WJ et al. The effect of spironolactone on morbidity and mortality in patients with severe heart failure. Randomized Aldactone Evaluation Study Investigators. *N Engl J Med* 1999; **341:** 709–17.

57 The Digitalis Investigation Group. The effect of digoxin on mortality and morbidity in patients with heart failure. *N Engl J Med* 1997; **336:** 525–33.

58 MERIT Investigators. Effect of metoprolol CR/XL in chronic heart failure: metoprolol CR/XL Randomised Intervention Trial in Congestive Heart Failure (Merit-HF). *Lancet* 1999; **353:** 2001–7.

59 Packer M, Poole-Wilson PA, Armstrong PW et al. Comparative effects of low and high doses of the angiotensin converting enzyme inhibitor, lisinopril, on morbidity and mortality in chronic heart failure. *Circulation* 1999; **100:** 2312–18.

60 SOLVD Investigators. Natural history and patterns of current practice in heart failure. *J Am Coll Cardiol* 1993; **4A:** 14A–19A.

61 Bart BA, Ertl G, Held P et al. Contemporary management of patients with left ventricular systolic dysfunction. Results from the study of patients intolerant of converting enzyme inhibitors (SPICE) registry. *Eur Heart J* 1999; **20:** 1182–90.

62 Ho KKL, Anderson KM, Karmel WB et al. Survival after the onset of congestive heart failure in the Framingham Heart Study subjects. *Circulation* 1993; **88:** 107–15.

63 Senni M, Tribouilloy CM, Rodeheffer RJ, Jacobsen EJ, Evans JM et al. Congestive heart failure in the community – trends in incidence and survival in a 10-year period. *Arch Intern Med* 1999; **159:** 29–34.

64 Cowie MR, Wood DA, Coats AJS et al. Survival of patients with a new diagnosis of heart failure: a population based study. *Heart* 2001; **83:** 505–10.

65 Stewart S, MacIntyre K, Hole DA, Capewell S, McMurray JJV. More malignant than cancer? Five-year survival following a first admission for heart failure in Scotland? *Eur J Heart Failure* 2001; **3:** 315–22.

66 Peeters A, Mamun AA, Willekens F, Bonneux L for NEDCOM. A cardiovascular life history: a life course analysis of the original Framingham Heart Study cohort. *Eur Heart J* 2002; **23:** 458–66.

67 Jong P, Vowineckel E, Liu PP, Gong Y, Tu JV. Prognosis and determinants of survival in patients newly hospitalised for heart failure: a population based study. *Arch Intern Med* 2002; **162:** 1689–94.

68 Petrie MC, Berry C, Stewart S, McMurray JJV. Failing ageing hearts. *Eur Heart J* 2001; **22:** 1978–90.

69 Petrie MC, Dawson NF, Murdoch DR, Davie AP, McMurray JJV. Failure of women's hearts. *Circulation* 1999; **99:** 2334–41.

70 Swedberg K, Kjekshus J, Snapinn S. Long-term survival in severe heart failure in patients treated with enalapril. Ten-year follow-up of CONSENSUS 1. *Eur Heart J* 1999; **2:** 136–9.

71 Murdoch DR, Love MP, Robb SD, McMurray JJV. Importance of heart failure as a cause of death: contribution to overall mortality and coronary heart disease mortality in Scotland 1979–1992. *Eur Heart J* 1998; **19:** 1829–35.

72 Stewart AL, Greenfield S, Hays RD et al. Functional status and well-being of patients with chronic conditions – results from the medical outcomes study. *JAMA* 1989; **262:** 907–13.

73 Fryback DG, Dasbach EJ, Klein R et al. The Beaver Dam Health Outcomes Study – initial catalog of health-state quality factors. *Med Des Making* 1993; **13:** 89–102.

74 Juenger J, Schellberg D, Kraemer S et al. Health related quality of life in patients with congestive heart failure: comparison with other chronic diseases and relation to functional variables. *Heart* 2002; **87:** 235–41.

75 Koenig HG. Depression in hospitalized older patients with congestive heart failure. *Gen Hosp Psych* 1998; **20:** 29–43.

76 Berry C, McMurray JJV. A review of quality of life evaluation in patients with congestive heart failure. *Pharmacoeconomics* 1999; **16:** 247–71.

77 Levenson JW, McCarthy EP, Lynn J, Davis RB, Phillips RS. The last six months of life for patients with congestive heart failure. *J Am Geriatr Soc* 2000; **48:** S101–9.

78 Krumholz HM, Phillips RS, Hamel MB et al. Resuscitation preferences among patients with severe congestive heart failure: results from the SUPPORT project. *Circulation*. 1998; **98:** 648–55.

79 Steward S, McMurray JJ. Palliative care for heart failure? *BMJ* 2002; **325:** 929–30.

80 Murray SA, Boyd K, Kendall M et al. Dying of lung cancer or cardiac failure: A community-based, prospective qualitative interview study of patients and their carers. *BMJ* 2002; **325:** 929–33.

81 Gibbs JS, McCoy AS, Gibbs LM, Rogers AE, Addington-Hall JM. Living with and dying from heart failure: the role of palliative care. *Heart*. 2002; **88(S2):** ii36–9.

82 Hanratty B, Hibbert D, Mair F et al. Doctors' perceptions of palliative care for heart failure: focus study group. *BMJ* 2002; **325:** 581–5.

83 Bonneux L, Barendregt JJ, Meeter K et al. Estimating clinical morbidity due to ischaemic heart disease and congestive heart failure: the future rise of heart failure. *Am J Public Health* 1994; **84:** 20–8.

84 Stewart S, MacIntyre K, Capewell S, McMurray JJV. An ageing population and heart failure: An increasing burden in the 21st century? *Heart* 2003; **89:** 49–53.

85 Shapiro BP, Chen HH, Burnett JC, Redfield MM. Use of plasma brain natriuretic peptide concentration to aid in the diagnosis of heart failure. *Mayo Clin Proc* 2003; **78:** 481–86.

86 Nielsen OW, McDonagh TA, Robb SD, Dargie HJ. Retrospective analysis of the cost-effectiveness of using plasma brain natriuretic peptide in screening for left ventricular systolic dysfunction in the general population. *J Am Coll Cardiol* 2003; **41:** 113–20.

2 From the individual to the health care system: measuring the burden of heart failure

Simon Stewart and David R Thompson

Introduction

As discussed in Chapter 1, heart failure is a nebulous condition. Similar to the ripples emanating from a stone dropped into a still pond, heart failure is rarely an isolated event, but rather a syndrome whose effects reach out to disrupt the lives of individuals and the capacity of the local health care system to cope with other health priorities. As can be appreciated from the previous chapter, the individual 'ripples' from an increasing number of cases of heart failure in older individuals has created a signal of 'tsunami' proportions in the health care systems of developed countries.[1]

The temptation, of course, is simply to measure an epiphenomenon like heart failure using basic epidemiological parameters. For example, as described in Chapter 1, it is important to quantify the incidence (the number of new cases arising each year) and prevalence (total number of cases within the population at any one time) of heart failure. However, it is also important to measure the burden of heart failure in a number of different ways to truly understand how both the individual and the health care system in which they are managed are affected. This chapter examines the different ways heart failure can be measured and the limitations that must be critically examined and acknowledged when interpreting such data.

Representing the norm: a case history in heart failure

Figure 2.1 is a schematic representation of the case history (see accompanying description) of a real patient, Mr S, in whom the trajectory of heart failure was typically convoluted and difficult to predict,[2] but which was also typically associated with significant morbidity and death.[3] Through this case history, the full spectrum of data that can be collated and interpreted (either singularly, or collectively

when combined with data from other cases) can be explored. It clearly demonstrates that a number of important parameters, including those listed below, need to be considered when attempting to measure the burden of heart failure (the first few being predominantly related to the individual and the latter becoming increasingly relevant to the operational performance and burden placed on the health care system in which they are managed):

- overall health status (e.g. physical, mental and social) and quality of life (including the patient's family/carer);
- capacity to undertake activities of daily living;
- discrete morbid events (e.g. hospitalization – type, length of stay, case-fatality, readmission status);
- pattern of health care utilization (e.g. community vs hospital-based)
- fatal events (e.g. type, survival, premature, etc.);
- cost of health care;
- overall trajectory/pattern of discrete heart failure and non-heart failure events.

From the individual to the health care system

The case study underlying Figure 2.1 is typically complicated and the potential to identify a myriad of parameters to quantify the burden of heart failure in this case (and others typical of this case history) is clearly evident. Conversely, the path of least resistance would involve a simple tabulation of how many admissions Mr S experienced before he died and this 'simplistic' approach is evident throughout the literature. However, in the process of being assessed for a clinical trial and participating in a longitudinal follow-up of typically old and fragile heart failure patients, the following parameters, all of which are relatively easy to measure specifically or are available from

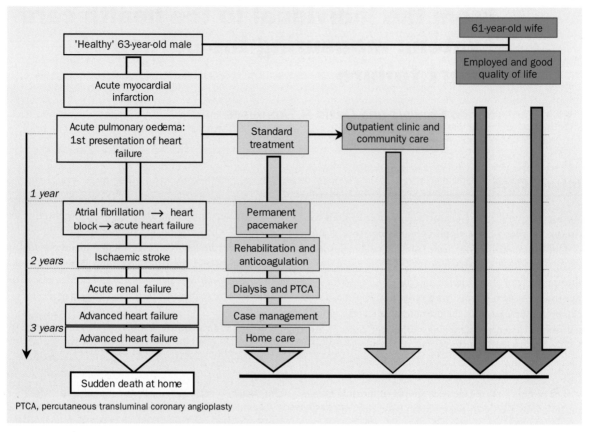

Figure 2.1. *Measuring the burden of heart failure from detection to death: three and a half years in the life of a 63-year-old man. (See Case history of Mr S overleaf).*

pre-existing datasets, were documented. It is important to note that this list does not include those parameters that specifically reflect extent of cardiac dysfunction (e.g. left ventricular ejection fraction). Rather, they reflect the 'visible' impact of heart failure.

New York Heart Association (NYHA) class

The most recognized and utilized grading system used to describe the effect of heart failure on the physical capacity of individual patients is NYHA class. Ranging from NYHA class I (presence of cardiac disease but without resulting limitations of physical activity) to NYHA class IV (cardiac disease resulting in an inability to perform ordinary physical activity due to persistent fatigue and dyspnoea) is extremely easy to remember and apply.[4] Patients with heart failure (by their very definition) are usually in NYHA class II–IV. However, assessing NYHA status requires a subjective assessment of functional status and is open to interpretation (particularly when differentiating between NYHA class II, III or the subcategories (e.g. IIIb) that have gained popularity in clinical trials (e.g. the COPERNICUS Study).[5]

Six-minute walk test

In addition to asking patients about their physical limitations and classifying their responses according to an agreed formula (e.g. NYHA class), it clearly desirable to gain a more objective measure of their functional capabilities. In this respect, the easiest, most tolerated and realistic test of a patient's ability to carry out activity daily living is the 'six-minute walk test'.* As simple as it sounds, the test only requires someone to measure how far a patient can

---

* An excellent review of the purpose and application of the six-minute walk test was produced by the American Thoracic Society in March 2002. The review can be found at: http://www.dolphinmedical.com/papers/ats-statement-smwt-rccm–2002.pdf

Case history of Mr S

Mr S was a 63-year-old man in good health prior to his acute myocardial infarction affecting the anterolateral wall of his left ventricle. A coronary angiogram revealed an occlusion to the distal portion of his left anterior descending artery and smaller branches distal to the occlusion but with largely intact cardiac function (left ventricular ejection fraction > 55%) and no other lesions likely to produce symptoms of ischaemia in the immediate future. Being largely fit and active, Mr S was surprised to find out that he was hypertensive and required pharmacotherapy, although he had no other obvious risk factors for heart disease. He was discharged from hospital, therefore, on routine medication (antiplatelet, a beta-blocker and angiotensin-converting enzyme inhibitor) and received a limited form of cardiac rehabilitation. It was at this point that Mr S decided to semi-retire (he needed some form of income) and become more socially active and travel more extensively with his wife who was in good health.

For 6 months, Mr S enjoyed relatively good health and good quality of life with routine follow-up for his heart disease. In the middle of winter, however, he developed what appeared to be a chest infection and found it difficult to breathe. In the middle of the night he found he could only breathe when he was sitting-up and was admitted to hospital as an emergency with acute pulmonary oedema secondary to moderate left ventricular systolic dysfunction (his left ventricular ejection fraction now 35%).

After, 7 days in hospital (two of which were spent in a Coronary Care Unit) Mr S was discharged from hospital with standard treatment for heart failure (a diuretic being added to his previous treatment with his dose of angiotensin-converting enzyme inhibitor increased). Following his discharge, Mr S was relatively stable and suffered shortness of breath only when performing moderate exercise (New York Heart Association Class II), but was still mentally agile and enjoyed an independent and socially active lifestyle with his wife, although he was forced to retire and the couple had to make financial adjustments accordingly to their lifestyle.

It was almost a year before Mr S had another acute event. This time, however, it was more serious with greater residual consequences. Initially, Mr S was admitted (once again in winter) with increasing fatigue and breathlessness secondary to atrial fibrillation. Before definitive treatment could be instigated however, Mr S developed a complete heart block leading to acute pulmonary oedema. This was diagnosed as sick sinus syndrome and a permanent pacemaker was inserted to stabilize his cardiac rhythm and output. Following this event, with a prolonged hospital admission to stabilize his cardiac function and to manage an emerging problem of mild renal failure, Mr S's mental and physical status was noticeably impaired. He now experienced breathlessness on mild exertion (NYHA III) and relied more heavily on his wife to assist him in his activities of daily living and manage his treatment. Naturally, he required more medical follow-up while the couple's social activity and overall quality of life decreased.

Approximately 6 months later Mr S suffered an ischaemic cerebral infarction and was once again readmitted to hospital for a prolonged time. Not qualifying for thrombolysis, Mr S was managed on a conservative basis and was discharged from hospital following this stroke with residual hemiplegia and dysphasia requiring intensive rehabilitation and long-term anticoagulation monitoring and titration in addition to his other medication. Mr S was found to have a number of other conditions that now required treatment. Firstly, Mr S had developed Type II diabetes mellitus and required oral hypoglycaemic agents and regular blood glucose monitoring. Secondly, a pulmonary function test showed that Mr S had borderline pulmonary disease (potentially due to micro-emboli) that was likely to deteriorate in the future. Clearly, this put Mr S's wife under considerable strain and her own health suffered accordingly.

After 5 months of rehabilitation, Mr S had regained most of his physical faculties but had deteriorated overall in terms of his overall functional, mental and social status. At this point in time he was once again admitted to hospital as an emergency. This time it was for acute renal failure – his renal function having progressively worsened over the course of his continued regimen of diuretics and an angiotensin-converting enzyme inhibitor. After a programme of renal dialysis was implemented, renal angiography revealed a proximal stenosis of his left renal artery that was treated with balloon angioplasty. Mr S's renal function subsequently stabilized, although he could no longer tolerate an angiotensin-converting enzyme inhibitor and was discharged from hospital to home in poor physical and mental condition.

Not surprisingly, Mr S's condition worsened rapidly and his final few months were punctuated by two emergency admissions for acute pulmonary oedema and an extremely poor quality of life at home with continuous symptoms of fatigue and dyspnoea (NYHA Class IV) requiring constant support via a case-management team approach in the absence of formal palliative care services for patients with heart failure. Not surprisingly, Mr S's wife suffered accordingly.

Approximately, 4 weeks following his final admission, Mr S died 'suddenly' whilst sitting upright in his permanent home – a recliner chair in his living room. Mr S had survived for approximately 3 years with heart failure, but had died approximately 8 years prior to his predicted life-expectancy. Mr S's wife was naturally exhausted and depressed at the time of her husband's death. Her health had also suffered with the emergence of symptomatic heart disease and she was forced to sell their home in order to consolidate her financial position due to her husband's premature retirement and the cost of 3 years' intensive treatment.

walk over a flat surface during the pre-defined time-frame of 6 minutes.[6] Although this test is not specific to the influence of underlying heart failure to exercise intolerance (e.g. underlying pulmonary disease and/or cardiac cachexia affecting peripheral muscle groups may be major factors in limiting exercise capacity), this simple walk test is sensitive to changes in cardiac function and can predict subsequent morbidity and mortality.[7] Once again, like NYHA class, the results of this walk test may vary so it is important to examine historical trends in patients rather than rely on a single test (i.e. using the patient as their own control).

As the level of exercise in the six-minute walk test is often submaximal and the measurement is relatively crude, patients with heart failure often undergo more sophisticated exercise tests that not only monitor their ability to sustain physical activity but measure changes in their cardiac and pulmonary function (e.g. peak oxygen uptake and metabolic equivalents) at the same time. Cynthia Adams, in Chapter 10, describes the role of exercise testing more eloquently and in greater detail.

Health-related quality of life

Whilst exercise testing and determining NYHA class provides a degree of objectivity in determining the individual burden of heart failure, simply quantifying, for example, the fact that someone is unable to walk far may not be of great importance to the patient. Health professionals tend to become excited about numbers and concepts that assist them to 'benchmark' patients and place them within the whole spectrum of heart failure patients through the revolving door of the health care system. To the individual patient, of course, the most important issues are likely to be highly personalized and based upon an entirely different perspective. For example, it has become increasingly clear that while survival (see below) represents an important clinical endpoint in the large-scale clinical trials, prolonged life, particularly if associated with a miserable existence characterized by extreme dyspnoea, pain and depression,[8] may be seen as a curse rather than a blessing.

The World Health Organization defines health as a 'state of complete physical, mental and social well-being and not merely the absence of disease'.[9] Prior to his heart attack, and indeed immediately following, Mr S and his wife described a good quality of life with their only concerns being the loss of income likely to impinge on their ability to socialize and travel. Clearly this situation changed as Mr S's heart failure emerged and progressed and his wife suffered accordingly as the burden of care increased (at no stage was Mr S admitted to long-term institutional care). Not surprisingly, heart failure (particularly secondary to ischaemic heart disease) is often associated with a degree of poor quality of life that is worse than any other common disease state.[10,11]

Measuring changes in health-related quality of life in a meaningful and consistent manner is a difficult task. However, over the past decade there have been a number of excellent 'generic' instruments developed in addition to those that specifically examine the impact of heart failure and the symptoms and problems it typically engenders. Before covering some of the specific issues that impact upon the relevance and quality of collected data, it is important to acknowledge that the broad complexity of issues surrounding the development and application of health-related quality of life instruments is beyond the scope of this chapter. A number of excellent articles, including a comprehensive overview of the problems inherent in measuring quality of life in congestive heart failure by Berry and McMurray,[12] represent a good start to understanding the complexity of developing, applying and interpreting health-related quality of life instruments.

There are a number of key ingredients to a clinically useful instrument. These include the following:

- It should be able to accurately evaluate an individual's physical, emotional and social well-being;
- It should be reliable and reproducible (an associated Cronbach's $\alpha > 0.7$ is usually accepted in this regard).[13]
- The instrument should have various forms of validity. Criterion validity refers to comparable results using other instruments measuring the same variable. Content validity is the appropriateness of items to the purpose of the instrument (e.g. measuring the impact of heart failure). Face validity represents being consistent with current knowledge and expert opinion. Construct validity is the ability of the instrument to be sensitive to different levels of quality of life in a variety of patient groups. Discriminative validity is the instrument's ability to detect changes in the observed variable without provoking a 'floor' or 'ceiling' effect that reflects an inability to detect clinically significant changes at the lower or higher spectrum of quality of life.
- Preferably, the instrument should have the above comprehensibly documented for the patient population of interest and a large amount of reference data with which to compare current data (e.g. population norms and other disease states).

- The instrument should be easy to complete, irrespective of whether it is self-completing or administered by the health professional with measures to reduce inter-rater and intrasubject variation.
- Finally, the results of the instrument should be easy to interpret.

Health-related quality of life instruments are either 'generic' or 'disease-specific'. Generic questionnaires focus on general issues of health rather than the specific features of a particular disease: the role of disease-specific instruments. Ideally, any evaluation of a patient's quality of life will involve both, a generic instrument being useful for evaluating the quality of life of significant others/carers.

A number of generic instruments are commonly used in studies of heart failure patients.[14–17] Two commonly used instruments of this type are:

- *Sickness Impact Profile.* This instrument involves 136 questions relating to 12 'domains' of health (mobility, ambulation, domestic affairs, social interaction, behaviour, communication, recreation, eating, work, sleep, emotions and self-care).[14] This instrument was used in the Study to Understand Prognosis and Preference for Outcomes and Risks of Treatments (SUPPORT).[18] Although useful in the setting of heart failure, there are probably more appropriate instruments available (see below).
- *The Medical Outcome Study 36-item Short Form Health Survey (SF–36).* This study was designed in a health insurance study – the Medical Outcome Study – and involves 36 questions covering eight domains (physical functioning, social functioning, physical impairment, emotional impairment, emotions, vitality, pain and global health.)[15] A shorter form, the SF–12, is also available and widely used.[19] Both have been used successfully to describe quality of life in patients with heart failure.

Recently, a number of instruments have been designed to specifically examine the typical impact of heart failure on quality of life (e.g. paroxysmal nocturnal dyspnoea and associated sleep disturbance). Two commonly used instruments of this type are:

- *The Minnesota Living With Heart Failure Questionnaire.* This instrument comprises 21 questions with a range of 6-item responses ranging from no, very little, to very much to produce a range of scores of 0 (no disability) to 105 (maximal disability) in relation to signs and symptoms typical of heart failure, physical activity, social interaction, sexual activity, work and emotions.[20] This instrument has been utilized extensively in studies of heart failure patients and, overall, is extremely useful in this regard.
- *The Quality of Life in Severe Heart Failure Questionnaire.* This instrument has 26-items with a Likert scale to quantify physical activities and a visual analogue scale to assess life satisfaction, social and emotional parameters with a combined global score (higher scores reflecting poorer health).[21] As the name suggests it was developed in a patient cohort with severe heart failure and has also proved to be a useful instrument in this particular context.[12]

Clearly, there are a number of instruments available. In the case of Mr S, both the SF–36 and the Minnesota Living With Heart Failure questionnaires reflected the changes in his quality of life as his heart failure worsened; the former was also sensitive to changes in the quality of life of Mr S's wife.

Pattern of health care utilization

Like most individuals who develop a chronic disease late in life, Mr S spent the majority of life in good health and 'avoiding doctors' before experiencing a frustrating inability to sever his dependence on the health care system. The pattern of Mr S's contacts with, and uptake of, the various components of the health care system can be formally measured and provide extremely important data to design more effective health care strategies for future heart failure patients.

Before considering specific components of health care, however, a number of important issues need to be addressed. The first of these relates to how events are measured. In this respect it is extremely important to describe the 'pattern' of events rather than simply counting events. For example, a patient with chronic heart failure may survive for 5 years with the syndrome and, during this period, be admitted to hospital on an emergency basis on four occasions. Compare this to the patient of similar age who survives for 1 year but who is admitted on only three occasions before they die. If both patients were followed for 5 years and hospitalization data were compared without correction for the 'intensity' and overall pattern of events (e.g. admissions per year of follow-up) it may be assumed that the former patient fared worse than the patient who had four fewer years of life and less time in hospital relative to survival time (see below). Unfortunately, misrepresentation of such comparative data is common in the literature. In an excellent review of the type of hospitalization, data are presented in clinical studies of heart failure. Metcalfe and colleagues from the Institute of Public Health at Cambridge University outlined the current inadequacies and misconceptions associated with the reporting of such data in the literature to date.[22]

Community care

Despite the 'high' profile of hospital care (it certainly costs more), the vast majority of health care occurs in the primary care setting. In describing such care it is important to account for all components of community care within a specific health care system and how it is utilized. For example, in the case of Mr S the following components of health care were utilized:

General practitioner (primary care physician): Importantly, after each hospitalization a cluster of consultations took place in order to provide routine post-discharge care and to adjust medical treatment (particularly pharmacotherapy) accordingly. Initially, between hospital admissions the intensity of such visits decreased markedly. However, as Mr S's condition worsened and his treatment became more complex, the intensity of visits increased to those equivalent to 'routine post-discharge care' (e.g. once a week). They also changed from brief clinic visits to more prolonged domiciliary visits involving a case-management approach utilizing a range of health care professionals to provide a limited form of 'palliative care'.

Community pharmacist: At first, Mr S had no need for regular consultations with his community pharmacist. However, following his admission for atrial fibrillation/complete heart block, he had difficulty with his pharmacotherapy and his wife assumed greater responsibility. At the same time, Mr S was provided with a domiciliary pharmacist service, where his medications were delivered each week and his response to these monitored. This continued until his death.

Community nurse: As above, initially, Mr S had no need for domiciliary visits by a community health care nurse. However, as his condition worsened he required regular visits to monitor his anticoagulation and diabetes therapy, in addition to those required to assist in his essential activities of daily living (e.g. hygiene).

Hospital activity

As indicated, this represents the most visible (and costly) impact of heart failure. Despite the fact that the majority of time patients with heart failure are managed in the community, like Mr S, studies confirm that despite increasing treatment options, hospital admissions are almost inevitable before death.[23,24] As such, a number of specific characteristics of hospital activity need to be considered:

Emergency vs elective: The majority of admissions in patients with heart failure are 'unplanned' and occur on an emergency basis. Emergency admissions by their very nature are of longer duration and require admission to more expensive units. It important to differentiate these types of admissions, remembering that in many cases hospital admissions are 'therapeutic' and eliminating *all* admissions in heart failure is unrealistic. Moreover, if a patient's condition improves, they are more likely to qualify for elective procedures that were cancelled because of their anaesthetic risk and this will 'artificially' increase their hospital use.

Heart failure specific?: A common mistake in measuring the impact of treatment strategies in heart failure is to focus solely on those admissions caused *primarily* by heart failure. Whilst this may be a legitimate outcome for younger individuals in whom heart failure is a 'discrete' syndrome (i.e. nearly all admissions are for heart failure), with increasing age the level of comorbidity in such patients increases[25] as does the proportion of admissions where heart failure is a contributory rather than primary cause (i.e. 50–75% of admissions in those aged 75 years or more).[25,26] Recent UK data suggest that the profile of these two types of admissions is becoming increasingly similar. For example, an admission primarily for renal failure is likely to reflect an adverse effect of heart failure treatment.[25] It would appear prudent therefore that 'all-cause' admissions (particularly those that occur on an emergency basis) be measured.

Length of stay: Studies from nearly all developed countries have shown that average length of stay is progressively falling,[27] despite the direct correlation between length of stay and increasing age and the increasing age of admitted patients.[25] However, overall length of stay in heart failure remains prolonged relative to other conditions[27] and the presence of other significant diagnoses (e.g. stroke and renal dysfunction)[28,29] require particularly prolonged hospitalization.[25,26] It is important to note that reporting mean length of stay (as is common) is extremely misleading given the skewed distribution of such data. For example, in the UK mean length of stay for heart failure is approximately 7 days. Alternatively, the median length of stay is approximately 12 days with an interquartile range of 4–21 days.[25] Clearly, median length of stay plus interquartile range is a much more meaningful figure in this regard.

Unit-specific data: Not unexpectedly, patients admitted to general medical units cost far less than those who require intensive medical and nursing therapy in more expensive coronary and intensive care units.[30] Apart from providing important data for costing purposes (see below), determining length of stay on a unit-specific basis provides important clues, in addition to length of stay, as to the severity of the event.

Procedures. For the majority of heart failure patients, 'active' treatment is confined to titration of pharmacotherapy. However, there is an increasing trend towards more invasive procedures in heart failure (e.g. extending the umbrella of coronary artery bypass procedures to treat hibernating or stunned myocardium contributing to heart failure,[31] prophylactic implantation of defibrillators to prevent fatal ventricular arrhythmias[32] and 'cardiac resynchronization' with the insertion of right and left ventricular pacing leads designed to overcome inter- and intraventricular conduction delays and therefore optimize cardiac output.)[33] All of these procedures are costly and consume significant health care resources, as well as having the potential to impact negatively on the patient's quality of life.[34] In Mr S's case, a pacemaker was inserted to treat his complete heart block and this obviously required a prolonged stay plus regular pacemaker checks thereafter.

Outpatient management: As with primary care visits, post-discharge management usually involves a 'cluster' of out-patient clinic visits followed by a less intensive schedule of visits to specialist care in between. As with primary care visits, it important to document the type (e.g. specialist cardiology vs a nurse-led clinic) and duration of outpatient contacts.

Pattern of hospitalization: As indicated above, it is extremely useful to determine the pattern of hospitalization relative to survival time and other events (e.g. first recorded admission for heart failure). The following parameters are therefore extremely important in this regard:

- readmission rate (typically within 28 days, 3, 6 and 12 months of the last admission);
- total admissions and hospital stays;
- frequency of admissions and hospital stays per month of follow-up.

Survival

Although survival status may appear to be a clear-cut issue, there are a number of parameters that need to be considered (including a combined analysis of morbidity and mortality data). These include:

All-cause mortality: The simplest approach to survival data is determining whether the patient has survived a particular period of follow-up and if not, when they died.

Cause-specific: A more sophisticated approach involves determining the cause of death. This usually depends on official coding data. However, it should be noted that in many countries, legal constraints prevent certifying officers identifying the syndrome of heart failure as the primary cause of death.[35] Moreover, deaths in elderly individuals are less likely to be the subject of a post-mortem and the listed causes of death become far less accurate.

Location of death/case-fatality: It is well known that there is a dichotomy in the way individuals with heart failure die. In almost one-half of cases, patients with heart failure die suddenly from a ventricular arrhythmia in the community (hence the clinical utility of implantable defibrillators).[32] Alternatively, a large proportion of patients die in hospital as a result of an acute myocardial infarction, stroke or, worst of all from a quality of life perspective, from progressive heart failure.[36,37]

Survival Time: In Chapter 1, Figures 1.3 and 1.4 show the 5 year survival curves for a large cohort of patients with a range of conditions (including heart failure) using life-table/Kaplan–Meier analysis. A more detailed description of this approach is available at the following website: http://www.medcalc.be/manual/mpage01–04.html (accessed June 2003). However, in simple terms, this approach reflects the proportion of patients who survive to reach certain time points (e.g. 50% alive at 2 years) and a key parameter – median survival (e.g. 50% of a total heart failure cohort dead within 36 months). On an individual basis, survival data provide the duration of survival relative to either potential follow-up or 'life expectancy'. For example, the cohort in which Mr S was being studied had a maximum of 72 months of follow-up but Mr S survived only to approximately 36 months (50% of potential follow-up) and, more importantly, died 9 years sooner than his predicted life expectancy.

Event-free survival: The same type of data analysis may be used to determine a combined endpoint of 'event-free survival' using both hospitalization and mortality data. Event-free survival usually refers to the duration of time (usually expressed as a median and plotted as an event-free survival curve when a cohort analysis is available) an individual avoids either hospitalization or death. Naturally, event-free survival (as a composite event) is always shorter in duration that survival alone.

Cost of health care

As indicated above, when considering the overall cost of heart failure, hospital costs represent the predominant component of expenditure in developed countries (usually more that 70% of expenditure).[38,39] Given the increasing complexity and cost of invasive procedures directed towards heart failure (e.g. resynchronization therapy and implantable defibrillators)[32,33] this component of expenditure is likely to increase rather than decrease. Figure 2.2 shows how the cost of health care can be calculated for an

individual patient or within a whole cohort – in this instance it reflects the average cost per heart failure patient in the UK based on a recent analysis of the economic burden of heart failure that examined the following important components of health care expenditure:

- prescribed pharmacotherapy (the cost of the drug plus dispensing costs);
- primary care consultations;
- unit-specific, per diem cost of hospitalization (inclusive of procedures);
- outpatient consultations;
- long-term institutional care.[39]

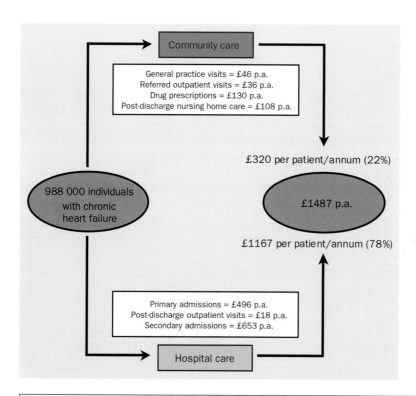

General practice visits = £46 p.a.
Referred outpatient visits = £36 p.a.
Drug prescriptions = £130 p.a.
Post-discharge nursing home care = £108 p.a.

£320 per patient/annum (22%)

988 000 individuals with chronic heart failure

£1487 p.a.

£1167 per patient/annum (78%)

Primary admissions = £496 p.a.
Post-discharge outpatient visits = £18 p.a.
Secondary admissions = £653 p.a.

Figure 2.2. The total direct cost of heart failure management in the UK: community vs hospital-based expenditure.

These data show the average cost of care per patient per annum in the UK for 1995. They were derived from a recent analysis of the economic burden of heart failure in the UK and are expressed in pounds sterling.[39]

It is important to note that these are overall figures from the estimated number of patients (approximately 1 million in 1995) who were being treated for heart failure in some way. For example, from the overall patient population of approximately 1 million individuals, it was further estimated that approximately one quarter were admitted during the calendar year 1995. Consistent with previous reports from other developed countries, therefore, approximately a relatively small proportion of patients consumed the major proportion of health care expenditure devoted to heart failure. Those patients who are managed in the community and avoid hospitalization (for the time being) cost the health care system far less. It is important to note that these are extremely conservative figures.

Creating an overall snapshot of the burden of heart failure

The above list, whilst fairly comprehensive, is also complex and may appear to be difficult to interpret. However, it is possible to utilize all these data to create an overall picture of the burden of heart failure within the patient population. Consider Figure 2.3. These data were generated from a similar cohort of older patients with heart failure who had divergent paths with respect to the pattern of morbidity and mortality dependent on whether they were exposed to a nurse-led,

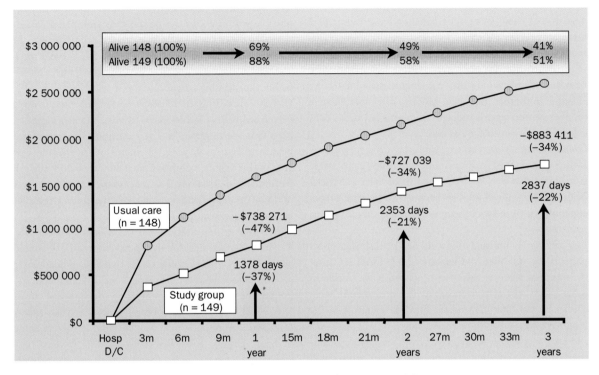

Figure 2.3. Combined outcome data from a cohort of 297 older patients with heart failure.

These data were generated from the 100% follow-up of 297 patients who participated in a recently reported study of the effects of a nurse-led, multidisciplinary home-based intervention following an acute hospital admission (hence the control and study groups).[40]

The horizontal axis shows that 100% follow-up was completed at 3 years following the index hospitalization. On the vertical axis is the cost of 'all-cause' hospital admission during this period (in this case AUD $). The two plots of the increasing cost of accumulated admissions over the 3-year period show that overall expenditure in the study group was far less at 1 (47% less relative to a usual care group of similar size), 2 (34% less) and 3 years (34% less). Importantly, if the relative number of days of hospitalization in the study group (37%, 21% and 22% less at 1, 2 and 3 years relative to usual care) were reported without being plotted on such a graph and without considering the absolute figures, generated cost-savings and patient survival, one might assume that the study intervention was of marginal benefit over a prolonged period with the greatest (relative) benefits occurring within 1 year (a period that is clearly too short to fully evaluate the effect of the intervention).

As these data show, however, the study intervention overall was successful in prolonging life without exposing patients to increased hospital admissions in the medium term and the health care system to increased costs. Alternatively, the study does not provide data on quality of life in surviving patients (crucially, these data were not collected). Other study data did show, however, that the cost of community care was comparable for the two groups over 3 years.

The data show the relative number of days.

The text box at the top of the figure shows the all-cause survival rates in the two groups at 1, 2 and 3 years following the index hospital admission.

multidisciplinary intervention following an 'index' hospital admission.[40]

As can be appreciated, despite surviving longer (with more patients surviving to 3 years), intervention patients still accumulated less 'all-cause' days of hospitalization, a similar quantity of community-based care and lower health care costs. However, despite the apparently better health outcomes, a number of issues require comment. The first of these is 'survival benefit'. Despite our best intentions, given sufficient follow-up and current treatment options, patients with heart failure will die sooner than if they did not have heart failure. Therefore, if a treatment does prolong life (e.g. angiotensin-converting enzyme inhibitors and beta-blockers) it may have a number of unintended 'side-effects' that need to be considered and, if possible, measured:

Quality of life of the patients (and carers if appropriate). Living an average of six more months may not be palatable if it means that it is six more months of extremely poor quality of life. Indeed, studies demonstrate that our preoccupation with survival benefit is not often shared by our patients.[8]

Cost shifting. By limiting follow-up to a period when most patients are still alive and healthy (i.e. before they enter the terminal phase of their heart failure), it is possible to inflate the 'cost-effectiveness' of the treatment. Most studies do not look 'beyond the horizon' to factor in the long-term cost of health care (see below).

Increased health care utilization. Given an increased lifespan, it is possible that patients with heart failure will consume a greater proportion of health care resources. Certainly, they will still require continuous treatment and community-based management. As indicated by the case history of Mr S, they are also likely to enter a 'hot' phase where their heart failure is terminal and they require intensive (and costly) treatment – usually in hospital.

It is for these reasons that a comprehensive picture of the pattern and burden of heart failure, both on the individual level and from an overall health care system perspective needs to be attained. The final section of this chapter discusses briefly major factors that might also provide misleading data and the danger of applying individual or localized data to the wider heart failure patient population.

Figure 2.3 combines some of these data to show the potential interrelationships between the various parameters that can be measured and how isolated data (especially when misrepresented) can be taken out of context.

Important caveats

The serial data presented in Figure 2.3 provide suitable warning with respect to 'when and how' the burden of heart failure is measured and presented. For example, when describing the utility of the NYHA classification it is especially important to remember that heart failure is a dynamic and 'fluid' syndrome with major fluctuations possible within a 24-hour period. For example, a patient may experience paroxysmal nocturnal dyspnoea overnight with dyspnoea at rest (NYHA class IV), take his/her medications in the morning and perform moderate exercise before experiencing fatigue and dyspnoea (NYHA class II). Clearly, recording the history of NYHA class over a prolonged period is extremely useful. The same type of problems are inherent in the six-minute walk test and health-related quality of life instruments that do not account for a 'fluid' condition such as heart failure and ask the individual questions that are extremely hard to answer in a non-specific manner – hence the need for a comprehensive overview of the individual's status.

It is within this context that the recent update of the AHA/ACC guidelines for the management of HF should be considered.[41] In response to the evolving epidemiologic profile of cardiovascular disease and the difficulty in determining the status of the patient using conventional means (e.g. NYHA class) at any one point in time, this expert committee proposed a new way of defining the epidemic of heart failure. In a new classification system, they identified four stages of heart failure with relevant features (see Table 2.1). Whilst in no way perfect, such a classification system acknowledges our current limitations in measuring and defining the impact of heart failure.

Table 2.1. *Stages of heart failure[41]*

Stage A	Individuals at high risk of developing heart failure, e.g. those with pre-existing hypertension, coronary artery disease and diabetes
Stage B	Individuals with previous acute myocardial infarction, asymptomatic valvular disease and/or asymptomatic left ventricular systolic dysfunction
Stage C	Individuals who have developed symptomatic heart failure
Stage D	Patients with chronic heart failure who have reached the stage where they require at least one hospitalization[41]

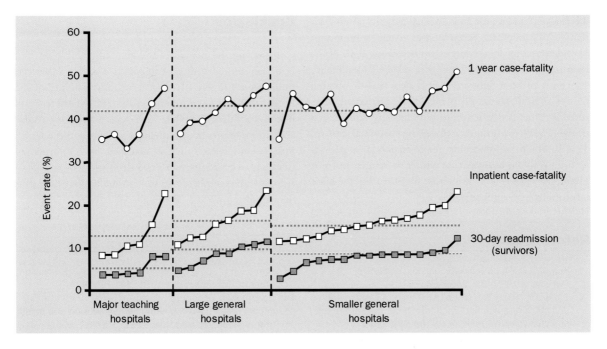

Figure 2.4. *Variations in readmission and case-fatality rates according to hospital of admission in Scotland (adapted from original data).*[48]

Each symbol (same order for each parameter) represents a hospital. The grey dotted lines show the average for each hospital (e.g. 12% inpatient case fatality in major teaching hospitals versus 16% in large general hospitals).

Apart from the uncertain trajectory of illness inherent to heart failure, there are other factors that have the potential to influence the individual patient and the overall burden of heart failure. For example, whilst clinical trials typically enrol patients in their thousands to demonstrate statistically significant differences between 'standard management' and new pharmacological modalities, it is clear that individualized pharmacological management is extremely important. Unfortunately, it is clear that despite clear guidelines[42] many patients do not receive gold-standard therapy. Quite apart from the issue of patient mismanagement in the setting of chronic disease and the need for greater empowerment to promote effective self-care behaviours,[43] it is clear that there are important national[44] and specialist-related[45] differences in the management of heart failure.

Even within a relatively homogeneous country with standard treatment guidelines and a uniform health care system, large variations in health outcomes are evident.[25] Figure 2.4 shows the large variation in morbidity and mortality rates following incident admissions for heart failure to three types of hospital in Scotland. Even when accounting for a number of important parameters (age, sex, deprivation, comorbidity and length of stay) these variations persisted.[46] Another important phenomenon, seasonal variations in heart failure-related morbidity and morbidity, was first reported in France[47] and subsequently Scotland.[48] In both studies from markedly different climates (predominantly Mediterranean vs cold temperate), it was evident that heart failure-related events, both in terms of hospital admissions and deaths, were markedly elevated in winter compared with months with variations as high as 40% in peak vs summer months. Older individuals with heart failure appear to be at greatest risk for such variation, with chronic lung disease representing an important contributor to the observed seasonal variations observed in these two countries.[47,48] What are the major implications of these large variations when attempting to measure accurately the individual and overall burden of heart failure? Firstly, it is clear that taking 'snapshots' of heart failure in the individual and the health care system is clearly inferior to obtaining detailed historical (even if this means over 1 month for an individual patient) trends for a number of parameters. Secondly, it is extremely important to understand the local context and determine some of the factors and issues (confounders) that are likely to influence the course of heart failure (e.g. it is clear that the natural history of heart failure often includes exacerbations triggered by other concurrent disease states). If performing a study of a therapeutic strategy using historical control data, it would be important not to match time periods according to the seasons (i.e. winter vs winter and not summer vs winter) and ensure that patients from the same institutions were compared.

Conclusion

Considering the nebulous and unpredictable nature of heart failure, measuring its impact is not easy. However, undertaken properly, with a clear understanding of the limitations of the commonly measured parameters and instruments used to collate such data, it provides invaluable information about individual patients and the health care system in which they are managed. Such information can be used to design more effective treatment and management strategies by determining whether they have produced substantive and meaningful changes.

References

1 Kelly DT. Our future society: a global challenge. *Circulation* 1997; **95:** 2459–64.

2 Gibbs JS, McCoy AS, Gibbs LM, Rogers AE, Addington-Hall JM. Living with and dying from heart failure: the role of palliative care. *Heart.* 2002; **88(S2):** 36–9.

3 McKee PA, Castelli WP, McNamara PM, Kannel WB. The natural history of congestive heart failure: the Framingham study. *N Engl J Med* 1971; **285:** 1441–6.

4 The New York Heart Association. Diseases of the heart and blood vessels; nomenclature and criteria for diagnosis. 6th ed. Boston: Little Brown and Co., 1964.

5 Packer M, Coats AJS, Fowler MB et al, for the Carvedilol Prospective Randomized Cumulative Survival (COPERNICUS) Study Group. *N Engl J Med* 2001; **344:** 1651–8.

6 Fletcher GF, Baladay G, Froelicher VF et al. Exercise standards: a statement for healthcare professionals from the American Heart Association writing group. *Circulation* 1995; **91:** 580–615.

7 Bittner V, Weiner DH, Yusuf S et al. Prediction of mortality and morbidity with a 6-minute walk test in patients with left ventricular dysfunction. *JAMA* 1993; **270:** 1702–7.

8 Levenson JW, McCarthy EP, Lynn J, Davis RB, Phillips RS. The last six months of life for patients with congestive heart failure. *J Am Geriatr Soc* 2000; **48:** S101–9.

9 Calman KC. Quality of life in cancer patients: a hypothesis. *J Med Ethics* 1984; **10:** 124–7.

10 Stewart AL, Greenfield S, Hays RD et al. Functional status and well-being of patients with chronic conditions: results from the Medical Outcomes Study. *JAMA* 1989; **262:** 907–13.

11 Juenger J, Schellberg D, Kraemer S et al. Health related quality of life in patients with congestive heart failure: comparison with other chronic diseases and relation to functional variables. *Heart* 2002; **87:** 235–41.

12 Berry C, McMurray JJV. A review of quality of life evaluations in patients with congestive heart failure. *Pharmacoeconomics* 1999; **16:** 247–71.

13 Cronbach LJ. Coefficient alpha and the internal structure of tests. *Psychometrika* 1951; **16:** 297–334.

14 Bergener M, Bobbitt RA, Carter WB et al. The sickness impact profile: development and final version of a health status measure. *Med Care* 1981; **19:** 787–805.

15 Ware J, Sherbourne C. The MOS 36-item short-form health survey (SF-36): conceptual framework and item selection. *Med Care* 1992; **30:** 473–83.

16 Hunt SM, McKenna SP, McEwen J et al. A quantitative approach to perceived health status: a validation study. *J Epidemiol Commun Health* 1980; **34:** 281–6.

17 Anderson JP, Kaplan RM, Berry CC et al. Interday reliability of functional assessment for a health status measure: the Quality of Well-being scale. *Med Care* 1989; **27:** 1076–84.

18 Wu AW, Damiano AM, Lynn J et al. Predicting future functional status for seriously ill hospitalised adults: the SUPPORT prognostic model. *Ann Intern Med* 1995; **122:** 342–50.

19 Ware JE, Kosinki M, Keller SD. A 12-item short-form health survey: construction of scales and preliminary tests of reliability and validity. *Med Care* 1995; **34:** 220–33.

20 Rector TS, Kubo SH, Cohn JN. Validity of the Minnesota Living with Heart Failure Questionnaire as a measure of therapeutic response to enalapril of placebo. *Am J Cardiol* 1993; **71:** 1106–7.

21 Wiklund I, Lindvall K, Swedberg K et al. Self-assessment of quality of life in severe heart failure. *Scand J Psychol* 1987; **28:** 220–5.

22 Metcalfe C, Thompson SG, Cowie MR, Sharples LD. The use of hospital admission data as a measure of outcome in clinical studies of heart failure. *Eur Heart J* 2003; **24:** 105–12.

23 Clarke KW, Gray D, Hampton JR. Evidence of inadequate investigation and treatment of patients with heart failure. *Br Heart J* 1994; **71:** 584–7.

24 Cowie MR, Fox KF, Wood DA et al. Hospitalization of patients with heart failure: a population-based study. *Eur Heart J* 2002; **23:** 842–5.

25 Stewart S, MacIntyre K, McCleod ME, Bailey AE, Capewell S, McMurray JJ. Trends in heart failure hospitalisations in Scotland, 1990–1996: an epidemic that has reached its peak? *Eur Heart J* 2001; **22:** 209–17.

26 Haldeman GA, Croft JB, Giles WH, Rashidee A. Hospitalization of patients with heart failure: national hospital discharge survey 1985–1995. *Am Heart J* 1999; **137:** 352–60.

27 Westert GP, Lagoe RJ, Keskimäki, Leyland A, Murphy M. An international study of hospital readmissions in Europe and the USA. *Health Policy* 2002; **61:** 269–78.

28 Brown A, Cleland J. Influence of concomitant disease on patterns of hospitalization in patients with heart failure discharged from Scottish hospitals in 1995. *Eur Heart J* 1998; **19:** 1063–9.

29 Jaagosild P, Dawson N, Thomas C et al. Outcomes of acute exacerbation of severe congestive heart failure. *Arch Intern Med* 1998; **158:** 1081–9.

30 National Health Service in Scotland. Scottish Health Service Costs *1995/96*. Edinburgh: Information and Statistics Division, 1995.

31 Lorusso R, La Canna G, Ceconi C et al. Long-term results of coronary artery bypass grafting procedure in the presence of left ventricular dysfunction and hibernating myocardium. *Eur J Cardiothorac Surg* 2001; **20:** 937–48.

32 Moss AJ Zareba W, Hall J et al. Prophylactic implantation of a defibrillator in patients with myorcardial infarction and reduced ejection fraction. *N Engl J Med* 2002; **346:** 877–83.

33 Cohen TJ, Klein J. Cardiac resynchronization therapy for treatment of chronic heart failure. *J Invasive Cardiol* 2002; **14:** 48–53.

34 Hsu J, Uratsu C, Truman A et al. Life after a ventricular arrhythmia. *Am Heart J* 2002; **144:** 404–12.

35 Murdoch DR, Love MP, Robb SD. Importance of heart failure as a cause of death: contribution to overall mortality and coronary heart disease mortality in Scotland 1979–1992. *Eur Heart J* 1998; **19:** 1829–35.

36 Burns RB, McCarthy EP, Moskowitz MA, Ash A, Kane RL, Finch M. Outcomes for older men and women with congestive heart failure. *J Am Geriatr Soc* 1997; **45:** 276–80.

37 Cowie MR, Wood DA, Coats AJS et al. Survival of patients with a new diagnosis of heart failure: a population based study. *Heart* 2001; **83:** 505–10.

38 Rydén-Bergsten T, Andersson F. The health care costs of heart failure in Sweden. *J Intern Med* 1999; **246:** 275–84.

39 Stewart S, Jenkins A, Buchan S, Capewell S, McGuire A, McMurray JJ. The current cost of heart failure in the UK – an economic analysis. *Eur J Heart Failure* 2002; **4:** 361–71.

40 Stewart S, Horowitz JD. Home-based intervention in congestive heart failure: long-term implications on readmission and survival. *Circulation* 2002; **105:** 2861–6.

41 ACC/AHA Guidelines for the Evaluation and Management of Chronic Heart Failure in the Adult. Executive Summary. A Report of the American College of Cardiology/American Heart Association Task Force on Practice Guidelines (Committee to Revise the 1995 Guidelines for the Evaluation and Management of Heart Failure): Developed in Collaboration with the International Society for Heart and Lung Transplantation; Endorsed by the Heart Failure Society of America. *Circulation* 2001; **104:** 2996–3007.

42 Remme WJ, Swedberg K. Guidelines for the diagnosis and treatment of chronic heart failure. *Eur Heart J* 2001; **22:** 1527–60.

43 Tattersall RL. The expert patient: a new approach to chronic disease management for the twenty-first century. *Clin Med* 2002; **2:** 227–9.

44 Cleland JG, Armstrong P, Horowitz JD et al. Baseline clinical characteristics of patients recruited into the assessment of treatment with lisinopril and survival study. *Eur J Heart Fail* 1999; **1:** 73–9.

45 Reis SE, Holubkov R, Edmundowicz D et al. Treatment of patients admitted to hospital with congestive heart failure: specialty-related disparities in practice patterns and outcomes. *J Am Coll Cardiol* 1997; **30:** 733–8.

46 Stewart S, Demers C, Murdoch DR et al. Substantial between-hospital variation in outcome following acute admission with heart failure. *Eur Heart J* 2002; **23:** 650–7.

47 Boulay F, Berthier F, Sisteron O, Gendreike Y, Gibelin P. Seasonal variation in chronic heart failure hospitalizations and mortality in France. *Circulation* 1999; **3:** 280–6.

48 Stewart S, MacIntyre K, Capewell S, McMurray JJV. Heart failure in a cold climate: seasonal variation in heart failure-related morbidity and mortality. *J Am Coll Cardiol* 2002; **39:** 760–6.

3 The pathophysiology of acute heart failure

Mary A Woo

Introduction

Heart failure has a devastating impact on quality of life, morbidity, and mortality and is one of the few cardiovascular diseases which is increasing in incidence and mortality.[1,2] If health care providers are to reverse this trend, they must provide timely and appropriate heart failure assessment and treatment. However, pathophysiology, symptoms, and treatment options can differ dramatically depending upon the acuity of heart failure. Acute heart failure is associated with a sudden onset initiated by a precipitating event that diminishes cardiac or hemodynamic function, and the usual compensatory mechanisms for inadequate cardiac output have not yet taken effect. Chronic heart failure occurs after an acute heart failure incident or when the precipitating event for the heart failure takes place over a longer period of time, allowing for partial compensatory mechanisms for inadequate cardiac output. Thus symptoms in acute heart failure often are more severe and underlying pathophysiology different in comparison with chronic heart failure.[3]

This chapter will concentrate on the pathophysiology of acute heart failure to provide the reader with baseline information for understanding other sections in this book on the pathophysiology of chronic heart failure and pharmacologic and non-pharmacologic interventions. However, before we can explore some of the specific pathophysiologic factors that precipitate acute heart failure, it might be of assistance to review briefly the general physiology of heart failure.

General physiology of heart failure – a brief review

Cardiac output is fundamentally altered in heart failure. Cardiac output is determined by heart rate and stroke volume. Heart rate largely is determined by the autonomic nervous system. Stroke volume is determined by preload, afterload, and contractility (Figure 3.1). A definition of these terms that every clinician should understand follows:

- *Preload*: the amount of end-diastolic fiber stretch in the heart caused by the end-diastolic volume. Within normal range, increased preload results in increased stroke volume and cardiac output. However, in the presence of abnormal cardiac tissue and when preload or end-diastolic fiber stretch (sarcomere length) increases excessively, higher than normal preload situations can cause a decrease in cardiac output. Clinically, preload can be evaluated using mean pulmonary capillary wedge pressure and the calculated pulmonary vascular resistance.

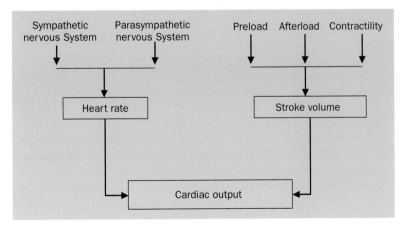

Figure 3.1. *Determinants of cardiac output.*

- *Frank–Starling principle*: describes the relationship between end-diastolic fiber stretch (preload) and cardiac contractility. Under normal physiologic conditions, as preload increases, cardiac contractility and cardiac output increases. However, in heart failure, the Frank–Starling curve is depressed. This means that in heart failure, increasing preload has a less positive relationship and impact on cardiac contractility and cardiac output.
- *Afterload*: this is the force that resists myocardial contraction and is influenced by blood pressure, blood volume, and cardiac wall thickness. Normally, cardiac output does not depend greatly on afterload. However, in heart failure, cardiac output is highly dependent on afterload. If afterload becomes too high, ventricular muscle strength/contractility will have difficulty overcoming the resistive force and will have increasingly limited ability to eject blood into the circulation. As a result, cardiac output decreases. Clinically, afterload can be estimated by systemic blood pressure or the calculated systemic vascular resistance.
- *Inotropy*: this ability to have variable contractility (changes in stroke volume and ejection force) is a unique characteristic of cardiac tissue. Inotropy is a complex process and is regulated to a great extent by the autonomic nervous system (Figure 3.2). Unfortunately, there is no direct clinical measure for contractility in intact, living organisms, and its impact on cardiac output must be estimated from measures of the other factors that influence cardiac output: heart rate, stroke volume, preload, and afterload.

When considering the pathophysiology of heart failure, it is important to remember that any factor that causes a fall in cardiac output or creates a situation in which cardiac output does not meet the demands of the body can precipitate heart failure. A decrease in cardiac function leads to a series of immediate systemic responses designed to improve perfusion to essential body organs (Figure 3.3). While these initial systemic responses can temporarily improve cardiac function and heart failure symptoms, if these systemic responses become chronic they can lead to further deterioration in cardiac function and the return of heart failure symptoms (Table 3.1).[4] Specific heart failure symptoms exhibited by patients will depend on the site of the cardiac failure (left vs right ventricle) and the form of cardiac dysfunction (systolic vs diastolic).

Impairment of the left vs right ventricle will give a different clinical spectrum of heart failure symptoms and treatments.[3] Left ventricular failure is the most common primary site of cardiac deterioration and is commonly caused by myocardial infarction and hypertension. When left ventricular performance is impaired, there is a drop in cardiac output and a sudden increase in pulmonary artery pressure (pulmonary capillary wedge pressure). As pulmonary pressure increases, it can overcome the oncotic pressure of the plasma proteins, thus causing pulmonary vascular congestion and edema, dyspnea, and pulmonary hypertension.

Failure of the right ventricle most commonly is due to left ventricular failure.[3] As the left ventricle fails, pulmonary pressure increases, which in turn increases right ventricular myocardial oxygen demand and workload, leading to eventual right ventricular dysfunction. Other causes of right ventricular failure include right ventricular myocardial infarction, primary pulmonary hypertension, pulmonary emboli, and mitral stenosis.[3,4] As right ventricular dysfunction becomes more pronounced, systemic venous congestion manifests and symptoms of hepatic and splanchnic enlargement and dysfunction, as well as peripheral edema (frequently seen in the ankles, legs and abdomen) are seen. Unfortunately, both left and right ventricles are often involved in heart failure. Yet the primary or principle ventricular failure site must be kept in mind and treated aggressively for optimal heart failure outcome.

Cardiac dysfunction can manifest as systolic or diastolic failure, or as a combination of both (often seen during coronary atherosclerosis and acute myocardial infarction). Systolic dysfunction is the more classic form of heart failure and primarily is associated with ventricular contractile (inotropic) abnormalities or physical loss of cardiac contractile tissue.[3,5] The ability of the heart to contract and mechanically eject blood into the systemic circulation is greatly diminished. Thus there is a net effect of decreased stroke volume and ejection fraction. Systolic dysfunction can occur from a variety of causes, including hypertension, severe pulmonary emboli, and dilated cardiomyopathy. Systolic heart failure can affect either or both ventricles.

Diastolic dysfunction is not as widely recognized by clinicians as systolic dysfunction, yet it is estimated to occur in 20–40% of heart failure patients.[4] The primary abnormalities in diastolic dysfunction are decreased ability of the heart to accept blood (increased stiffness) and decreased relaxation of the heart muscle. The stiffness is associated with diminished ventricular compliance (decreased end diastolic volume and shorter sarcomere length) and dramatically increased ventricular diastolic

Table 3.1. Acute vs chronic effects of systemic responses to decreased or impaired cardiac function

Systemic responses	Acute effects	Chronic effects
Sympathetic stimulation	Increases heart rate and cardiac contractility – this increases cardiac output by improvements in ejection fraction and heart rate	Increases myocardial oxygen demand, which can cause increased myocardial damage and dysfunction
Salt and water retention	Increases preload/ventricular myofibril stretch to increase cardiac output	Pulmonary and systemic venous congestion – increases systemic vascular resistance and creates excessive pulmonary vascular resistance – leads to decreased cardiac output
Vasoconstriction	Increases blood pressure to maintain perfusion to important body organs	Increases myocardial oxygen demand, which can cause increased myocardial damage and dysfunction

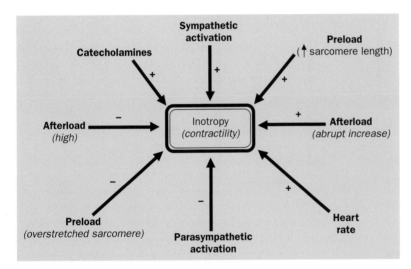

Figure 3.2. Elements that regulate and influence inotropy. + indicates elements increase inotropy; – indicates elements decrease inotropy.

pressure.[6,7] The end result is less ventricular filling and decreased stroke volume. Diastolic dysfunction also can occur by impairment in ventricular muscle relaxation. Relaxation can be diminished through abnormalities in calcium uptake by the sarcoplasmic reticulum or other mechanisms that reduce the rate of unbinding of actin from myosin.[5–7] Both of these forms of diastolic dysfunction can be caused by replacement of the heart's normally flexible tissue with nondistensible fibrous scar, ischemic myocardium, amyloid infiltration, or during conditions of ventricular hypertrophy.

Regardless of the site or form of cardiac dysfunction, when cardiac output decreases a variety of neurohormonal and hemodynamic responses occur immediately (see Figure 3.3). Neurohormonal activity is initiated when changes in cardiac output are detected in the ventricular stretch receptors and pressure receptors in the aortic arch and carotid artery.[3] Sympathetic nervous system and renin–angiotensin–aldosterone reflexes are triggered. These in turn initiate the release of antidiuretic hormone and natriuretic peptides.[3,8] In the short term, these neurohormonal responses cause arterial vasoconstriction

33

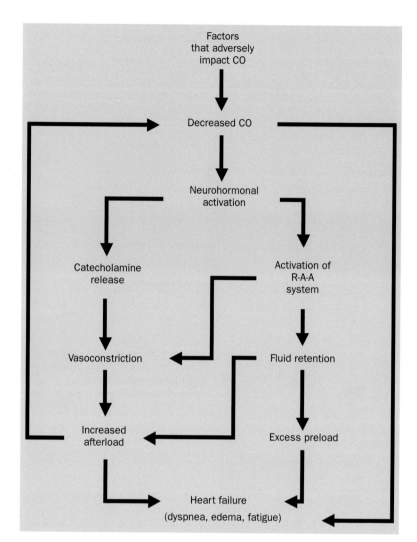

Figure 3.3. *General sequence of events leading to acute heart failure. CO, cardiac output; R-A-A, renin–angiotensin–aldosterone.*

(increased blood pressure), venous vasoconstriction (increased preload to the heart), and greater blood volume (increase in both blood pressure and preload).

Hemodynamic responses to a decrease in cardiac output are initiated by neurohormonal reflexes as well as by reduction in tissue oxygen delivery. The primary hemodynamic response is increased blood pressure owing to compensatory increase in blood volume. This increase in blood volume is accomplished through a variety of mechanisms. As renal perfusion decreases, urine output declines, fluid is retained, and blood volume increases. In addition, renin is released, which in turn activates the renin-angiotensin-aldosterone system (Figure 3.4) and enhances antidiuretic hormone secretion. All of these factors contribute to greater reabsorption of sodium and water by the kidneys.[9] This hemodynamic response will temporarily improve cardiac output and blood pressure. However, chronic activation of this system can lead to excessive preload, increased afterload, and elevated myocardial oxygen demand. All of these effects of chronic activation of hemodynamic responses to low cardiac output can lead to further myocardial injury, pulmonary and systemic edema, dyspnea and fatigue.

Pathophysiology of acute heart failure

Virtually anything that can create a situation in which cardiac output suddenly becomes inadequate to meet the body's needs can cause acute heart failure. However, the most common underlying causes for acute heart failure can be broadly classified into four areas:

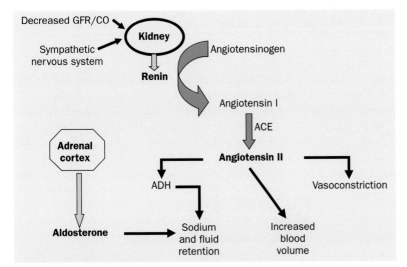

Figure 3.4.
Renin–angiotensin–aldosterone system response to decreased cardiac output. GFR, glomerular filtration rate; CO, cardiac output; ACE, angiotensin-converting enzyme; ADH, antidiuretic hormone.

- structural abnormalities;
- neurohormonal conditions;
- hemodynamic factors; and
- precipitating causes.

Structural abnormalities

Structural abnormalities induce acute heart failure by interfering with cardiac function to the extent that cardiac output is diminished. These conditions include acquired or congenital abnormalities that affect cardiac tissue, heart valves, and peripheral or cardiac blood vessels (Table 3.2). Probably the most common acquired structural abnormality is acute myocardial infarction. Acute myocardial infarction or myocardial ischemia can dramatically impact cardiac output and thus induce acute heart failure through loss of functional cardiac tissue.[10–12] Loss of cardiac tissue owing

to infarction/cell death or cell ischemia adversely affects cardiac contractility, stroke volume, and ejection fraction.[4]

In addition to the physical loss of functional myocardium, myocardial infarction can also induce heart failure through cardiac rupture or valvular impairment. Cardiac rupture is an actual tear in cardiac tissue, often at the site of the myocardial infarction. This can occur between heart chambers or even between the heart and the outside/pericardial sac. It is life-threatening and typically occurs several days after the acute myocardial infarction. Cardiac rupture can induce acute heart failure either through the shunting of blood to lower-pressure chambers in the heart or by hemorrhage into the pericardial sac. Both of these conditions divert blood from the systemic circulation and significantly decrease stroke volume.

Table 3.2. *Examples of underlying structural causes for acute heart failure*

Factor	How it causes heart failure
Myocardial infarction	Decreased stroke volume and ejection fraction by one or more of the following: • loss of functional myocardium • valvular dysfunction • cardiac rupture
Cardiac tamponade	Decreased stroke volume and ejection fraction by external compression of the heart
Congenital heart defects (valvular atresia; hypoplastic left heart syndrome)	Decreased stroke volume and ejection fraction; or excessive workload of the heart through abnormal vascular shunting

A common form of serious valvular dysfunction due to an acute myocardial infarction is papillary muscle rupture. While less common than cardiac rupture, its clinical presentation time is similar, in that it often occurs several days after the acute myocardial infarction. It is more frequent in patients who have an inferior wall myocardial infarction secondary to occlusion of the posterior descending artery of the right coronary artery.[3] With papillary muscle rupture, the heart valve can no longer close or remain closed during systole. As a result, significant valvular regurgitation (backward flow of the blood through the malfunctioning valve) can occur, thus decreasing forward flow/ejection fraction and if the regurgitation is severe, causing acute heart failure.

Cardiac tamponade is pericardial hemorrhage (leakage into the pericardial sac) secondary to cardiac rupture or pericarditis. It can induce acute heart failure by markedly restricting end-diastolic volume, thus decreasing stroke volume and limiting preload.

Congenital heart defects are the most common of the major birth defects (incidence is 8 cases out of every 1000 live births in the United States).[1] While most congenital heart defects are mild and unnoticed at birth, in some cases the abnormality is so severe that acute heart failure can quickly develop in the perinatal period. Some of the more severe congenital heart defects that can cause acute heart failure include valvular atresia and hypoplastic left heart syndrome. In valvular atresia, there is complete closure of the four heart valves. Of course if a heart valve doesn't open, then blood cannot progress through the heart. This can quickly induce heart failure through a lack of cardiac output. In the case of hypoplastic left heart syndrome, the chambers, valves, and related vessels on the left side of the heart are so underdeveloped that they cannot generate sufficient cardiac output.

Patients with structural abnormalities should be evaluated closely for early signs and symptoms of acute heart failure. Treatment should be targeted at alleviating the underlying structural defect. Closely linked to this phenomenon are the neurohormonal factors that both are triggered by, and contribute to, the impact of structural abnormalities on acute heart failure.

Neurohormonal conditions

When acute heart failure occurs, the neurohormonal system is rapidly activated in order to increase cardiac output. While neurohormonal system activation is often thought of as a response to heart failure, it also can trigger an acute heart failure event. Some examples of neurohormonal conditions that can cause acute heart failure are anxiety and stress, thyroid dysfunction, and medications or procedures that alter autonomic nervous system activity (Table 3.3).

Anxiety, stress, hyperthyroidism, and sympathomimetic medications can dramatically increase sympathetic activity. Increases in sympathetic tone can elevate myocardial and systemic oxygen demand, as well as raise heart rate and afterload.[5] These conditions set up a situation in which cardiac dysrhythmias and myocardial tissue damage can

Table 3.3. *Examples of underlying neurohormonal causes for acute heart failure*

Factor	How it causes heart failure
Anxiety/stress	Increased sympathetic activation (increased heart rate, increased myocardial oxygen demand, activation of the renin–angiotensin–aldosterone system)
Thyroid	Hyperthyroid – increased sympathetic activity and myocardial oxygen demand Hypothyroid – decreased heart rate and cardiac output

Medications/procedures
  Sympathetic stimulation
  (examples: cocaine, epinephrine, atropine)
	Increased myocardial oxygen demand, activation of renin–angiotensin–aldosterone system; if excessive sympathetic stimulation, damage to myocardial tissue and loss of functional myocardium

Parasympathetic stimulation/block sympathetic activity (examples: barbiturates, beta-blockers, calcium-channel blockers, carotid/vagal stimulation)	Decreased stroke volume and/or cardiac output

occur easily. As heart rate increases, preload is decreased to suboptimal levels and if there is excessive afterload, stroke volume and cardiac output also can be diminished.

The opposite situation, in which there is inadequate sympathetic stimulation or high parasympathetic activity, also can trigger acute heart failure.[3] Cases of significant hypothyroidism or medications and procedures that stimulate parasympathetic activity or block sympathetic tone, can dramatically lower heart rate and contractility. In such situations of diminished heart rate and contractility, stroke volume and cardiac output can drop to the extent that acute heart failure is induced. The risk of acute heart failure can be exacerbated if hemodynamic systems also begin to malfunction.

Hemodynamic factors

Hemodynamic factors that can produce acute heart failure are those primarily concerned with gas (oxygen and carbon dioxide) and nutrient delivery between the heart and tissues. Characteristics of the blood vessels and blood components are also of concern in this area. There are a variety of ways that abnormalities in these hemodynamic factors can induce acute heart failure (Table 3.4).

Situations that decrease oxygen and nutrient supply to the tissues can increase risk for acute heart failure. This decrease in oxygen and nutrient supply can occur due to lack of adequate blood (because of hemorrhage or excessive vasodilation due to septic or neurogenic shock). When this occurs, cardiac output may be unable to increase sufficiently to meet metabolic demands. As a result, acute heart failure can occur.

Another hemodynamic situation that can increase risk for acute heart failure is elevated preload. This can happen when there is excessive amounts of fluid in the intravascular spaces (example: renal failure, excess intravenous fluid administration) or when forward blood flow is impeded (as when there is massive pulmonary emboli that elevates right ventricular pressures).[3] When preload becomes too high in these cases, the sarcomeres become overstretched and stroke volume and cardiac output falls.

Hypertension is the most frequent antecedent to heart failure.[3,4] While it often is associated with chronic heart failure, if it develops quickly and reaches extremely high levels ('malignant hypertension') it can cause acute heart failure. What happens in such cases is that as the heart attempts to eject blood into the systemic circulatory system against the sudden high afterload produced by markedly elevated blood pressure, the heart can fail and cardiac output can decrease.[13] This dramatically increases myocardial oxygen demand, which can lead quickly to myocardial cell ischemia or death and thus further cardiac dysfunction and decreased cardiac output.

Precipitating causes

The factors in this category, dysrhythmias and inappropriate therapy, can cause acute heart failure in very different ways (Table 3.5). Cardiac dysrhythmias most often occur in persons with abnormal cardiac tissue/structure or excessive neurohormonal activation. Thus, dysrhythmias can be seen as a marker for the existence of other underlying causes of acute heart failure. Yet by themselves they can induce acute heart failure through a variety of

Table 3.4. *Examples of underlying hemodynamic causes for acute heart failure*

Factor	How it causes heart failure
Hemorrhage	Reduced oxygen delivery to tissues, causing increased myocardial oxygen demand and ischemic injury to the myocardium
Excess intravenous fluids	Excessive preload and venous congestion
Renal failure	Excessive preload and venous congestion
Hypertension	Increased afterload and increased myocardial oxygen demand
Vasodilation (septic or neurogenic shock)	Reduced oxygen delivery to tissues, causing increased myocardial oxygen demand and ischemic injury to the myocardium
Pulmonary emboli	Increases right ventricular systolic pressures thus heightening myocardial oxygen demand and increasing myocardial cellular damage

Table 3.5. *Examples of underlying precipitating causes for acute heart failure*

Factor	How it causes heart failure
Dysrhythmias	Can cause heart failure through: • tachycardia (high heart rates, decreased stroke volume) • bradycardia (decreased cardiac output) • dissociation between atria and ventricles (loss of 'atrial kick'/ventricular preload) • loss of ventricular contraction coordination (less efficient contraction and decreased stroke volume)
Inappropriate therapy (clinician error or patient non-compliance)	Multiple ways that this can cause heart failure, either related to increased myocardial workload and oxygen demand, decreased stroke volume, or decreased ejection fraction. Examples include: • excessive sodium intake • missed/deleted heart failure medications (such as diuretics) • excess medications which adversely impact cardiac function (examples: antidysrhythmics; calcium-channel blockers; beta-blockers)

mechanisms: decreased preload, decreased stroke volume, and low heart rates.[3] Tachycardias decrease the time allowed for ventricular filling, thus diminishing sarcomere stretch and lowering preload. As a result, stroke volume can be decreased dramatically. Additionally, tachycardias will greatly increase myocardial oxygen demand and ischemia, thereby inducing further impairment to inotropy and coordinated cardiac function.

The opposite condition, bradycardia, also can induce acute heart failure if there is a significant drop in cardiac output secondary to a very low heart rate. Another dysrhythmia that can drop preload to dangerously low levels is atrial fibrillation, particularly if the heart already has structural abnormalities and decreased ejection fraction. The loss of coordinated atrial contraction of blood into the ventricles ('atrial kick') can decrease end-diastolic ventricular volume (preload) and significantly lower cardiac output.

Inappropriate therapy can occur over a wide selection of treatment types and for numerous reasons.[14,15] A few examples of inappropriate therapy include patient non-compliance with dietary sodium restriction or medication regimens (e.g. missing diuretic doses) and clinician error (excessive amount of intravenous fluid or beta-blocker medication). Inappropriate therapy is extremely frequent and is a major cause of heart failure patient morbidity and mortality.[3,15] With such a wide range of possibilities, the ways that inappropriate therapies can induce acute heart failure appear almost endless. They include excessively high preload and afterload (high sodium intake; missed diuretic medication doses) as well as cardiac tissue depression/diminished contractility (excess beta-blocker, calcium-channel blocker, or antidysrhythmic medications). Fortunately, factors are often amenable to prevention and correction (please see the chapters on patient management and education).

Summary

It would be simplistic to view these underlying causes of acute heart failure (structural abnormalities, neurohormonal conditions, hemodynamic factors, and precipitating causes) in isolation. As with most pathophysiologic mechanisms, these factors often overlap and interact. Also, their relationships may not remain stable during the heart failure process. For example, noncompliance with diuretic medication may be the initial cause for an acute heart failure event, but neurohormonal and hemodynamic factors may be emphasized for treatment by clinicians.

To provide optimal care for heart failure patients, clinicians need to understand the pathophysiology of both acute and chronic heart failure. This knowledge will provide them with the tools to plan appropriate care for the heart failure patient. It also will allow them to objectively evaluate current therapies and judge or develop future therapeutic options for heart failure management.

References

1 American Heart Association. 2001 Heart and Stroke Statistical Update. Dallas, TX: American Heart Association, 2000.

2 National Heart, Lung and Blood Institute. Mortality and Morbidity: 2000 Chart Book on Cardiovascular, Lung, and Blood Diseases. Bethesda, MD: National Institutes of Health, 2000.

3 Colucci WS, Braunwald E. Pathophysiology of heart failure. In: E. Braunwald (ed). *Heart Disease: A Textbook of Cardiovascular Medicine*, 6th edition. Philadelphia, PA: W.B. Saunders, 2001:534–61.

4 Katz AM. *Physiology of the Heart*, 3rd edition. Philadelphia, PA: Lippincott, Williams & Wilkins, 2001.

5 Carelock J, Clark AP. Heart failure: pathophysiologic mechanisms. *Am J Nurs* 2001; **101:** 26–33.

6 Vasan RS, Benjamin EJ. Diastolic heart failure – no time to relax. *N Engl J Med* 2001; **344:** 56–9.

7 Philbin E, Rocco T, Lindenmuth N, Ulrich K, Jenkins P. Systolic versus diastolic heart failure in community practice: clinical features, outcomes, and the use of angiotensin-converting enzyme inhibitors. *Am J Med* 2000; **109:** 605–13.

8 Stevenson LW. Natriuretic peptides and CHF. *Cardiology Rev* 1999; **16:** 38–41.

9 Stowasser M. New perspectives on the role of aldosterone excess in cardiovascular disease. *Clin Exp Pharmacol Physiol* 2001; **28:** 783–91.

10 Marino P, Destro G, Barbieri E, Bicego D. Reperfusion of the infarct-related coronary artery limits left ventricular expansion beyond myocardial salvage. *Am Heart J* 1992; **123:** 1157–65.

11 Solomon SD, Glynn RJ, Greaves S, Ajani U, Rouleau J et al. Recovery of ventricular function after myocardial infarction in the reperfusion era: the healing and early afterload reducing therapy study. *Ann Intern Med* 2001; **134:** 451–8.

12 Gadsboll N, Torp-Pederson C, Hoilund-Carlsen P. In-hospital heart failure, first-year ventricular dilation, and 10-year survival after acute myocardial infarction. *Eur J Heart Failure* 2001; **3:** 91–6.

13 Gandhi S, Powers J, Nomeir A, Fowle K, Kitzman D et al. The pathogenesis of acute pulmonary edema associated with hypertension. *N Engl J Med* 2001; **344:** 17–22.

14 Miura T, Kojima R, Mizutani M, Shiga Y, Takatsu F, Suzuki Y. Effect of digoxin noncompliance on hospitalization and mortality in patients with heart failure in long-term therapy: a prospective cohort study. *Eur J Clin Pharmacol* 2001; **57:** 77–83.

15 Evangelista LS, Dracup K. A closer look at compliance research in heart failure patients in the last decade. *Progress Cardiovasc Nurs* 2000; **15:** 97–103.

4 The pathophysiology of chronic heart failure

Mariann R Piano

Introduction

The purpose of this chapter is to provide an overview of the pathophysiology of chronic heart failure and to specifically detail how the progression of heart failure is linked to the process of ventricular remodeling. The syndrome of chronic heart failure is no longer conceptualized as a hemodynamic disorder due to changes in renal and neurohormonal function. Instead, heart failure is a syndrome that begins at the cellular level and is characterized by abnormal myocyte growth (hypertrophy), changes in the extracellular matrix protein composition and myocyte cell loss, all of which culminate in significant structural ventricular remodeling of the heart and loss of ventricular function. In this chapter, also reviewed are the different pathophysiologic signals (neurohormones, peptides, cytokines, growth factors) that are activated in the syndrome of heart failure. Insight into the pathophysiologic mechanisms and signals that underlie the development and progression of heart failure will provide the clinician with a better understanding of pharmacologic approaches in the treatment of heart failure. In addition, the clinician will better understand how certain signs and symptoms are linked to the development of heart failure.

Definition and classification of chronic heart failure: systolic vs diastolic heart failure

Chronic heart failure is not a disease. Chronic heart failure is a syndrome that is preceded by an initiating cardiovascular event such as myocardial infarction (MI), hypertension or cardiomyopathy. Therefore, in the continuum of cardiovascular disease, chronic heart failure is viewed as an end event and represents the most severe manifestation of cardiovascular disease. However, even though chronic heart failure is viewed as an end event, it is a progressive syndrome that develops over the course of many years.

The definition and classification of chronic heart failure has changed over the years. In the past, most definitions emphasized secondary alterations in hemodynamics; consequently heart failure was defined as a circulatory disorder secondary to systolic dysfunction.[1] However, it is well recognized that more than 40% of adult patients with heart failure have preserved systolic function with diastolic dysfunction.[2–4] Consequently, two separate definitions have emerged. Systolic heart failure is defined as an inability of the left ventricle to contract against a load and eject blood volume into the aorta.[5] A hallmark sign of systolic heart failure is a reduced stroke volume and ejection fraction.[5] Diastolic heart failure is defined as the inability of the left ventricle to accommodate blood volume during diastole at low to normal filling pressures.[6–8] In other words, the left ventricle is less accommodating and normal end-diastolic volumes are associated with high end-diastolic pressures. Patients with diastolic heart failure have signs and symptoms of pulmonary congestion, in the presence of normal or near normal left ventricular function.[6–8] These designations have been important to delineate, since patient outcomes, signs and symptoms and treatment options are different depending upon the presence of systolic vs diastolic heart failure. The differences between systolic and diastolic heart failure are presented in Table 4.1 and Figure 4.1.

In the past, the classifications of heart failure have been linked to the side of the heart affected (left vs right), direction of blood flow (backward vs forward) or the underlying condition (abnormal cardiac muscle contraction and relaxation and/or both, excessive pressure or volume overload or limited ventricular filling). Currently, however, the definition and classification of heart failure are essentially the same, in that heart failure is classified as systolic vs diastolic heart failure or heart failure with preserved (usually defined as ejection fraction (EF) ≥ 40%) vs non-preserved (usually defined as EF ≤ 40%) left ventricular function.[9] Based upon these designations, it has become apparent that these two types of heart failure differ in terms of underlying pathophysiology, initiating events, risk factors and clinical characteristics (Table 4.1). In

Table 4.1. *Differentiating systolic vs diastolic heart failure*

	Systolic HF (EF ≤ 39%)	Diastolic HF (EF ≥ 40%)
Clinical correlates	History of HF, cardiomegaly, history of ischemic heart disease, male gender, lower body index	Older age, diabetes (early stage), systolic hypertension, female gender, greater body mass index
Associated conditions	Ischemic heart disease Idiopathic CM Hypertension	Hypertrophy or restricted CM Valvular etiology of HF
Annual mortality rate	15–30%	5–12%
Length of hospitalization	Same	Same
Distinguishing diagnostic features	↓ EF (<39%) ↑↑ intraventricular diastolic pressure and volumes	Normal EF Presence of increased diastolic filling pressure or impaired filling due to decreased ventricular compliance ↑ LV filling pressures ↑ Pulmonary pressures during exercise
Remodeling characteristics	Eccentric hypertrophy LV dilatation and wall thinning, ↑ myocardium size Imbalance between collagen breakdown and accumulation Myocyte hypertrophy ↑ Compliance	Concentric hypertrophy ↑ Wall thickness and interstitial fibrosis (↑ collagen deposition) ↑ fibrosis and ↓ compliance Delayed relaxation (↓ SERCA2 function) Myocyte hypertrophy Subendocardial ischemia
Echo-derived correlates	↓ EF ↓ Wall thickness and ↑ EDD and ESD	↔ EF ↑ Wall thickness and ↓ EDD and ESD Early-to-late filling ratio (E/A) < 1.0* ↑ Deceleration time and Isovolumic relaxation time

CM, cardiomyopathy; EF, ejection fraction; EDD, end-diastolic dimension; ESD, end-systolic dimension; SERCA2, sarcoplasmic reticulum Ca^{2+}-activated ATPase pump; LV, left ventricle; HF, heart failure; E/A, early diastolic (E) and atrial filling velocity (A).

* Indicates that with progression of disease there can be a pseudonormalization of the E/A ratio (E/A > 1.0)

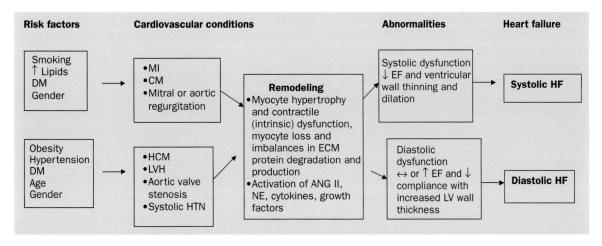

Figure 4.1. *Differences between diastolic and systolic heart failure. CM, cardiomyopathy; MI, myocardial infarction; LVH, left ventricular hypertrophy; HCM, hypertrophic cardiomyopathy; DM, diabetes mellitus; HF, heart failure; EF, ejection fraction; LV, left ventricle. DM can be associated with the development of both systolic and diastolic heart failure. However, more often in the early stages of diabetes, patients have diastolic dysfunction. As the diseases progresses, patients develop enlarged LV chambers and wall thinning and at this point patients are considered to have DM cardiomyopathy. Adapted and used with permission from Mandinov et al.[6]*

terms of clinical characteristics, Devereux et al[4] (the Strong Heart Study) reported that patients with heart failure and normal left ventricular EF (EF ≥ 40%), more frequently had the following characteristics:

- female gender;
- older age;
- increased body mass;
- increased systolic blood pressure;
- renal dysfunction;
- concentric left ventricular geometry; and
- impaired early diastolic left ventricular relaxation.[4]

In a multivariate analysis the strongest predictors were renal dysfunction and older age.[4] The Strong Heart Study was a population-based survey of cardiovascular risk factors and cardiovascular disease in American Indian communities in Arizona.[4] Investigators have confirmed these findings in other populations. For example, Philbin et al found older age, female sex, greater body weight and valvular heart disease occurred more often in patients with EF > 50%.[3] In this latter study there was no difference in the occurrence of hypertensive disease between the two groups of heart failure patients. Philbin et al also compared readmission for heart failure, time to first heart failure-related hospital readmission between patients with diastolic (EF > 50%) and systolic (EF < 39%) dysfunction and found no differences in these outcome variables.[3]

However, total mortality was significantly greater in the heart failure patients with systolic dysfunction (EF < 39%) compared with those with diastolic dysfunction (EF > 50%).[3]

Ventricular remodeling: definition and gross structural changes

Definition

As noted above, the progression of heart failure is linked to the process of ventricular remodeling. The term ventricular remodeling refers to progressive changes in the size and shape of the myocardium.[10,11] As discussed in more detail below, the process of ventricular remodeling is due to changes that begin at the cellular level and involve both the myocyte and non-myocyte cell types. Specifically, there are alterations in molecular events regulating the gene expression of various cardiac proteins that affect the following:

- myocyte growth (hypertrophy);
- intrinsic myocyte function;
- myocyte loss (apoptosis/necrosis); and
- proliferation/degradation of proteins in the extracellular matrix.

It is important to note that the changes and involvement of the specific cell types one finds in the remodeled myocardium may depend on the initial etiopathology, the stage of remodeling and the area of the myocardium evaluated. These cellular mechanisms underlie the progressive global cardiac dysfunction and transition toward end-stage heart failure, which makes the remodeling process a cause rather than consequence of heart failure. In addition, at least in post MI patients, left ventricular remodeling was associated with higher morbidity and mortality rates.[12,13] Lamas et al[14] found that after MI, patients with a spherical shaped ventricle had lower ejection fractions, decreased exercise tolerance and increased incidence of heart failure.

These data further support the idea that left ventricular remodeling contributes to the development of heart failure.

Gross structural changes

Initially the term ventricular remodeling was used to describe changes in ventricular size and geometry that occurred after MI. This term has become more encompassing and is used to describe changes in ventricular geometry and shape that occur in association with other cardiovascular events, such as long-standing hypertension

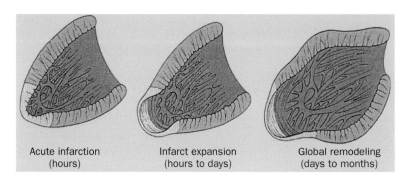

Acute infarction
(hours)

Infarct expansion
(hours to days)

Global remodeling
(days to months)

Figure 4.2. *Cardiac remodeling associated with myocardial infarction. Used with permission from Pfeffer.[16]*

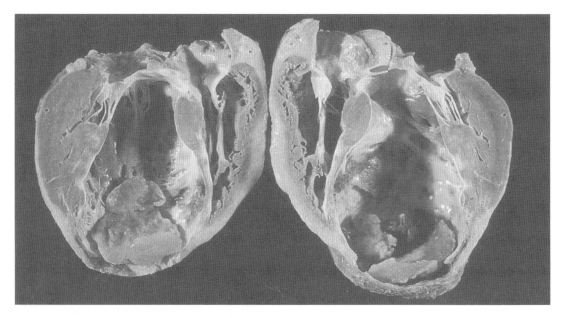

Figure 4.3. *Cross-sectional view of a heart from a cardiac transplant patient who survived a large transmural anterior/septal myocardial infarction. There is thinning and elongation of the infarcted region and cavity enlargement and hypertrophy in the remaining section. Used with permission from Pfeffer.[16]*

and cardiomyopathies.[11] However, the changes that occur in ventricular size/shape and function are dependent in part on the initiating condition. As detailed below, ventricular remodeling after MI is characterized by profound ventricular dilation, wall thinning, increased heart size, eccentric hypertrophy, and systolic dysfunction.[11,15] Ventricular remodeling associated with long-standing hypertension is characterized by left ventricular hypertrophy (concentric hypertrophy), increased myocardial mass and diastolic dysfunction (at least in the early stages) (Table 4.1).[11,15,16]

To date, researchers have most extensively studied the time course, pathophysiology and clinical correlates of postinfarction ventricular remodeling. Postinfarction remodeling has been divided into two phases: early (within 72 hours of infarct) and late remodeling (> 72 hours after infarct).[15] In the immediate time frame after the infarct (early phase), remodeling changes are limited to the area surrounding the infarct (Figure 4.2).[16] In brief, during this time frame the process of cell necrosis is associated with activation of a local inflammatory response, in which numerous cell types (monocytes, macrophages, neutrophils) are activated and recruited to this region of myocardium.[15] Neutrophils release matrix metalloproteinases (MMPs) which degrade the supporting fibrillar collagen network that weaves around and connects the myocytes. However, over the course of months to years there is involvement of the entire ventricle, such that the entire ventricle becomes dilated and globular in shape (late remodeling). In this setting, ventricular thinning and elongation are due in part to misalignment and slippage of the myocytes and occurs in the area close to the infarct.[10] The non-infarcted area of the myocardium dilates and hypertrophies (Figures 4.2 and 4.3).

As noted above, remodeling also occurs in association with hypertensive heart disease although the overall shape and size of the myocardium are different, in that left ventricular hypertrophy and extensive interstitial fibrosis are prominent clinical features (Figure 4.4).[11] In the early stages patients are usually asymptomatic, however diastolic filling abnormalities may be present, such as a decrease in the E/A wave ratio, and an increase in deceleration time and isovolumic relaxation time (Figure 4.4). In the later stages of hypertensive heart disease, patients become symptomatic and develop diastolic heart failure.[11]

Does remodeling occur in all patients with cardiovascular disease? Several cardiac conditions are associated with ventricular remodeling. However, not all patients (even in the absence of specific pharmacologic therapies, e.g. angiotensin-converting enzyme inhibitors) with these conditions experience ventricular remodeling. For example, ventricular remodeling does not occur in all patients experiencing MI.[17,18] In both animal models of MI and in humans, extensive collateral circulation, small transmural MIs and non-Q-wave MIs are less often associated with remodeling.[17,18] Gaudron et al found the following factors were associated with an increased risk for remodeling and progressive left ventricular dysfunction: ventriculographic infarct size, EF at day 4 (EF ≤ 39%), and anterior transmural MIs and TIMI grade flow (rate of arteriographic contrast flow in the infarct artery).[18] The predictive value of these factors was highest when all four factors were used together. In general, others have corroborated these findings. However, results of more recent investigations suggest that ventricular function evaluated later after MI (2 weeks' pre-discharge) was more predictive of remodeling.[19] Therefore, based on these findings, Solomon and Pfeffer recommend that later rather than early assessment of left ventricular function may be a better predictor of ventricular function and remodeling.[17]

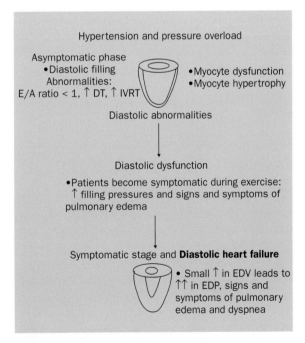

Figure 4.4. Changes in myocardial structure associated with diastolic heart failure. E/A, early diastolic (E) and atrial filling velocity (A); DT, deceleration time; IVRT, isovolumic relaxation time; EDV, end-diastolic volume; EDP, end-diastolic pressure.

Cellular changes involved in remodeling

The remodeling process that ensues after a MI or long-standing hypertension is due to events that originate at the cellular level and involve changes in the both myocyte and non-myocyte cell types. The non-myocytes include fibroblasts that secrete collagen, endothelial cells, and vascular smooth muscle cells. With regard to the non-myocytes, the discussion in this chapter is limited to the fibroblasts. This is not to underemphasize the importance of changes in the coronary vessels, such as impaired angiogenesis and endothelial cell dysfunction; however, the latter is an extensive topic and would require a separate full review.

Myocyte hypertrophy and intrinsic myocyte dysfunction

One of the best-characterized cellular changes in the remodeling process is myocyte hypertrophy. This is defined as an increased myocyte size in the absence of cell division. Under conditions of physiologic demand, such as increased pressure or stretch, the myocyte will hypertrophy to maintain contractile force.[20] Hypertrophy occurs due to a coordinated increase in protein synthesis, which is primarily the result of the increased expression of the genes that encode for the contractile proteins.[21] Some of the contractile proteins that have been shown to increase in myocyte hypertrophy include β-myosin heavy chain and troponin T.[21] There are many other changes in the cell that accompany the process of hypertrophy. As shown in Figure 4.5, there is an increase in the number of mitochondria, the sarcoplasmic reticulum enlarges and there are changes in many of the membrane-bound transport pumps, ion channels and receptors.[22] For example, there is a decrease in the number of β-adrenergic receptors. In addition, the gene expression and protein levels of non-contractile proteins, atrial natriuretic peptide (ANP) and brain natriuretic peptide (BNP) have been shown to be increased in myocyte hypertrophy.[23]

Along with myocyte hypertrophy, the myocardial remodeling process is also associated with changes in intrinsic myocyte function. Intrinsic myocyte dysfunction arises from within the cell and therefore can be attributed to either alterations in the structure or function of intracellular organelles, in particular, intracellular organelles that are critical to excitation–contraction (EC) coupling. Changes in any of the events involved in the EC process could alter calcium homeostasis, myocardial contraction and relaxation. Almost every aspect of EC coupling has been studied in the setting of both human and animal heart failure. The number of published studies is immense; therefore a summary of the changes in EC coupling mechanisms is presented in Table 4.2.[24] It is important to note that EC alterations have not been found consistently in

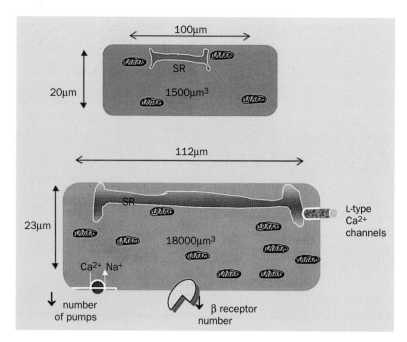

Figure 4.5. Myocyte changes in hypertrophy. See text for explanation. SR, sarcoplasmic reticulum. Adapted with permission from Chevalier et al.[22]

Table 4.2. Changes in excitation–contraction (EC) coupling

	Sarcolemmal channels/Pumps	Change in heart failure
L-type calcium channel	ECF Ca^{2+} entry through these voltage activated channels stimulates Ca^{2+} release from SR[20]	$\downarrow$ and $\leftrightarrow$ channel number[25–30] Potential effect on peak Ca^{2+} current, $\downarrow$ SR Ca^{2+} release–these changes could influence systolic force development
Na–Ca exchanger	Bidirectionally transports three Na^+ ions for one Ca^{2+} ion[20]	$\uparrow$ Na–Ca protein levels and mRNA levels[31,32] May be adaptive mechanism that facilitates Ca^{2+} removal during diastole
β_1-adrenergic receptors	Activation of these receptors is associated with an $\uparrow$ in myocardial force, rate of relaxation and heart rate[20]	Downregulation of β receptors[33] Attenuated affect of β agonists
Intracellular organelles		
SR–CRC	The SR is the major site for Ca^{2+} storage and release. Ca^{2+} is released from the CRC[20]	$\downarrow$CRC number and mRNA levels[34–36] $\downarrow Ca^{2+}$ release from SR and $\downarrow$ in peak Ca^{2+} transients and therefore force production
SERCA2	This is a Ca^{2+}-activated ATPase protein which is responsible for the re-uptake of Ca^{2+} into the SR during diastole[20]	$\downarrow$ SERCA2 levels and mRNA levels[37–41] $\downarrow Ca^{2+}$ uptake into SR and therefore a $\downarrow$ in the rate of relaxation
Phospholamban	Protein co-localized with SERCA2, which regulates SERCA2 activity. Phospholamban phosphorylation increases SERCA2 activity and therefore increases Ca^{2+} uptake into SR[20]	$\downarrow$ and $\leftrightarrow$ in phospholamban protein and mRNA levels[39,40] $\downarrow Ca^{2+}$ uptake into SR and therefore a $\downarrow$ in the rate of relaxation

ECF, extracellular fluid; SR, sarcoplasmic reticulum; mRNA, messenger ribonucleic acid; CRC, calcium release channel; SERCA2, sarcoplasmic reticulum Ca^{2+}-activated ATPase pump.
Used with permission from Piano et al.[24]

47

human heart failure or animal models of heart failure. For example, both increases and no change in the number of L-type calcium channels have been found in the setting of heart failure.[25–30] On the other hand, one of the most consistent findings has been a decrease in the activity, protein quantity and messenger ribonucleic acid (mRNA) quantity of the sarcoplasmic reticulum Ca^{2+}-activated ATPase (SERCA2) pump (Table 4.2).[31–41] As noted in Table 4.2, the primary function of the SERCA2 pump is to pump calcium back into the sarcoplasmic reticulum during diastole. Recent findings from del Monte et al underscore the importance of the SERCA2 pump in heart failure. These investigators used an adenoviral gene transfer technique to overexpress SERCA2 protein into myocardial tissue from non-failing and failing human myocardial tissue.[42] The overexpression of SERCA2 was associated with a significant improvement in diastolic and systolic function.[42]

The above results suggest, at least in failing end-stage hearts, the restoration of SERCA2 function can improve both diastolic and systolic function and therefore intrinsic myocyte function is in part an important determinant of contractile dysfunction. However, it is not known if changes in intrinsic myocyte function precede the remodeling process or are a late finding in the setting of remodeling and heart failure. In addition, the changes found may relate to the stage/severity of left ventricular remodeling, as well as the etiology of the remodeling process. Recently, Gupta et al evaluated myocyte intrinsic function 1 week and 5 weeks after the experimental induction of a MI in a rat.[43] Interestingly, these authors found that myocytes isolated from a remote non-infarcted area of the myocardium had normal intrinsic contractile function (evaluated in isolated myocytes), even though there was significant ventricular dilation, wall thinning and global ventricular dysfunction (as measured in the whole heart, as well as papillary muscle preparations).[43] Furthermore, these myocytes were hypertrophied and there were significant changes in gene expression (i.e. an increase in BNP mRNA and decrease in SERCA2 mRNA). These findings suggest, in an animal model of MI, that myocardial remodeling and global functional abnormalities have occurred in the absence of intrinsic myocyte dysfunction. These authors concluded that, at least in the early stages after a MI, non-myocyte factors, such as loss of myocytes due to apoptosis may be more important in the generation of contractile dysfunction in the remodeled heart.[43] Finally, in terms of the significance of these changes, some experts have suggested that these changes are adaptive and

serve to protect the already damaged myocyte; however, these damaged and weakly contracting myocytes can further contribute to reduced myocardial performance and the process of ventricular remodeling.

Changes in gene expression

Many of the changes noted above in intrinsic myocyte function are due to increases or decreases in the expression of various proteins, such that there is the emergence of a new myocyte phenotype.[44] Interestingly, some genes that were present in embryonic or fetal life are re-expressed, whereas the gene expression of other proteins, such as the SERCA2, phospholamban and calcium release channel (Table 4.2) are decreased. Genes that are upregulated include those encoding for the fetal protein isoforms of β-myosin heavy chain and α-skeletal actin.[44] In contrast, genes which encode for the adult isoforms of α-myosin heavy chain and α-cardiac actin are downregulated.[44] As noted earlier, one of the most ubiquitous findings in human heart failure and animal heart failure models is the increased expression of ANP and BNP mRNA and protein levels in ventricular tissue.[44] How these changes contribute to the process of left ventricular remodeling and progression of heart failure is not completely understood.

Apoptosis: cell death

Another process that may be involved in remodeling is cell death due to apoptosis. Apoptosis is a process whereby cells undergo a 'programmed' genetically-determined cell death.[45] Apoptosis of cardiomyoctyes and non-myocytes have been found in the biopsy specimens of patients in heart failure associated with ischemic and idiopathic dilated cardiomyopathy as well as in the setting of acute MI.[46–51] In some ways this was not a surprising finding because the process of apoptosis can be stimulated by stress conditions such as ischemia, cytokines (tumor necrosis factor-α or TNF-α), angiotensin II, and norepinephrine, all of which are activated or increased in the setting of heart failure.

Apoptosis is one of two very different modes of cell death that occur in physiologic systems; the other is necrosis. As shown in Figure 4.6, these two modes of cell death differ in many ways.[52] However, it is important to first note that apoptosis is a critical physiologic mechanism by which cells are deleted during normal development and other stages of life to regulate cell mass and organ architecture.[45] In later stages of life, apoptosis may play a role in maintaining health by eliminating malignant, infective or

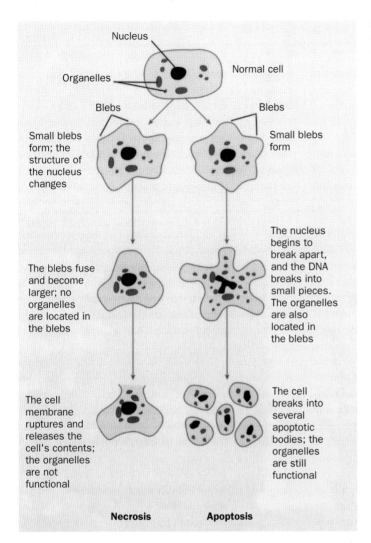

Figure 4.6. Cellular differences between apoptosis and necrosis. From Nanji and Hiller-Strumhofel.[52]

redundant cells. However, excessive and unbalanced apoptotic cell death can lead to disease or organ failure.

Cell necrosis occurs in response to a physical or chemical injury, such as ischemia or toxins. In necrosis, there is cell swelling, clumping of the nuclear chromatin, disruption of intracellular organelles and eventual rupture of the membrane and calcium overload, all of which occur over the course of 20–30 minutes.[45,52] The cell contents are released into the surrounding tissue, initiating an inflammatory response. In contrast, the process of apoptosis is initiated by activation of caspase enzymes, which belong to a family of intracellular proteases.[45] The activity of capsase enzymes is regulated by the expression of genes (bcl-2) that encode for pro-apoptotic (e.g. BAX) and anti-apoptotic (e.g. bcl-2) proteins.[45,52] Normally, these proteins are associated with the mitochondria, but when they detach from the mitochondria, they activate caspase enzymes.[45] The time course of apoptosis is about 12–24 hours and the cell characteristics include shrinkage of the cell, condensation of the cytoplasm, nuclear deoxyribonucleic acid (DNA) fragmentation and membrane blebbing. As shown in Figure 4.6 the cell breaks into metabolically active apoptotic bodies, which are evenly absorbed (phagocytosed) by neighboring cells and this process does not elicit an inflammatory response.[52] In the heart, the functional consequences of apoptosis may include electrical heterogeneity which gives rise to arrhythmias, myocyte misalignment and ventricular wall thinning and dilation.[53]

As noted above, there are several reports of apoptosis occurring in the setting of MI and idiopathic dilated cardiomyopathy.[49–51,54,55] In the setting of MI, human and animal studies have shown that in addition to necrosis, in both early and late stages of infarction there is also cell death due to apoptosis.[50,51] Others have shown in rodent models of experimental MI, that there is increased apoptosis in the myocardial tissue remote to the infarct both at 5 weeks and 6 months post MI.[43,56] In patients who died of MI, Saraste et al[50] and Olivetti et al[51] found evidence of apoptotic cell death in tissue obtained from the infarct border zone, compared with tissue remote from the infarct area. In the setting of dilated cardiomyopathy, there is variability among studies, in terms of the number of apoptotic cells and the specific regions of the myocardium that are affected by apoptotic death.[57] For example, Gorza et al[58] reported that 0–0.16% of myocyte loss was due to apoptotic cell death in patients with idiopathic cardiomyopathy. In contrast, Olivetti et al[48] reported an apoptotic rate around 0.23% (i.e. 2318 cells with apoptotic nuclei per 10^6 myocytes) in myocardial tissues samples obtained at transplant from patients with ischemic and idiopathic dilated cardiomyopathy (CM). Possible discrepancies among the studies may relate to the patient population and etiology of heart failure and apoptotic quantification method (there are currently six different techniques available to measure apoptosis). Nevertheless, data from both animal and human studies provide evidence for a role of apoptosis in the setting of MI and CM. However, it remains to be determined if apoptosis plays a significant role in the remodeling process and the transition from compensated to decompensated heart failure.

Even though the importance of apoptosis in the transition from compensated heart failure to cardiac failure remains unknown, there are many pathological stimuli in heart failure that can activate apoptosis. For example, angiotensin II (ANG II),[59] TNF-α,[60] norepinephrine (NE),[61] and ventricular dilatation/stretching[62] are linked to apoptotic cell death. In heart failure, the occurrence of apoptosis may also be influenced by the production of bcl-2 proteins. As noted above, the bcl-2 protein has anti-apoptotic effects, whereas other bcl-2-like proteins, BAK and BAX, are pro-apoptotic. In heart failure patients,

Olivetti et al[48] examined the rate of apoptosis and the quantities of these proteins. These investigators, using the the DNA laddering technique, found a marked increase in apoptotic cell death and a higher level of bcl-2 expression in failing myocytes compared to non-failing myocytes. BAX levels were unchanged between failing and non-failing myocytes. This was an unexpected finding since, bcl-2 proteins protect cells from apoptosis, whereas BAX proteins are pro-apoptotic.[48] Latif et al also determined the levels of bcl-2 proteins in patients with dilated and ischemic CM.[63] They found an increased rate of apoptosis (exemplified by higher percentage of TUNEL-positive cells) in both CM groups compared to normal donor hearts, as well as an increase in levels of the pro-apoptotic proteins, BAK and BAX.[63] However, they also found increased levels of the anti-apoptotic proteins, bcl-2 and bcl-xL.[63] These latter findings suggest that there may be an imbalance between production of pro- and anti-apoptotic proteins in the setting of CM.

Extracellular matrix remodeling

As noted above, non-myocytes, specifically the fibroblasts, are involved in the remodeling process. Fibroblasts synthesize and secrete collagen, the major structural protein of the extracellular matrix (ECM).[64] The ECM is primarily composed of fibrillar collagen proteins, such as type I and III collagen.[64] In the heart, type I collagen is the most abundant of the collagens and has the tensile strength of steel.[64] Type I collagen forms a two-dimensional extracellular scaffold-like structure that weaves around and tethers myocytes and other cell types together (Figure 4.7).[65] The collagen component of the ECM is very important in maintaining myocyte alignment, transducing force generated by the myocytes, preventing myocyte slippage and overstretching during the cardiac cycle.[66] Collagen is also a major determinant of myocardial compliance.

The ECM also contains important non-fibrillar collagen proteins, such as fibronectin, laminin, cell adhesion molecules and integrins.[67] Fibronectins within the ECM serve to adhere the myocytes to collagen. Cardiac laminin is found predominantly in the basal membrane (a thin sheet-like network of ECM proteins linked to the cell membrane) and also binds collagen.[67] Collectively, these non-collagen proteins function as anchors and also guide or facilitate different processes such as cell migration and proliferation. A loss of these non-collagen fibers could result in myocyte detachment to the basal membrane and a loss of ventricular force transmission from the myocyte to the ECM.[68] Finally, the integrins located in the cell

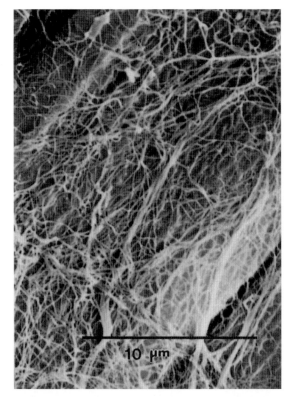 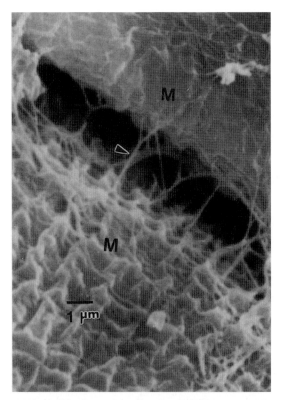

Figure 4.7. *Scanning electron micrograph at × 5200 (left) and × 10 000 (right) of normal rat extra cellular matrix (ECM). As shown, the collagen fibers weave around the myocytes and at the higher magnification, collagen struts can be seen between adjacent myocytes. Used with permission from Caulfield et al.[65]*

surface are very important in mediating cell–cell interactions and communication between the ECM and cytoskeleton.[67] (Integrins form a physical link between the ECM and the cytoskeleton [intracellular scaffold of connective proteins].)[67] Myocardial integrins also play a role in transmitting and distributing mechanical force generated by the myocyte to the ECM.[67]

During the remodeling process, fibroblasts proliferate and increase their production of collagen, as well as the non-collagen proteins, fibronectin, and laminin.[69] This, along with myocyte hypertrophy, contributes to the increase in cardiac mass and size. In the area of cardiac ECM remodeling, most of the investigations to date have focused on the collagen component of the ECM and the development of cardiac fibrosis. Cardiac fibrosis is defined as an increase in collagen synthesis and deposition within the cardiac interstitium, as well as a change in the type of collagen synthesized, the organization and cross-links among collagen fibers types.[70] Fibrosis may occur in response to a direct injury, such as MI (*reparative* fibrosis),

or *reactive* fibrosis may occur due to the presence of stimuli such as angiotensin II, aldosterone, immune complexes, and increased stretch.

Cardiac fibrosis may be preceded by enhanced breakdown of the fibrillar collagen network. As noted earlier, in the early phase following MI, neutrophils release MMPs, which degrade the supporting fibrillar collagen network.[15] Loss of the supporting fibrillar collagen network is shown in Figure 4.8.[65] Loss of the collagen tethers leads to myocyte slippage, ventricular wall thinning and enlargement.[15,16] However, over the course of months to years in areas remote to the infarct there is a disproportionate increase in collagen type III relative to type I and myocyte hypertrophy.[15] This leads to ventricular dilatation, increased wall stress, increased compliance) and systolic dysfunction.

With hypertensive heart disease, excessive collagen deposition predominates.[64,68] In the early stages there is collagen accumulation, myocyte hypertrophy, and microvascular alterations. The primary stimulus for

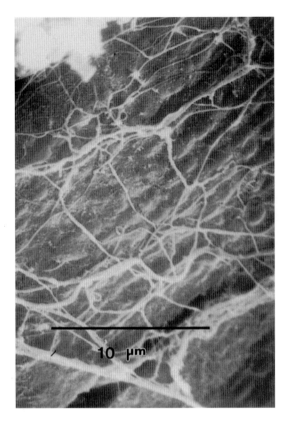
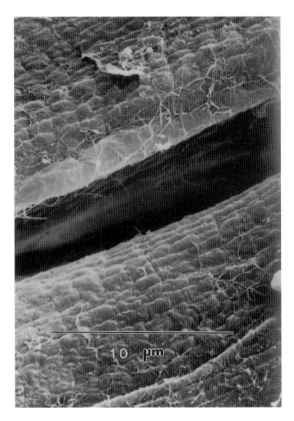

Figure 4.8. *Scanning micrographs of the extracellular matrix obtained from rat myocardium 5 weeks after the administration of an oxidized glutathione, an agent which activates collagenolysis, possibly by activating matrix metalloproteinases. As shown in both panels, there is a loss of the fibrillar network and tethers between the myocytes. Used with permission from Caulfield et al.*[65]

increased fibroblast collagen production is pressure, regardless of whether the increased pressure is a result of longstanding hypertension or valvular heart disease. Interestingly, when there is increased pressure due to volume, there is no increase in collagen accumulation.[64,68] In the later stages there is loss of myocytes, which are progressively replaced with dense fibrous tissue. Myocardial fibrosis contributes to the increase in myocardial mass, decreased myocardial compliance and diastolic dysfunction, and abnormalities in electrical conduction (Figure 4.4).[69,70]

As noted above, in some situations the process of fibrosis is preceded by small cuts or breaks in the fine fibrillar collagen that weaves around the myocyte due to activation of the MMPs.[71] There is another group of related endogenous proteins, the tissue inhibitors of matrix metalloproteinases (TIMPS) which control/inhibit the activity of the MMPs.[72] Therefore, the structural integrity of the ECM is influenced by the balance between TIMP and MMP activity. Recently, Li et al[73] found decreased gene expression and protein quantities of TIMP-1 and TIMP-3 and increased protein quantities and activity of MMP-9 in ventricular tissues of patients with ischemic and dilated cardiomyoapthy. (As a point of clarification, there are several TIMP and MMP proteins [usually designated as TIMP-1, TIMP-2, MMP-1, MMP-2, etc.] and their role, as well as level of expression, is probably tissue specific.) In another study, Thomas et al[74] found increased quantities of several MMPs, as well as increased MMP activity, in the hearts of patients with end-stage dilated cardiomyopathy (DCM) compared with controls; however, this was accompanied by increased quantities of TIMP-1 and TIMP-2. Although further research is warranted in this area, data from these investigations suggest an imbalance in MMP and TIMP activity may be involved in the left ventricular remodeling process.

Mechanical and chemical signals involved in stimulating myocyte and non-myocyte changes

The above changes in the biology of the myocyte and non-myocyte components of the heart are stimulated by a multitude of signals that are classified as mechanical/hemodynamic (pressure, volume, stretch) or chemical (neurohormones, peptides, growth factors).[75] Blocking these signals has become the major goal of pharmacologic therapy. For example, renin angiotensin-converting enzyme (ACE) inhibitors and angiotensin II receptor blockers are used to attenuate the effects of ANG II. In the section below several well-established signals are reviewed, along with their role in the remodeling process.

Pressure and stretch

It is well established that mechanical signals such as pressure and stretch are involved in the evolution of cardiac remodeling.[76] Under normal physiologic circumstances, pressure is important in maintaining heart weight. However, sustained increases in pressure, due to increased blood pressure (afterload) or increased intraventricular pressure (due to left ventricular dilation or increased diastolic filling pressure) stimulate an increased expression of a variety of cardiac genes and proteins. In addition, via mechanical stretch there is increased release of tissue ANG II and growth factors and activation of signal transduction pathways which are linked to increased protein synthesis and cell proliferation mechanisms (e.g. phosphoinositide signal transduction system and protein kinase C).[77]

Mechanical stretch also affects the ECM. As noted above, the integrins are important in communicating outside signals from the ECM into the cell and therefore may play a role in stimulating the changes in fibroblasts. Only recently has the role of the cell surface integrins been investigated and some data support the idea that physical stimulation of the integrins may activate intracellular signals, that impact cell growth and proliferation.[78]

Norepinephrine

Norepinephrine (NE) is a neurohormone released from sympathetic post ganglionic nerve terminals and increased plasma levels are found after sympathetic activation, which occurs in response to a decrease in cardiac output, renal hypoperfusion and arterial underfilling.[79] In 1984, Cohn et al established that increased plasma NE levels were associated with an increased mortality rate in heart failure patients.[80] In the setting of heart failure there is increased sympathetic activity to the myocardium and there is increased NE levels in the vicinity of the myocyte as well as in the circulation.[79] NE stimulates a variety of pathologic events in the remodeling process such as myocyte hypertrophy, fibroblast proliferation (increased collagen production), activation of fetal-gene programs, downregulation of β receptors, and apoptosis.[81,82] NE also produces arterial vasoconstriction (increased afterload), redistribution of regional blood flow and arrhythmias.[79]

Renin–angiotension–aldosterone system

ANG II is the effector hormone of the renin–angiotensin system (RAS). There are two pathways or sources of ANG II formation: circulating, and tissue-derived.[83] In the circulation, ANG II is produced via ACE-stimulated conversion of ANG I to ANG II. ANG I is derived from angiotensinogen (renin substrate).[83] Renin released from the kidney stimulates the conversion of angiotensinogen to ANG I. It is also important to note that ACE (or kininase II) breaks down bradykinin.[83] Bradykinin has many effects that oppose ANG II, some of which include vasodilatation, anti-growth and anti-apoptotic effects (effects attenuating the remodeling process).[84] Therefore, it has been speculated that the beneficial effects of ACE inhibitors are due to both a decrease in ANG II formation, as well as an increase in bradykinin levels. ANG II is also produced within the myocardial tissue (i.e. tissue-derived) and several of the circulating components, such as renin and angiotensinogen are involved in tissue ANG II formation.[85] However, at least in the human heart, ANG II is formed by non-ACE dependent mechanisms involving different enzyme systems (e.g. cathepsin G, chymostatin-sensitive ANG II-generating system, heart chymase).[85] Once ANG II is secreted from the cell, it acts in a paracrine manner to stimulate neighboring myocytes and fibroblasts.

What are the consequences of ANG II production? Data from human pharmacologic clinical trials, as well as recent experiments in transgenic animals has established ANG II as a key player in the remodeling process and progression of heart failure. In fact, similar to increased NE plasma levels, increased plasma levels of ANG II correlate with increased morbidity and mortality.[86] Circulating ANG II stimulates vasoconstriction, aldosterone secretion, increased reabsorption of sodium, and presynaptic release of NE from post ganglionic nerve terminals.[85] Tissue-derived ANG II plays a role in stimulating myocyte hypertrophy, apoptosis, and fibroblast proliferation with subsequent production of collagen.[87] In addition, in other in vitro cell studies, others found that ANG II enhanced the production of local superoxides.[88] Collectively, these observations suggest circulating, as well as tissue-derived, ANG II are involved in stimulating the remodeling process.

What stimulates the production of ANG II during the remodeling process? Depending on the initiating condition there could be different stimulants. For example, after a MI, there is renal hypoperfusion and arterial underfilling, which stimulates renin release from the renal afferent arteriole and NE release from noradrenergic nerve terminals.[89] NE also stimulates β1 adrenoreceptors in the juxtaglomerular apparatus to secrete renin.[89] In terms of tissue ANG II production, activation of serine proteases (enzymes) are associated with an increase in angiotensinogen gene expression, and stretch due to increased wall stress increases the release of ANG II from cytoplasmic (within the cell) granules.[15,76]

Another key component of this system is aldosterone. Aldosterone is a mineralocorticoid synthesized in the zona glomerulosa of the adrenal cortex.[90] The main function of aldosterone is to stimulate distal renal tubule reabsorption of sodium (a process coupled to secretion of potassium and hydrogen ion). In the setting of heart failure, plasma aldosterone levels are much greater than physiologic levels.[91] The increased aldosterone levels may be due to ANG II-stimulated aldosterone release, as well as decreased hepatic clearance.[91] In addition, fibroblasts that have been transformed into myofibroblasts (via transforming growth factor β) secrete aldosterone.[78] In terms of the remodeling process, aldosterone stimulates fibroblast proliferation and collagen accumulation and is therefore thought to be a key contributor in ECM remodeling.[78] Aldosterone, via increased sodium reabsorption also contributes to edema formation.

Cytokines

Over the last decade, others have established that TNF-α and ET-1 may play a significant role in the development and pathogenesis of left ventricular dysfunction and heart failure.[92,93] Plasma levels of ET-1 and TNF-α are elevated in patients with left ventricular dysfunction and are correlated to worsening New York Heart Association (NYHA) functional class, EF and exercise capacity.[94–97] Cytokines are proteins released by immune cells, such as macrophages and monocytes, which in turn stimulate and regulate a variety of immune responses.[92] For example, proinflammatory cytokines such as TNF-α, stimulate via an autocrine or paracrine manner, the synthesis of other inflammatory mediators, such as platelet-activating factor, eicosanoids and oxidative radicals.[92] Furthermore, TNF-α stimulates fibroblasts to release MMPS while inhibiting the secretion of TIMPs and TNF-α also stimulates the fibroblast to express adhesion molecules.[98]

A major source of TNF-α production is macrophages, and the myocardium, similar to other organs, contains resident macrophages. However, it is well established that myocytes also produce TNF-α and others have shown that the myocardium produces more TNF-α per gram of tissue in response to endotoxin compared with the liver and spleen.[99] Bozkurt et al showed that a continuous infusion of TNF-α in rats led to a time-dependent decrease in left ventricular function that was accompanied by left ventricular dilation.[100] Additional work has shown that TNF-α stimulates a number of processes such as hypertrophy, apoptosis and fibroblast proliferation that are key cellular events in the remodeling process.[101] In animal models of heart failure several investigators have demonstrated that physiologic concentrations of TNF-α (i.e. concentrations found in heart failure patients) are associated with the development of left ventricular hypertrophy and dilation.[100,102] In further support of the role of TNF-α in left ventricular remodeling, Kubota et al found that transgenic mice that overexpress TNF-α progressively developed left ventricular dysfunction and remodeling, similar to what is found in heart failure.[103] In addition, some of the other signs and symptoms in heart failure, such as decreased contractility, pulmonary edema, decreased peripheral organ perfusion, and anorexia and cachexia have been attributed to increased cytokine levels.[104]

TNF-α primarily exerts its effects via two TNF-α receptor subtypes: TNF-R1 and TNF-R2; however, most of the effects of TNF-α are mediated via the TNF-R1 receptor subtype.[92] The biology of TNF-α receptor is interesting because mammalian cells shed the TNF-α receptors under the influence of various stimuli, such as prolonged exposure to TNA-α. Some studies have shown that once the TNF-α receptors are cleaved (and shed) from the cell membrane, they exist in the blood as circulating, soluble receptors.[92] Soluble TNF-α receptors retain their ability to bind to TNF-α and inhibit the cytotoxic effects of this cytokine in cell culture. The soluble TNF-α receptors may serve as a biological buffer, since the receptor can bind and neutralize the cytotoxic activities of TNF-α.[92] Increased plasma levels of the TNF-α receptors have been found in hospitalized heart failure patients.[105] The TNF-α receptors may have an immediate benefit of buffering the potentially untoward effects of TNF-α.

However, most investigators believe that over time, the increased levels of the receptors are maladaptive and actually stabilize biologically-active TNF-α to slowly release the cytokine into the circulation.[92] Recently, Bozkurt et al reported significant improvement in left ventricular structure and function in heart failure patients (NYHA III/IV, n = 15–16) treated twice daily with etanercept (Enbrel) for 3 months.[106] Etanercept is a soluble TNF receptor antagonist that binds and inactivates TNF-α. However, the large randomized clinical trial, Randomized Etanercept North American Strategy to Study Antagonism of Cytokines, which was designed to examine the effect of etanercept on mortality, demonstrated no benefit.[107] In some patients, etanercept induced or exacerbated heart failure.[107] There may be a multitude of reasons for the poor clinical outcomes, however, at this time the cytokine hypothesis, as well as the role of anticytokine medications, requires further investigation in the context of heart failure.

Similar to TNF-α, increased plasma levels of endothelin have been found in heart failure patients; however, increased plasma levels are primarily found in patients with severe heart failure (NYHA class IV).[95] In severe heart failure, increases in plasma big-ET and ET-1 have been found (big-ET is the biologically inactive precursor to ET-1). A major source of ET-1 are endothelin cells; however, levels of ET-1 are also found in the myocardium (it is unknown whether the myocytes take up ET-1 or are an actual source of ET-1) and ET-1 rather than big-ET is found in the myocardium.[95] In a rat MI model of heart failure, Kobayashi et al found an increase in myocardial tissue ET-1 content, as well as an increase in ET-1 receptors.[108] ET-1 is a potent vasoconstrictor and many of its effects on the myocardium may be exerted indirectly by way of its effects on afterload and the pulmonary vasculature. Also ET-1 stimulates the conversion of ANG to ANG II and may potentiate some of the effects of ANG II.[109]

Growth factors

Also released along with cytokines from injured or necrotic myocytes, is the growth factor peptide, transforming growth factor β1 (TGFβ1). Similar to other growth factor peptides, TGFβ1 exerts a spectrum of effects during normal cardiac growth and development; some of these effects are in part mediated by TGFβ1 effects on the production of other growth factors, extracellular matrix proteins and cell-adhesion molecules.[78] TGFβ1 is highly expressed in fetal atria and ventricles, but downregulated in adult ventricular tissue.[110] However, in animal models of MI and pressure overload (hypertrophy), there is an

upregulation of TGFβ1 gene expression.[111,112] Moreover, Boluyt et al have shown that there is increased TGFβ1 gene expression during the development of heart failure in spontaneously hypertensive rat, suggesting this growth factor may be involved in the remodeling process.[113] Specifically in vitro, TGFβ1 stimulates myocyte hypertrophy and fibroblasts proliferation. Cardiac fibroblasts are a principle source of TGFβ1.[114] TGFβ1 in turn increases collagen gene expression in fibroblasts.[114] Interestingly, ANG II (in cell culture) stimulates TGFβ1 gene expression, suggesting a mechanism whereby ANG II stimulates the development of cardiac fibrosis.[114]

Conclusion

Chronic heart failure is an end event that can be initiated by a number of cardiovascular conditions such as hypertension, MI or CM. Heart failure is defined and classified as either diastolic or systolic heart failure. Findings from recent investigations suggest that there are differences between the two types of heart failure, in terms of myocardial structure, performance, signs and symptoms. The development of systolic and diastolic heart failure is linked to the process of ventricular remodeling which is due to numerous changes in myocyte and nonmyocyte cell types. Initially these changes represent a general process of adaptation. For example, after a MI, there is myocyte dropout due to necrosis. As a means of adaption, neighboring viable cells surrounding the necrotic area change their phenotype (e.g. hypertrophy, decreased expression of SERCA2, increased Na–Ca exchanger) which sustains force production, while conserving energy.[115] At the same time there is activation of various neurohormones and peptide systems that act as 'signals' to further stimulate changes in the myocyte and fibroblasts. However, eventually there is excessive myocyte hypertrophy, imbalances in collagen degradation and production, further myocyte dropout, ventricular wall thinning and enlargement. These latter changes are associated with heart failure.

Signals such as ANG II are thought to play a key role in the remodeling process. In support of this, Harada et al have shown that transgenic mice lacking the AT_1 receptor have less left ventricular remodeling and improved survival after an experimentally induced MI.[116] These results suggest a very important role for ANG II in the left ventricular remodeling process. However, on the other hand, these results also suggest that since the effect of left ventricular remolding was not totally abolished in this transgenic model lacking the AT_1 receptor, other systems may be involved as well, such as NE, cytokines and growth factors. There are many redundant and backup systems in physiology; therefore, it is not unlikely that many systems must fail and or be activated for the myocardium itself to fail and lose its ability to maintain cardiac output. Therefore, preventing or attenuating the remodeling process has become the major objective of pharmacologic therapy.

References

1 Katz AM. *Heart Failure*. Philadelphia: Lippincott Williams & Wilkins, 2000.

2 Senni M, Tribouilloy CM, Rodeheffer RJ et al. Congestive heart failure in the community. *Circulation* 1998; **98:** 2282–9.

3 Philbin EP, Rocco TA, Lindenmuth NW, Ulrich K, Jenkins PL. Systolic versus diastolic heart failure in community practices: clinical features, outcomes, and the use of angiotensin-converting enzyme inhibitors. *Am J Med* 2000; **109:** 605–13.

4 Devereux RB, Roman, MJ, Liu JE et al. Congestive heart failure despite normal left ventricular systolic function in a population-based sample: the Strong Heart Study. *Am J Cardiol* 2000; **86:** 1090–6.

5 Goldsmith SR, Dick C. Differentiating systolic from diastolic heart failure: pathophysiologic and therapeutic considerations. *Am J Med* 1993; **95:** 645–55.

6 Mandinov L, Eberli FR, Seiler C, Hess OM. Diastolic heart failure. *Cardiovasc Rev* 2000; **45:** 813–25.

7 Lenihan DJ, Gerson MC, Hoit BD, Walsh RW. Mechanisms, diagnosis and treatment of diastolic heart failure. *Am Heart J* 1995; **130:** 153–66.

8 Stork T, Mockel M, Danne O, Voller, Eichstadt H, Frei U. Left ventricular hypertrophy and diastolic dysfunction: their relation to coronary artery disease. *Cardiovas Drugs Ther* 1995; **9:** 533–7.

9 Heart Failure: evaluation and care of patients with left-ventricular systolic dysfunction. Rockville, MD: U.S. Department of Health and Human Services. Agency for Health Care Policy and Research, June 1994 (AHCPR Pub. No. 94–0612).

10 Goldstein, S, Ali AS, Sabbah H. Ventricular remodeling. *Cardiol Clin* 1998; **16:** 623–32.

11 Maisch B. Ventricular remodeling. *Cardiology* 1996; **87(suppl 1):** 2–10.

12 White HD, Norris RM, Brown MA, Brandt PWT, Whitlock RML, Wild CJ. Left ventricular end-systolic volume as the major determinant of survival after recovery from myocardial infarction. *Circulation.* 1987; **76:** 44–51.

13 Pfeffer MA, Pfeffer JM. Ventricular enlargement and reduced survival after myocardial ionfarction. *Circulation.* 1987; **75(suppl):** IV93–IV97.

14 Lamas GA, Vaughan DE, Parisi AF et al. Effects of left ventricular shape and captopril therapy on exercise capacity after anterior wall acute myocardial infarction. *Am J Cardiol* 1989; **63:** 1167–73.

15 St John Sutton MG, Sharpe N. Left ventricular remodeling after myocardial infarction. *Circulation* 2000; **101:** 2981–8.

16 Pfeffer MC. Cardiac remodeling and its prevention. In: Braunwald E, ed. *Atlas of Heart Diseases*. Heart Failure: Cardiac Function and Dysfunction. New York, NY: Mosby Year Book;1995.

17 Solomon SD, Pfeffer MA. The decreasing incipience of left ventricular remodeling following myocardial infarction. *Basic Res Cardiol* 1997; **92:** 61–5.

18 Gaudron P, Eilles C, Kugler I, Ertl G. Progressive left ventricular dysfunction and remodeling after myocardial infarction: potential mechanisms and early predictors. *Circulation* 1993; **97:** 755–63.

19 Pfeffer MA, Greaves SC, Arnold JMA et al. Early versus delayed angiotensin converting enzyme inhibition therapy in acute myocardial infarction: in the Healing and Early Afterload reducing Therapy Trial. *Circulation* 1997; **95:** 2643–51.

20 Berne RM, Levy MN. *Physiology*. Fourth Edition. St. Louis: Mosby, 1998.

21 Lowes BD, Minobe W, Abraham WT, Rizeg MN, Bohlmeyer TJ. Changes in gene expression in the intact human heart. *J Clin Invest* 1997; **100:** 2315–24.

22 Chevalier B, Charlemagne D, Callens-el Amrani F, et al. The membrane proteins of the overloaded and senescent heart. Basic Res Cardiol 1992; **87:** S187–97.

23 de Bold AJ, Bruneau BG, Kuroski-de Bold MK. Mechanical and neuroendocrine regulation of the endocrine heart. *Cardiovasc Res* 1996; **31:** 7–18.

24 Piano MR, Kim SD, Jarvis C. Cellular events linked to cardiac remodeling in heart failure: targets for pharmacologic intervention. *J Cardiovasc Nurs* 2000; **14:** 1–23.

25 Li GR, Ferrier GR, Howlett SE. Calcium currents univentricular myocytes of prehypertrophic cardiomyopathic hamsters. *Am J Physiol* 1995; **268:** H999–H1005.

26 Colston JT, Kumar P, Chamber JP, Freeman GL. Altered sarcolemmal calcium channel density Ca^{2+}-ATPase activity in tachycardiac-induced heart failure. *Cell Calcium* 1994; **16:** 349–56.

27 Rasmussen RP, Minobe B, Bristow MR. Calcium antagonist binding sites in failing and nonfailing human ventricular myocardium. *Biochem Pharmacol* 1990; **39:** 691–6.

28 Sen L, Smith TW. T-type Ca^{2+} channels are abnormal in genetically determined cardiomyopathic hamster hearts. *Circ Res* 1994; **75:** 149–55.

29 Gomez AM, Valdivia HH, Cheng H et al. Defective excitation–contraction coupling in experimental cardiac hypertrophy and heart failure. *Science* 1997; **276:** 800–6.

30 Takahashi T, Allen PD, Lacro RV et al. Expression of dihydropyridine receptor (Ca^{2+} channel) and calsequestrin genes in the myocardium of patients with end-stage heart failure. *J Clin Invest* 1992; **90:** 927–35.

31 Studer R, Reinecke H, Vetter R, Holtz J, Drexler H. Expression and function of the cardiac Na^+/Ca^{2+} exchanger in postnatal development in the rat, in experimental-induced cardiac hypertrophy and in the failing human heart. *Basic Res Cardiol* 1997; **92(suppl):** 53–8.

32 Hasenfuss G, Schillinger W, Lehnart SE et al. Relationship between $Na^+–Ca^{2+}$-exchanger protein levels and diastolic function of failing human myocardium. *Circulation* 1999; **99:** 641–8.

33 Bristow MR, Ginsburg R, Minobe W et al. Decreased catecholamine sensitivity and β-adrenergic receptor density in failing human hearts. *N Engl J Med* 1982; **307:** 205–11.

34 Kim DH, Mkparu F, Kim C-R, Caroll RF. Alteration of Ca^{2+} release channel function in sarcoplasmic reticulum of pressure-overload-induced hypertrophic rat heart. *J Mol Cell Cardiol* 1994; **26:** 1505–12.

35 Naudin V, Oliviero P, Rannou F, Sainte Beuve C, Charlemagne D. The density of ryanodine receptors decreases with pressure overload-induced rat hypertrophy. *FEBS Lett* 1991; **285:** 135–8.

36 Go LO, Moschella MC, Watras J, Handa KK, Fyfe BS, Marks AR. Differential regulation of two types of intracellular calcium release channels during end-stage heart failure. *J Clin Invest* 1995; **95:** 888–94.

37 de la Bastie D, Levitsky D, Rappaport L, Mercadier J-J et al. Function of the sarcoplasmic reticulum and expression of its Ca^{2+}-ATPase gene in pressure overload-induced cardiac hypertrophy in the rat. *Circ Res* 1990; **66:** 554–64.

38 Schwinger RHG, Bohm M, Schmidt U et al. Unchanged protein levels of SERCA II and phospholamban but reduced Ca^{2+} uptake and Ca^{2+}-ATPase activity of cardiac sarcoplasmic reticulum from dilated cardiomyopathy patients compared with patients with nonfailing hearts. *Circulation* 1995; **92:** 3220–8.

39 Hasenfuss G, Reinecke H, Studer R et al. Relation between myocardial function and expression of sarcoplasmic reticulum Ca^{2+}-ATPase in failing and nonfailing human myocardium. *Circ Res* 1994; **75:** 434–42.

40 Limas CJ, Olivari MT, Goldenberg IF et al. Calcium uptake by cardiac sarcoplasmic reticulum in human dilated cardiomyopathy. *Cardiovasc Res* 1987; **21:** 601–5.

41 de la Bastie D, Levitsky D, Rappaport L et al. Function of the sarcoplasmic reticulum and expression of its Ca^{2+} ATPase gene in pressure overload-induced cardiac hypertrophy in the rat. *Cir Res* 1990; **66:** 554–64.

42 del Monte F, Harding SE, Schmidt U et al. Restoration of contractile function in isolated cardiomyocytes from failing human hearts by gene transfer of SERCA2. *Circulation* 1999; **100:** 2308–11.

43 Gupta S, Prahash AJC, Anand IS. Myocyte contractile function in the post-infarct remodeled rat heart despite molecular alterations. *Cardiovas Res* 2000; **48:** 77–88.

44 Komuro I, Yazaki Y. Control of cardiac gene expression by mechanical stress. *Ann Rev Physiol* 1993; **55:** 55–75.

45 Haunstetter A, Izumo S. Apoptosis: basic mechanisms and implications for cardiovascular disease. *Circ Res* 1989; **82:** 1111–9.

46 Narula J, Haider N, Virmani R et al. Apoptosis in myocytes in end stage heart failure. *N Engl J Med* 1996; **335:** 1182–89.

47 Mallat Z, Tedgui A, Fontaliran F, Frank R, Durigon M, Fontaine G. Evidence of apoptosis in arrhythmogenic right ventricular dysplasia. *N Eng J Med* 1996; **335:** 1190–6.

48 Olivetti G, Abbi R, Quaini F et al. Apoptosis in the failing human heart. *N Engl J Med* 1997; **336:** 1131–41.

49 Rayment NB, Haven AJ, Madden B et al. Myocyte loss in chronic heart failure. *J Patholog* 1999; **188:** 213–19.

50 Saraste A, Pulkki K, Kallajoki M et al. Apoptosis in human acute myocardial infarction. *Circulation* 1997; **95:** 320–3.

51 Olivetti G, Quaini F, Sala R et al. Acute myocardial infarction in humans is associated with activation of programmed cell death in the surviving portion of the heart. *J Mol Cell Cardiol* 1994; **28:** 2005–16.

52 Nanji AA, Hiller-Strumhofel S. Apoptosis and necrosis: two types of cell death in alcoholic liver disease. *Alcohol Health Res World* 1997; **21:** 325–30.

53 Feuerstein GZ. Apoptosis in cardiac diseases-new opportunities for novel therapeutics for heart disease. *Cardiovasc Drugs Therapy* 1999; **13:** 289–94.

54 Valente M, Calabrese F, Thiene G et al. In vivo evidence of apoptosis in arrhythmogenic right ventricular cardiomyopathy. *Am J Pathol* 1998; **152:** 479–84.

55 Saraste A, Pulkki K, Kallajoki M, Heikkila P et al. Cardiomyocyte apoptosis and progression of heart failure to transplantation. *Eur J Clin Invest* 1999; **29:** 369–71.

56 Sam F, Sawyer DB, Chang D L-F, Eberli FR et al. Progressive left ventricular remodeling and apoptosis late after myocardial infarction in mouse heart. *Am J Physiol Heart Circ Physiol* 2000; **279:** H422–H428.

57 Schaper J, Meyer-Lorenz S, Suzuki K. The role of apoptosis in dilated cardiomyopathy. *Herz* 1999; **24:** 219–24.

58 Gorza L, Menabo R, Di Lisa F, Vitadello M. Troponion T in human apoptotic cardiomyocytes. *Am J Pathol* 1997; **150:** 2087–97.

59 Kajstura J, Cigola E, Mahorta A et al. Angiotensin II induces apoptosis of adult rat ventricular myocytes in vitro. *J Mol Cell Cardiol* 1997; **29:** 859–70.

60 Krwon KA, Page TM, Nguyen C et al. Tumor necrosis factor alpha-induced apoptosis in cardiac myocytes: involvement of the sphingolipid signaling cascade in cardiac cell death. *J Clin Invest* 1996; **98:** 2854–65.

61 Singh K, Communal C, Sawyer DB, Colucci WS. Adrenergic regulation of myocardial apoptosis. *Cardiovasc Res* 2000; **45:** 713–19.

62 Cheng W, Li B, Kajstura J, Li P et al. Stretch-induced programmed myocyte cell death. *J Clin Invest* 1995; **96:** 2247–59.

63 Latif N, Khan MA, Birks E et al. Upregulation of the Bcl-2 family of proteins in end stage heart failure. *J Am Coll Cardiol* 2000; **35:** 1769–77.

64 Campbell SE. *Collagen matrix in the heart.* Molecular Biology of Collagen Matrix in the Heart. TX: R.G. Landes Company, Austin, 1994:1–21.

65 Caulfield JB, Norton P, Weaver RD. Cardiac dilatation associated with collagen alterations. *Mol Cell Biochem* 1992; **118:** 171–9.

66 Pelouch V, Dixon IMC, Golfman L, Beamish RE, Dhalla NS. Role of the extracellular matrix proteins in heart function. *Mol Cell Biochem* 1994; **129:** 101–20.

67 Carver W, Terracio L, Borg TK. *Cell-matrix interactions: matrix receptors in the development and maintenance of the heart.* Molecular Biology of Collagen Matrix in the Heart. Austin, TX: R.G. Landes Company, 1994:41–59.

68 Agocha AE, Eghbali-Webb M. *Molecular mechanisms of the remodeling of collagen in the heart.* Molecular Biology of Collagen Matrix in the Heart. Austin, TX: R.G. Landes Company, 1994:1–21.

69 Weber KT, Sun Y, Tyagi SC, Cleutjens JP. Collagen network of the myocardium: functional, structural remodeling and regulatory mechanisms. *J Mol Cell Cardiol* 1994; **26:** 279–92.

70 Li YY, McTiernan CF, Feldman AM. Interplay of matrix metalloproteinases, tissue inhibitors of metalloproteinases and their regulators in cardiac matrix remodeling. *Cardiovasc Res* 2000; **46:** 214–24.

71 Mann DL, Spinale FG. Activation of matrix metalloproteinases in the failing human heart. *Circulation* 1998; **98:** 1699–702.

72 Jumd H, McDixon I. Extracellular matrix and cardiovascular diseases. *Can J Cardiol* 1996; **12:** 1259–67.

73 Li YY, Feldman AM, Sun Y, McTiernan CF. Differential expression of tissue inhibitors of metalloproteinases in the failing human heart. *Circulation* 1998; **98:** 1728–34.

74 Thomas CV, Coker ML, Zellner JL, Handy JR, Crumbley AJ. Increased matrix metalloproteinases activity and selective upregulation in LV myocardium from patients with end-stage dilated cardiomyopathy. *Circulation* 1998; **97:** 1708–15.

75 Molkentin JD, Dorn JW. Cytoplasmic signaling pathways that regulate cardiac hypertrophy. *Annu Rev Physiol* 2001; **63:** 391–426.

76 Yamazaki T, Komuro I, Yazaki Y. Molecular mechanisms of cardiac cellular hypertrophy by mechanical stress. *J Mol Cell Cardiol* 1995; **27:** 133–40.

77 Sadoshima J-I, Jahn L, Takahashi T, Kulik TJ, Izumo S. Molecular characterizations of the stretch-induced adaptation of cultured cardiac cells. An in vitro model of load-induced cardiac hypertrophy. *J Biol Chem* 1992; **267:** 10551–60.

78 Booz GW, Baker KM. Molecular signaling mechanisms controlling growth and function of cardiac fibroblasts. *Cardiovas Res* 1995; **30:** 537–43.

79 Mark AL. Sympathetic dysregulation in heart failure: mechanisms and therapy. *Clin Cardiol* 1995; **18:** I3–I8.

80 Cohn JN, Levine TB, Oivari MT et al. Plasma norepinephrine as a guide to prognosis in patients with congestive heart failure. *N Engl J Med* 1984; **311:** 819–23.

81 Simpson PC, Karija K, Karns LR, Long CS, Karliner JS. Adrenergic hormones and control of cardiac myocyte growth. *Mol Cell Biochem* 1991; **104:** 35–43.

82 Schaub MC, Hefti MA, Harder BA, Eppenberger HM. Various hypertrophic stimuli induce distinct phenotypes in cardiomyocytes. *J Mol Med* 1997; **75:** 901–20.

83 Dzau VJ, Pratt RE. Renin-angiotensins system. In: Fozzard HA et al (ed.). *The Heart and Cardiovascular System.* New York: Raven Press, 1992.

84 Linz W, Wiemer G, Gohlke P, Unger T, Scholkens BA. Contibution of kinins to the cardiovascular actions of angiotensin-converting enzyme inhibitors. *Pharmacol Rev* 1995; **47:** 25–49.

85 Simko F, Simko J. Heart failure and angiotensin converting enzyme inhibition: Problems and perspectives. *Physio Res* 1999; **48:** 1–8.

86 Swedberg K, Eneroth P, Kjekshus J, Wilhemsen L. Hormones regulating cardiovascular function in patients with severe congestive heart failure and their relation to morality (follow-up of the CONSENSUS trial). *Am J Cardiol* 1990; **66:** 40D–45D.

87 Annarosa YL, Baosheng L, Wang X. Angiotensin II stimulation in vitro induces hypertrophy of normal and postinfarcted cardiac myocytes. *Circ Res* 1998;82:1145–59.

88 Dzau VJ. Tissue renin-angiotensin system in cardiovascular homeostasis. *Arch Intern Med* 1993; **153:** 937–42.

89 Cody R. The integrated effects of angiotensin II. *Am J Cardiol* 1997; **79:** 9–11.

90 Greenspan FS, Strewler GJ. *Basic and Clinical Endocrinology.* 5th edn. Stamford, CT: Appleton and Lange, 1997.

91 MacFadyen RJ, Lee AFC, Morton JJ, Pringle SD, Struthers AD. How often are angiotensin II and aldosterone concentrations raised during chronic ACE inhibitor treatment in cardiac failure? *Heart* 1999; **82:** 57–61.

92 Torre-Amione G, Bozkurt B, Deswal A, Mann DL. An overview of tumor necrosis factor α and the failing human heart. *Curr Opin Cardiol* 1999; **14:** 206–10.

93 Suresh DP, Lamba S, Abraham WT. New developments in heart failure: role of endothelin and of endothelin receptor antagonists. *J Cardiac Failure* 2000; **6:** 359–68.

94 Torre-Amione G, Kapadia S, Benedict C. Proinflammatory cytokine levels in patients with depressed left ventricular fraction: a report from the Studies of Left-Ventricular Dysfunction (SOLVD). *J Am Coll Cardiol* 1996; **27:** 1201–6.

95 Wei C-M, Lerman A, Rodeheffer RJ et al. Endothelin in human congestive heart failure. *Circulation* 1994; **89:** 1580–6.

96 Krum H, Goldsmith R, Wilshire-Clement M, Miller M, Packer M. Role of endothelin in the exercise intolerance of chronic heart failure. *Am J Cardiol* 1995; **75:** 1282–3.

97 Cody RJ, Hass GJ, Binkley PF, Capers Q, Kelley R. Plasma endothelin correlates with extent of pulmonary hypertension in patients with chronic congestive heart failure. *Circulation* 1992; **85:** 504–9.

98 Tyagi SC. Proteinases and myocardial extracellular matrix turnover. *Mol Cell Biochem* 1997; **168:** 1–12.

99 Kapadia SR. Cytokines and heart failure. *Cardiol Rev* 1999; **7:** 196–206.

100 Bozkurt B, Kribbs S, Clubb FJ et al. Pathophysio-logically relevant concentrations of tumor necrosis factor α promote progressive left ventricular dysfunction and remodeling in rats. *Circulation* 1998; **97:** 1382–91.

101 Meldrum DR. Tumor necrosis factor in the heart. *Am J Physiol* 1998; **27:** R577–R595.

102 Kokoyama Y, Nakano M, Bednarczyk JL, McIntyre B, Entman M, Mann DL. Tumor necrosis factor α provides a hypertrophic growth response in adult cardiac myocytes. *Circulation* 1997; **95:** 1247–52.

103 Kubota T, McTiernan CF, Frye CS, Demetris AJ, Feldman AM. Cardiac-specific overexpression of tumor necrosis factor-alpha causes lethal myocarditis in transgenic mice. *J Cardiac Failure.* 1997; **3:** 117–24.

104 Ceconi C, Curello S, Bachetti T, Corti A, Ferrari R. Tumor necrosis factor in congestive heart failure: a mechanism of disease for the new millennium. *Prog Cardiovasc Dis* 1998; **41:** 25–30.

105 Ferrari R, Bachetti T, Confortini R. Tumor necrosis factor soluble receptors in patients with various degrees of congestive failure. *Circulation* 1995; **92:** 1479–86.

106 Bozkurt B, Torre-Amione G, Warren SM et al. Results of targeted anti-tumor necrosis factor therapy with Etanercept (ENBREL) in patients with advanced heart failure. *Circulation* 2001; **103:** 1044–7.

107 Anker SD, Coasts AJS. How to RECOVER from RENAISSANCE? The significance of the results or RECOVER, RENAISSANCE, RENEWAL and ATTACH. *Int J Cardiol* 2002; **86:** 123–130.

108 Kobayashi T, Miyauchi T, Sakai S et al. Expression of endothelin-1, ET_A and ET_B receptors, and ECE and distribution of endothelin-1 in the failing rat heart. *Am J Physiol* 1999; **45:** H1197–H1206.

109 Pedram A, Razandi M, Hu RM, Levin ER. Vasoactive peptides modulate vascular endothelial cell growth factor production and endothelial proliferation and invasion. *J Biol Chem* 1997; **272:** 17097–103.

110 Thompson NL, Flanders KC, Smith JM et al. Expression of transforming growth factor β1 in specific cells and tissues of adult and neonatal mice. *J Cell Biol* 1989; **108:** 661–9.

111 Villarreal FJ, Dillmann WH. Cardiac hypertrophy-induced changes in messenger RNA levels for TGF-beta, fibronectin and collagen. *Am J Physiol* 1992; **262:** H1861–H1866.

112 Thompson NL, Bazoberry F, Speir H et al. Transforming growth factor-beta in acute myocardial infraction in rats. *Growth Factors* 1988; **1:** 91–9.

113 Boluyt MO, O'Neil L, Meredith AI et al. Alterations in cardiac gene expression during the transition from stable hypertrophy to heart failure. Marked upregulation of genes encoding extracellular matrix components. *Circ Res* 1994; **75:** 23–32.

114 Eghbali-Webb M. *Cardiac Fibroblasts.* Molecular Biology of Collagen Matrix in the Heart. Austin, TX: R.G. Landes Company, 1994:23–40.

115 Houser SR, Lakatta EG. Function of the cardiac myocyte in the conundrum of end-stage, dilated human heart failure. *Circulation* 1999; **99:** 600–4.

116 Harada K, Sugaya T, Murakami K, Yazaki Y, Komuro I. Angiotensin II type 1A receptor knockout mice display less left ventricular remodeling and improved survival after myocardial infarction. *Circulation* 1999; **100:** 2093–9.

5 A new role for primary and secondary prevention in the 21st century: preventing heart failure

David R Thompson, Karen Smith and Simon Stewart

Introduction

As discussed in previous chapters, heart failure is a clinical syndrome caused by a reduction in the heart's ability to meet the metabolic demands of the body. It usually comprises a constellation of debilitating symptoms including breathlessness, fatigue and peripheral oedema. Epidemiological surveys indicate that heart failure affects 1–2% of the population in Europe and the USA, although it probably affects about 10% of individuals over the age of 80 years.[1] The incidence and prevalence of heart failure appear to be rising steeply, and this is likely to be due to the combination of an ageing population, fewer sudden cardiac deaths[2] and improved medical management of acute myocardial infarction both acutely and in the longer term.[3,4]

There is little doubt that heart failure represents a modern-day epidemic[5] associated with poor quality of life and an extremely poor prognosis[6,7] on an individual level and exerting a significant financial burden (directly consuming 1–2% of health care expenditure) in developed countries.[1] Despite being closely associated with advanced age, heart failure is still associated with a large number of premature deaths each year in developed countries and is comparable to many forms of cancer in this regard.[8] Moreover, although there is some evidence that modern-day treatments have had some impact on survival rates following an incidence admission for heart failure,[8] the prevailing wisdom that between 50% and 75% of all heart failure patients die within 5 years of diagnosis[6] and that such rates are seen within 1 year of hospital admission in those with severe heart failure, has remained constant for the past 10–20 years.[6,9] Given the personal and national impact of heart failure and the difficulty in dealing with the many complex problems derived from this modern-day epidemic, it would appear prudent that the best way to tackle heart failure is to actually prevent, rather than treat it. As such, there are two main areas of endeavour that have the potential to limit the overall burden of heart failure in the future:

- primary prevention involving individual and population screening to enable optimal treatment and management of hypertension and other precursors of coronary heart disease (e.g. hyperlipidaemia, smoking and obesity) before a major cardiovascular event occurs;
- secondary prevention involving the optimal treatment and management of patients who have already revealed themselves to have coronary heart disease and are at risk of developing or exacerbating pre-existing left ventricular dysfunction.

However, before these are described in more detail, it must be acknowledged that most of the strategies directed at reducing the risk of coronary heart disease (such as cessation of smoking or cholesterol lowering) should be regarded as means of 'postponing' disease onset rather than as 'vaccines' against eventual events.[10] Moreover, improved survival rates for patients with acute myocardial infarction with therapy such as thrombolytic agents,[11] coronary angioplasty,[12] beta-blockers[13] and angiotensin–converting enzyme (ACE) inhibitors[14] also leaves more individuals with a residual component of chronic heart disease. At this stage, therefore, it should be explicitly understood that although heart failure is the epidemic we had to have, in attempting to 'delay' its onset, we are certainly providing a greater window of opportunity to develop and apply a cure for heart failure.

It is within this context that this chapter outlines the increasing importance of primary and secondary prevention in actually delaying the onset and in some cases, preventing heart failure.

Primary prevention

Despite the magnitude of the health problem associated with heart failure there are limited data on its primary prevention. Since heart failure is a result of many predisposing conditions, it seems sensible that its primary prevention should focus on these. This could be achieved in many cases by the identification of risk factors, both in individuals and populations, and the implementation of strategies to avoid the development or retard the progression of coronary heart disease.

Many patients who have ultimately developed heart failure have a long history of an unhealthy lifestyle and with established modifiable risk factors that would have been sensitive to active intervention. Even when modifiable risk factors are identified patients are often treated inadequately to achieve optimal blood pressure and lipid goals.[15] There is considerable potential, over and above that already achieved through current efforts, to prevent heart failure through more effective lifestyle modification, control of risk factors and optimal use of prophylactic drug therapy.

Screening issues

Prevention can be targeted either at the high-risk individual or at a whole population. Screening programmes have been established with the rationale that early identification allows earlier treatment, which improves prognosis and may even prevent the development of overt disease.[16] However, the development of these preventive strategies has major financial and resource implications.

A recent study examining the value of monitoring risk factors for, and development of heart disease in the UK based on a number of different screening models employed in a range of developed countries, showed that the type of population screening employed in the international MONICA project[17] is probably the most cost-effective means for preventing (or at least delaying) future cardiovascular events.[18] It is likely, with the increasing financial burden imposed by coronary heart disease and emerging cardiac epidemics such as heart failure[19] and atrial fibrillation,[20] that the cost incentive to employ population screening will increase. There is little doubt that a cost-effective approach will involve an extension of current health screening practices performed at the general practitioner/primary care physician clinic level and require specialist nurses who are both skilled at assessing risk and employing state of the art strategies and treatments to minimize that risk.

Current recommendations for the primary prevention of coronary heart disease in groups at high risk are dependent upon screening through primary care and the provision of risk-related advice or treatment. These recommendations have been criticized because of the lack of evidence for the cost-effectiveness of multiple risk factor interventions delivered through primary care.[21] However, it is argued that rather than focusing on maximizing participation in screening, which emphasizes the benefits and neglects the possible harms and uncertainties that this entails, there should be more emphasis placed on informed participation. This may increase the effectiveness of interventions among those who choose to participate and may prove at least as cost-effective as current efforts.[22]

While on the periphery of current efforts to prevent future heart disease, it is clear that genetic screening and subsequent pharmacogenetic treatment strategies are likely to become increasingly important.[23] For example, while inherited conditions such as familial hypertrophic cardiomyopathy are well documented,[24] it is becoming increasingly evident that ventricular remodelling, particularly following an acute ischaemic insult[25] can be exaggerated in some individuals due to inherent genetic polymorphism.[26]

Risk factor targets

Greater efforts must be made to institute risk factor intervention in those individuals identified at being at risk of developing heart failure. In the short to medium term, the risk of an individual developing heart failure often depends on the probability of established left ventricular dysfunction, and the likelihood of acute cardiovascular events.[16] However, as noted in Chapter 1, it is easy to forget that antecedent hypertension, along with coronary heart disease is a powerful precursor to heart failure. In fact, these two related disease states have the highest associated population-attributable risks associated with heart failure.[27,28] In other words, their prevention would have the greatest impact on the development of heart failure.

On a practical basis this means directly targeting hypertension and the other well-known risk factors that contribute to a greater probability of developing coronary heart disease. Formal guidelines for the prevention of coronary heart disease in clinical practice are readily available and provide important therapeutic targets.[15,29]

Hypertension

Hypertension, even at moderate levels, increases risk in patients with other risk factors for heart failure, and left ventricular hypertrophy predicts the development of heart failure independently of hypertension. The effective treatment of hypertension can reduce the risk of heart failure by half.[30] Hypertensive patients who have well-controlled blood pressure, and have not had a myocardial infarction, are unlikely to suffer from heart failure. Current guidelines suggest a blood pressure target of < 140 mmHg systolic and < 85 mmHg diastolic,[15] although these targets are always under constant revision.

Cholesterol

Cholesterol has been implicated in the alteration of endothelial function, and elevated cholesterol, in particular triglycerides or the high density lipoprotein ratio, is associated with an increased incidence of heart failure. Lowering levels have been reported to reduce the risk of developing heart failure from 10.8% to 3.8% over 5 years.[31] As such, current guidelines suggest a target total cholesterol level of < 5.0 mmol/l and a low density lipoprotein level of < 3.0 mmol/l.[15]

Smoking

Smoking represents a powerful independent predictor of coronary heart disease while significantly increasing this risk in those patients who are also hypertensive. The population attributable risk of smoking in middle age, irrespective of blood pressure, for the development of heart failure over a 20-year period is about 25% overall.[28] The suggested reasons for a 'synergistic' effect between hypertension and smoking in this regard, in addition to the exacerbation of atherosclerosis, concentrate on a nicotine-mediated hormone release that increases blood pressure and heart rate. Importantly, therefore, cessation of smoking can potentially offer more benefit than any hypertensive agent.

Obesity

Obesity, although associated with hypertension, elevated lipids and hyperglycaemia, all of which can accelerate atherosclerosis, is an independent risk factor for heart failure and can directly affect left ventricular function.[32] Increasing activity and reducing body mass index is also likely to help with lipid management and reduce multiple risk. At present it is recommended that patients aim for a target weight that results in a body mass index of < 25 kg/m^2.[15] However, in nearly all developed countries there is increasing concern with the growing epidemic of obesity – particularly affecting children and adolescents.[33] This epidemic is likely to undo much of the good work in reducing age-adjusted coronary events, amongst the ageing post-war 'baby boomer' population cohort, particularly. It also has the potential to create a new generation at risk of diabetes (see below) and associated cardiovascular disease without a concerted effort to reduce current trends.

Diabetes

In recent years there has been increasing interest in the association between metabolic disorders, endothelial dysfunction and the risk of developing heart disease and, more specifically, heart failure.[34] Patients with diabetes represent a high-risk group of individuals for all forms of cardiovascular disease. Phenomena such as insulin resistance,[35] and indeed nitrate resistance,[36] appear to be closely related and may be the key to the recent HOPE study results that showed that ramipril reduced cardiovascular events in patients with diabetes.[30] In patients with a pre-existing ejection fraction of < 35%, diabetes is an independent predictor for mortality, the development of overt symptoms of heart failure and hospitalization.[6] Irrespective of future treatments, possibly targeting scavenging of oxygen free radicals in such individuals,[37] it is clearly important to maintain blood sugar levels < 7.0 mmol/l in diabetic patients.

Identifying 'high-risk' individuals

Fortunately, the major modifiable risk factors for coronary heart disease are easily established through a simple examination and a minimal number of blood tests. Moreover, with accurate risk estimates it is possible to provide individuals with a reasonably accurate estimate of their risk of future events if no modification to their lifestyle occurs.

The preventive strategy for each individual patient will be dictated by the initial assessment made of the patient's baseline risk of developing heart disease and, specifically, heart failure. Thus, there is a need for the prompt identification and management of correctable underlying problems and avoidance of precipitating factors. There is also a need to educate the public at large to reduce delay in seeking medical help and minimize the extent of myocardial damage. In the absence of systematic population screening programmes, it should be remembered that much preventive work by general practitioners and nurses may be provided by opportunistic consultation.

Secondary prevention

Given that it is impossible to prevent all individuals from developing symptomatic heart disease, cardiac rehabilitation and secondary prevention strategies should be central to the prevention and management of individuals at risk of developing heart failure secondary to pre-existing disease. Cardiac rehabilitation services aim to facilitate physical, psychological, and emotional recovery in patients with heart disease and enable them to achieve and maintain better health through exercise, education and help with psychological sequelae.[38] The evidence to date suggests that cardiac rehabilitation is an effective intervention that should be offered to all who are likely to benefit, ideally using a needs-led, menu-driven approach.[39] Unfortunately, many of those who are at increased risk of developing heart failure but who have not experienced a documented acute ischaemic events (e.g. those patients with chronic angina and/or hypertension) are not routinely offered or included in secondary prevention programmes. The case for a cardiac rehabilitation service as a vehicle for secondary prevention is a strong one.[40] Poor control of hyperlipidaemia or hypertension, and inadequate use of post-infarction beta-blockers or ACE inhibitors have been well documented.[41] Important factors in this lack of provision include division of responsibility and lack of communication.

Screening patients for secondary prevention

Although identifying all patients who have established heart disease at risk of subsequently developing heart failure, or even a pre-existing but mild form of heart failure, appears to be a simpler objective than implementing an effective primary prevention programme, it remains problematic.

Although most heart failure patients are diagnosed and treated in a primary care setting this requires objective analysis of ventricular function, which is not routine practice in primary care.[42] In recent years there has been an increasing interest in providing rapid echocardiography services to facilitate the diagnosis of asymptomatic or mildly symptomatic left ventricular systolic (and in some cases diastolic) dysfunction in a community setting.[43] There has also been much interest in the role of atrial (ANP) and brain naturietic peptide (BNP) in identifying three types of patients:

- those at risk of developing heart failure;[44]
- those with undiagnosed heart failure who would benefit from appropriate treatment;[44] and
- those patients with heart failure who would benefit from incremental therapy guided by ANP or BNP levels.[45]

As discussed above, the key issue for the future will be designing cheap and accurate strategies to identify 'at risk' individuals. Certainly, anyone who has pre-existing heart disease should be considered to be at risk of heart failure and therefore require some screening process to determine a patient's functional status.

Risk factor modification

Irrespective of whether it comes in the form of primary or secondary prevention, the same risk factors identified above need to be addressed. There is considerable potential to raise the standard of preventive care through more effective lifestyle change and the use of drug therapies with proven efficacy. Whilst primary prevention may, of course, involve mainly non-pharmacological intervention, secondary prevention often requires a more coordinated effort and the use of pharmacological agents (including aspirin, beta-blockers and, increasingly, ACE inhibitors).[15] In this context, shared care programmes are necessary to ensure the continuous, long-term support these patients need. Symptom control and secondary prevention of disease progression are essential, and though standards for risk reduction are included in guidelines, implementation of these in practice remains a challenge. Surveys of clinical practice have shown there is considerable potential to further reduce risk in patients with established coronary heart disease because many are not achieving their lifestyle and risk factor goals outlined earlier.[46]

Even when patients are accurately diagnosed with heart failure, recommended interventions to reduce the progression of disease and signs and symptoms of heart failure are often under-utilized.[41,47] For example, some reports suggest that only one-third of heart failure patients receive ACE inhibitors[41,47] and often in sub-optimal doses.[46] As well as drug therapy, many behavioural interventions (e.g. exercise, smoking cessation and diet) are under-utilized.[41]

As discussed in greater detail in Chapter 12, there is often no individual designated to take responsibility for risk management, and health care professionals may lack skills in risk assessment, behaviour modification and pharmacotherapy. Communication between primary and secondary care sectors can also be problematic. For these reasons, initiatives need to be developed to prevent rehospitalization by control of risk factors and optimizing medical treatment, thus improving the function of the failing heart and enhancing the quality of life of these patients.[48]

As a consequence, heart failure programmes staffed by physicians and nurses with special expertise have been recommended as a means of improving care.[48–50] They appear to be effective in improving patient adherence, functional status and quality of life and reducing readmissions to hospital. In addition to directly managing patients with 'end-stage' or severe heart failure, there is clearly scope for these services to be expanded to provide easy access to specialist knowledge and skills and provide screening, diagnostic and monitoring facilities, and also provide medical management and patient education about diet, activity and medication adherence.[51]

Recent evidence suggests that the beneficial effects of home-based interventions in reducing the frequency of unplanned readmissions in these patients persist in the long term and are associated with prolonging survival.[52]

Key considerations

In order to ensure that preventive strategies are delivered in a systematic way, but are targeted at individuals on a needs-led basis, the following factors need to be addressed:

Lifestyle modification

In practice, changing an individual's behaviour is notoriously difficult and is fraught with problems. Efforts are more likely to be successful in those patients who are willing and able to make changes to their lifestyle. It is important to acknowledge that many patients make spontaneous changes to their lifestyle when confronted with the knowledge that they are at risk of heart disease. Many others respond to brief advice or behaviour change counselling and it is only in the more 'resistant' instances that one needs to resort to other more specialized techniques, such as motivational interviewing.[53,54]

Brief advice consists of:

- asking permission;
- using open questions;
- demonstrating respect;
- providing clear information; and
- encouraging responsibility

Behaviour change counselling is more complex but consists of:

- establishing rapport;
- using empathy;
- setting the agenda;
- exchanging information;

- using open questions;
- listening with empathy; and
- rolling with resistance.

Thus, there will be issues such as assessing motivation and brainstorming solutions. The former can be assessed by questions such as:

- How important is it for you to . . .?
- How confident are you that you will succeed?

Whereas, the latter can be aided by statements such as:

- I have a number of ideas;
- I know about what worked for others.

However, there are numerous factors that inhibit patients and carers from making changes to their lifestyle, or result in lapses, and these should be acknowledged. It is difficult to change the behaviour of individuals through advice alone; there must be an incentive for change. Patient adherence to any measures instituted is more likely to be accomplished if health care professionals understand the principles of behaviour change and apply, where appropriate, such strategies. There are some notable examples of where such strategies have been successful in accomplishing lifestyle change, notably the MULTIFIT (multiple risk factor intervention) programme at Stanford University.[55] This is designed to facilitate patients' recovery in the first year following a myocardial infarction. However, many of the principles used in the programme can be applied to patients at high risk for developing cardiovascular disease. Some of the key elements of the lifestyle modification programme are described below.

Individuals are likely to change behaviour when they believe they are at risk of developing a problem, when they believe the recommended change will improve their condition or reduce their risk, and when they believe they have the ability to accomplish the desired changes.[56] It is, therefore, important to discuss the following with each patient (and carer) for each behaviour to be changed:[55]

- why the patient is at risk;
- how the recommended changes will improve the patient's condition or reduce his/her risk; and
- whether the patient has the confidence and resources to accomplish the change.

Individuals may be at different stages of readiness to change:[57]

> * pre-contemplation: considering change but not strongly committed;
> * contemplation: willing to change and can be influenced to do so;
> * action: highly committed to change and has begun process.

This can be assessed fairly easily by simply asking the patient if he or she intends to adopt a particular behaviour.

The following 11 principles are adopted by the Stanford programme in guiding lifestyle intervention:[55]

1. Build positive and accurate expectations.
2. Precisely define the behaviour to be changed.
3. Help patients set realistic goals.
4. Use contracts to enhance commitment.
5. Prepare for lapses/relapses.
6. Model the desired behaviour.
7. Use prompts to remind the patient of the desired behaviour.
8. Provide feedback about the patient's progress.
9. Teach problem solving.
10. Reward achievement.
11. Enlist appropriate social support as needed.

Accomplishing behaviour change is difficult but maintaining it is even more difficult. Behaviour strategies that are likely to affect this include:

> * contracting: written agreements about setting goals (which are well defined);
> * social support: partner, family, friend or health care professional;
> * self-monitoring and feedback: activity log, feedback in the form of praise; and
> * relapse prevention: warning signals/high-risk situations indicating relapse might occur.

Education, counselling and social support

Patients often have to alter their lifestyle by adhering to a complex medication regimen, changing their diet and fluid intake, adapting their activities and monitoring symptoms of worsening heart failure.[58] Patients and carers therefore need to be educated about medications, diet, alcohol consumption, physical activity and symptoms.

Once a diagnosis of heart failure has been established, they should be counselled regarding the nature of heart failure, drug regimens, dietary restrictions, symptoms of worsening heart failure and what to do if they occur, and prognosis. For some patients and carers social isolation or a perception of lack of support is a real danger and they will benefit from the provision of long-term social support, through either formal or informal networks.

Patients need to understand the nature of the underlying condition, the basis for the diagnosis, the maintenance of stable weight, the control of fluid intake and the avoidance of salt. The desirability of immunization against influenza and pneumonia should be stressed.

Education and support by themselves appear to be effective in reducing readmissions and in-hospital costs among heart failure patients.[59] Education of patient and carers about heart failure will include imparting knowledge about these aspects as well as skills training in monitoring and self-management (e.g. daily weighing and adjusting the dose of diuretics in response to changes in weight).[60]

A central facet of education and counselling is to emphasize the importance of adhering to medication regimes and attending follow-up clinics. Patients need to learn the names, dosages, effects and side-effects of medications, and the possibility of such side-effects. They also need to understand the significance of increasing weight, ankle swelling, breathlessness and fatigue.

Medication can reduce symptoms, improve exercise tolerance and enhance quality of life, yet non-adherence to drug therapy is a common cause of hospitalization.[61] It is important that the patient has a full understanding of his or her medication and a regimen that is easy to follow. Using the minimum amount of drug therapy and appropriate timing for drugs is likely to improve adherence.[62]

It is vital that patients understand their disease and be involved in developing the plan for their care. To reinforce this, family members and other carers should be included in education and counselling. Self-management is a primary goal of treatment for heart failure and, though challenging, self-care strategies can be effective in managing symptoms.[63] It seems that better educated and more symptomatic patients are more likely to engage in self-care.[64] Tools have been developed to assist clinicians in evaluating the self-management abilities of their patients with heart failure.[65] It appears that the most frequently performed self-care behaviours are related to taking prescribed medications and the least frequently performed are concerned with symptom monitoring or management.[66]

Therefore, there is a need to examine the personal and environmental factors that affect self-care behaviours in each individual patient.

Nevertheless, there is a need to recognize that self-care is difficult for many patients with heart failure because early symptoms are subtle and the treatment regimen is complex. In many instances, knowledge is often poor and misperceptions are evident, and patients often have low self-confidence in their ability to perform self-care.[67,68]

The partner plays an important role in the support of patients with heart failure and they should be included in the process of self-care. In order to do so in a positive way, they need to feel involved, valued and supported.[69]

Encouragement of self-monitoring involves patients in their own care and helps detect changes that may indicate an exacerbation of symptoms. Diaries are a useful way of monitoring change.

Practical advice is required, such as the importance of stopping smoking and restricting dietary salt to about 2 g per day. Many patients have inadequate knowledge regarding dietary salt intake.[70] Therefore, they need directed education focusing on salt intake. Alcohol should be discouraged, but those who drink alcohol should be advised to consume no more than one unit per day.

Patients should weigh themselves every morning (immediately after going to the toilet and before breakfast and dressing) and record the weight in their diary. Regular exercise such as walking or cycling should be encouraged for all patients with stable heart failure. Exercise should be of about 30 minutes at least five times per week. Patients should be reassured that they can exercise safely and that regular exercise may improve functional status and sense of well-being and decrease symptoms. The typical signs and symptoms of worsening heart failure (orthopnoea, paroxysmal dyspnoea, leg oedema, or exercise intolerance) should be explained to patients and carers. They should also be given an explanation of what the patient can expect to experience as this will help avoid anxiety over symptoms and prevent fear of performing daily activities that might provoke shortness of breath.

Sexual difficulties are common in these patients, and part of this arises from fear that exertion is detrimental. Sexual practices may need to be modified to accommodate patients with limited exercise tolerance.[71]

The importance of adherence should be emphasized at follow-up visits and practitioners should assist in removing barriers to adherence, such as cost, side-effects, or complexity of the medical regimen. A variety of factors influence adherence with prescribed treatments, especially dietary and exercise regimens, in patients with chronic heart failure, including personality, the disease and its treatment, social activities and relations, and health care professionals, and these should be recognized.[72,73]

There is some evidence that nurses may not be properly educated in heart failure self-management principles.[74] If nurses are to improve the quality and amount of information they offer to patients they must be provided with the right information themselves. They must have the knowledge and skills to assess self-care deficits and to develop and test innovative teaching approaches and educational plans. Novel approaches include the use of interactive education on CD-ROM, which appears to be rated positively by patients and nurses.[75]

Psychological state

The importance of psychological and spiritual well-being should not be overlooked in these patients. The impact of heart failure on a patient's life may be related as much to psychological adaptation to the disease as to impairment of physical functioning. Anxiety, depression, denial and fear are common reactions, and there should be some form of assessment and monitoring of these and, where appropriate, referral to expert treatment. Depression is particularly common in chronic heart failure,[76] which is not surprising when it has a worse prognosis than many cancers. Patients with heart failure who have more physical symptoms and less physical functioning report greater depression, although the depression is more strongly related to having more physical symptoms than having greater limitations in physical functioning.[77]

Patients with heart failure often experience confusion, short-term memory loss and fatigue, and these factors create barriers to communication.

Finally, the importance of the family should not be overlooked. Patients with heart failure and their family members often experience a process of disruption, incoherence and reconciling. Reconciling is often manifested as struggling, participating in partnerships, finding purpose and meaning in the illness experience, and surrendering.[78]

Quality of life

Heart failure imposes a significant impact on quality of life, particularly on functional abilities. It appears that women may have a poorer quality of life than men.[79] An important goal is to improve how patients feel and function during daily activities. It appears that individuals with worse functional status perceive their health to be worse.

As functional status increases an individual's mental health component of health-related quality of life improves.[80]

The improvement of aspects of a patient's quality of life may be as important as prolonging survival. A measure that comprehensively assesses the effects of treatments on a patient's lifestyle or quality of life is critical to the evaluation of treatments for heart failure.[81] Several health-related quality of life questionnaires have been developed specifically for patients with heart failure. One of the most widely used is the Minnesota Living with Heart Failure questionnaire (MLHFQ).[82] However, it might be best to use both a generic measure, such as the SF-36, with a disease-specific measure, such as the MLHFQ, as there is some evidence that the former is better able to differentiate physical and emotional aspects of quality of life in patients with chronic heart failure.[83]

The information obtained should be used to modify treatment and to guide additional patient and family teaching and counselling.

Rehabilitation

Many patients with heart failure have either not been offered access to or been excluded from cardiac rehabilitation due to a traditional fear of worsening cardiac function with exercise.[84] However, there is now ample evidence of the benefits of exercise training in patients with heart failure, especially for NYHA class I–III patients.[85]

Cardiac rehabilitation for chronic heart failure patients can improve functional ability, alleviate activity-related symptoms, improve quality of life, and restore and maintain physiological, psychological and social status.[86] The expansion of home care services and advances in technology allow cardiac rehabilitation to take place in the patient's home.[87] Indeed, home-based walking and resistance training reduces fatigue and breathlessness and improves quality of life.[88]

The patient with heart failure can be included safely in the exercise component of cardiac rehabilitation. The patient with mild-to-moderate heart failure (NYHA classes III and III) can expect to gain most from rehabilitation and, as a result, symptoms can be reduced and exercise tolerance and functional capacity, mood and morale improved. For these patients, home-based exercise can provide the same gains as a hospital-based programme.

Cardiac rehabilitation is much more than exercise: it also includes education, counselling and risk factor control. Participation in rehabilitation also offers peer support and professional advice and encouragement, improves confidence and reduces social isolation and anxiety and depression. It is multifaceted and multidisciplinary and is likely to improve morbidity and quality of life. It should be integrated with secondary prevention to provide comprehensive cardiac care for these patients.

The importance of family members, especially the partner, in the rehabilitation process should not be overlooked. They are often the key to the success of the whole rehabilitation enterprise.[89]

Aftercare and follow-up

Frequent follow-up ensures that regular contact and monitoring is maintained, enabling the nurse not only to act as a source of information and support but also to monitor progress.

To bridge the primary/secondary interface care can be offered in a variety of ways. This includes 'outreach' follow-up by specialist nurses of those admitted with heart failure to provide education and support begun before discharge from hospital and nurse-led, home-based multidisciplinary interventions with access to social care and palliative care for on-going support where necessary.

Modest reorganization of discharge procedures and the provision of counselling and education by nurses can have a significant effect on quality of life during the hospital to home transition.[90]

The evidence for nurse-led interventions in heart failure is positive.[48] Nurses' involvement in predischarge patient education and home visiting, concentrating on adherence to treatment and recognizing early signs of deterioration, has shown significant reductions in readmissions and improvements in quality of life as well as health care costs.[91–94] In addition, it can result in increased self-care behaviour.[95] There is promising evidence that such interventions can also improve survival;[52,96] however, the potential for such programmes to improve health outcomes in patients newly diagnosed with heart failure in the community is unknown.

What is clear from these studies is that such nurses need to be highly trained and appropriately qualified, have the authority to initiate and/or titrate drug therapy, be able to implement multifaceted educational strategies, liaise and consult with other members of the health care team, visit patients at home, and establish ongoing follow-up.[51]

Recent novel approaches to home intervention using the telephone have yielded promising results. For example, a potentially useful approach to improving health care professional and patient interaction and to achieving specific secondary prevention goals is coaching. Coaching is a method of training patients to take responsibility for the achievement and maintenance of the target levels for their particular modifiable risk factors. This approach via the telephone has been used successfully in patients with coronary heart disease to achieve the target cholesterol level.[97]

The use of other telecare interventions needs to be examined further, although it appears that video-based home telecare may not offer incremental benefits beyond those resulting from regular telephone follow-up in reducing frequent hospital readmissions and emergency department visits for patients with heart failure.[98]

A new paradigm for prevention: the continuum of cardiovascular health/disease

Given the limitations of what we have achieved thus far and the ground we have lost with respect to an increasing prevalence of diabetes and obesity in particular, it is worth considering cardiovascular health and disease throughout the entire lifespan. Rather than focus on individual stages of cardiovascular disease and narrow parts of treatment (e.g. medical treatment of acute crises), it would appear more prudent to take a more holistic view that considers the many determinants of cardiovascular health across the lifespan and how well cardiovascular disease, when it does develop, is subsequently diagnosed, treated and managed.

Figure 5.1 is a relatively uncomplicated representation of the continuum of cardiovascular health and the many determinants that may impact on the development of cardiovascular disease and ultimately heart failure. It shows, for example, that the combination of persuading patients to seek treatment earlier during the initial symptomatic phase of acute myocardial infarction[99] and providing for community-based, automated external defibrillators[100,101] to treat potentially life-threatening cardiac arrhythmias and induced hypothermia to provide cerebral protection[102] in order to reduce rates of out-of-hospital deaths[103] will increase the number of patients living with cardiac disease. Alternatively, it suggests that in the future we might be able to reduce the number of cases requiring such treatment via genetic screening,[104] optimizing fetal development[105] and delaying disease onset through more proactive prevention strategies in childhood.

Clearly, the best possible outcome is for each individual to reach their maximal potential lifespan having avoided cardiovascular disease altogether (or at least until the last possible moment). The reality suggests that until a 'vaccination' is developed, we will continue to strive to achieve the next best thing – delaying cardiovascular events and heart failure until very old age. As this is already occurring (to some extent), the health care system is already grappling with the issue of palliative care for patients with chronic heart failure (this is discussed in detail in Chapter 14) as opposed to the traditional model of caring for those with terminal cancer.

Conclusion

Education to help patients respond appropriately to signs and symptoms of heart failure and to improve adherence to pharmacotherapy, diet and lifestyle advice is important. So too is good discharge planning, prevention of respiratory infections, control of blood pressure and optimal and simplified drug regimens, especially when targeted at the elderly, as they are at increased risk of worsening heart failure.

Despite the growing body of evidence attesting to the benefits of primary and secondary prevention in patients at risk of developing heart failure, the practical implementation of measures is problematic. It is likely to be improved if a systematic approach to the screening, assessment, referral, treatment and follow-up of individuals is adopted. Monitoring and maintaining the practical implementation of preventive measures require the effective and efficient use of resources and more creative approaches to staff working across health care sectors. Improved methods of recording, monitoring and auditing data, and avoiding duplication of effort are required, and the use of novel modes of service delivery, such as nurse-led case management and clinics and routine telephone and home visit follow-up, should be considered. This depends on a willingness and ability of staff to be flexible and innovative and on organizations having sufficient resources and good management, information and quality improvement systems.

Finally, the prevention of heart failure may also require a new paradigm, one that acknowledges the whole life course, with risk-factor profiling based on genetic inheritance, programmes to promote nutritional supplements and healthy lifestyles in pregnancy to optimize fetal development and a focus on preventable risk factors throughout the human lifespan from childhood to old age. Such an approach is likely to be most cost-effective and reduce the economic burden of chronic disease in the future as most other options (e.g. genetic manipulation, synthetic organ transplantation and pharmacotherapy) are likely to be extremely costly and favour those who can afford to pay.

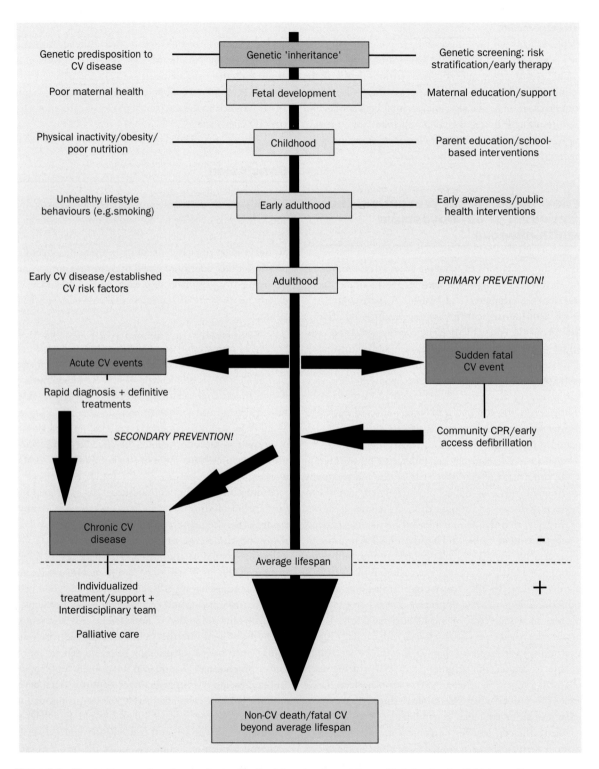

Figure 5.1. *The continuum of cardiovascular health, its determinants and the multiplicity of potential interventions throughout the lifespan. CV, cardiovascular; CPR, cardiopulmonary resuscitation.*

References

1 McMurray JJV, Stewart S. Epidemiology, aetiology and prognosis of heart failure. *Heart* 2000; **83**: 596–602.

2 Capewell S, MacIntyre K, Stewart S et al. Age, sex and social trends in out-of-hospital cardiac deaths in Scotland 1986–1995: a retrospective cohort study. *Lancet* 2001; **358**: 1213–17.

3 Capewell S, Livingstone BM, MacIntyre K et al. Trends in case-fatality in 117,718 patients admitted with acute myocardial infarction in Scotland. *Eur Heart J* 2001; **21**: 1833–40.

4 Morrison C, Woodward M, Leslie W, Tunstall-Pedoe H. Effect of socio-economic group on the incidence of management of, and survival after, myocardial infarction and coronary death; analysis of a community coronary event register. *BMJ* 1997; **314**: 541–6.

5 McCullough PA, Philbin EF, Spertus JA et al. Confirmation of a heart failure epidemic: findings from the Resource Utilization Among Congestive Heart Failure (REACH) study. *J Am Coll Cardiol* 2002; **39**: 60–9.

6 Ho KKL, Anderson KM, Karmel WB et al. Survival after the onset of congestive heart failure in the Framingham Heart Study subjects. *Circulation* 1993; **88**: 107–15.

7 Stewart S, MacIntyre K, Hole DA, Capewell S, McMurray JJV. More malignant than cancer? Five-year survival following a first admission for heart failure in Scotland? *Eur J Heart Failure* 2001; **3**: 315–22.

8 MacIntyre K, Capewell S, Stewart S et al. Evidence of improving prognosis in heart failure: trends in case-fatality in 66,547 patients hospitalised between 1986 and 1995. *Circulation* 2000; **102**: 1126–31.

9 Wolinski FD, Smith DM, Stump TE, Everhoge JM, Lubitz RM. The sequelae of hospitalization for congestive heart failure among older adults. *J Am Geriatr Soc* 1997; **45**: 558–63.

10 Horowitz JD, Stewart S. Heart failure in the elderly – the epidemic we had to have. *Med J Aust* 2001; **174**: 432–3.

11 Fibrinolytic Therapy Trialists' (FTT) Collaborative Group. Indications for fibrinolytic therapy in suspected acute myocardial: collaborative overview of early mortality and major morbidity results from all randomised trials of more than 1000 patients. *Lancet* 1994; **343**: 311–22.

12 Hasdai D, Granger CB, Srivatsa SS et al. Diabetes mellitus and outcome after primary coronary angioplasty for acute myocardial infarction: lessons from the GUSTO-IIb Angioplasty Substudy. Global use of strategies to open occluded arteries in acute coronary syndromes. *J Am Coll Cardiol* 2000; **35**: 1502–12.

13 MERIT Investigators. Effect of metoprolol CR/XL in chronic heart failure: Metoprolol CR/XL Randomised Intervention Trial in Congestive Heart Failure (Merit-HF). *Lancet* 1999; **353**: 2001–7.

14 Packer M, Poole-Wilson PA, Armstrong PW et al. Comparative effects of low and high doses of the angiotensin converting enzyme inhibitor, lisinopril, on morbidity and mortality in chronic heart failure. *Circulation* 1999; **100**: 2312–18.

15 British Cardiac Society, British Hyperlipidaemia Association, British Hypertension Society. Joint British recommendations on prevention of coronary heart disease in clinical practice. *Heart* 1998; **80**: 1–29.

16 Byrne J, Dargie HJ. Prevention of heart failure. In: Dargie HJ, McMurray JJV, Poole-Wilson PA, eds. *Managing Heart Failure in Primary Care*. London: Blackwell Healthcare, 1996: 172–91.

17 Tunstall-Pedoe H, Kuulasmaa K, Mahonen M et al. Contribution of trends in survival and coronary-event rates to changes in coronary heart disease mortality: 10 year results from 37 WHO MONICA Project populations. *Lancet* 1999; **353**: 1547–57.

18 Perry A, Capewell S, Walker A et al. Measuring the costs and benefits of heart disease monitoring. *Heart* 2000; **83**: 651–6.

19 Stewart S, MacIntyre K, McCleod ME, Bailey AE, Capewell S, McMurray JJ. Trends in heart failure hospitalisations in Scotland, 1990–1996: an epidemic that has reached its peak? *Eur Heart J* 2001; **22**: 209–17.

20 Stewart S, MacIntyre K, McCleod MC, Bailey AE, McMurray JJV. Trends in hospital activity, morbidity and case fatality related to atrial fibrillation in Scotland, 1986–1996. *Eur Heart J* 2001; **22**: 693–701.

21 Toop L, Richards D. Preventing cardiovascular disease in primary care. *BMJ* 2001; **323**: 246–7.

22 Marteau TM, Kinmonth AL. Screening for cardiovascular risk: public health imperative or matter for individual informed choice? *BMJ* 2002; **325**: 78–80.

23 Komajda M, Charron P, Frederique T. Genetic aspects of heart failure. *Eur J Heart Failure* 1999; **3**: 121–6.

24 Keeling PJ, Gang Y, Smith G et al. Familial dilated cardiomyopathy in the United Kingdom. *Br Heart J* 1995; **73**: 417–21.

25 Pinto YM, van Gilst WH, Kingma JH, Schunket H. Deletion-type allele of the angiotensin-converting enzyme gene is associated with progressive ventricular dilation after anterior myocardial infarction. Captopril and Thrombolysis Study Investigators. *J Am Coll Cardiol* 1995; **25**: 1622–6.

26 Adams TD, Yanowitz FG, Fisher AG et al. Heritability of cardiac size: an echocardiographic and electrocardiographic study of monzygotic and dizygotic twins. *Circulation* 1985; **71**: 39–44.

27 Ho KK, Pinsky JL, Kannel WB, Levy D. The epidemiology of heart failure: the Framingham Study. *J Am Coll Cardiol* 1993; **22**: 6–13A.

28 Stewart S, Hart CL, Hole DJ, McMurray JJV. The incidence and natural history of heart failure in 15,406

men and women over 20 years: the Renfrew/Paisley Study. *Eur Heart J* 2001; **22:** 208.

29 Pearson TA, Blair SN, Daniels SR et al. AHA guidelines for primary prevention of cardiovascular disease and stroke: 2002 update. Consensus panel guide to comprehensive risk reduction for adult patients without coronary or other atherosoclerotic vascular diseases. *Circulation* 2002; **106:** 388–91.

30 Yusuf S, Sleight P, Pogue J, Bosch J, Davies R, Dagenais G. Effects of an angiotensin-converting-enzyme inhibitor, ramipril, on cardiovascular events in high-risk patients. The Heart Outcomes Prevention Evaluation Study Investigators. *N Engl J Med* 2000; **342:** 145–53.

31 Kjekshus J, Pedersen TR, Olsson AG, Faergeman O, Pyorala K. The effects of simvastatin on the incidence of heart failure in patients with coronary heart disease. *J Card Fail* 1998; **3:** 249–54.

32 Hoffman RM, Psaty BM, Kronmal RA. Modifiable risk factors for incident heart failure in the coronary artery surgery study. *Arch Intern Med* 1994; **154:** 417–23.

33 Micic D. Obesity in children and adolescents – a new epidemic? Consequences in adult life. *J Pediatr Endocrinol Metab* 2001; **S5:** 1345–52.

34 Anker SD, Rachhaus M. Heart failure as metabolic problem. *Eur J Heart Failure* 1999; **1:** 127–31.

35 Swan JW, Anker SD, Walton C et al. Insulin resistance in chronic heart failure: relation to severity and etiology of heart failure. *J Am Coll Cardiol* 1997; **30:** 527–32.

36 Chirkov YY, Holmes AS, Wuttke RD et al. Resistance to anti-aggregatory effects of nitric oxide donors in platelets from patients with ischaemic heart disease. *J Am Coll Cardiol* 2001; **37:** 1851–7.

37 Ferrari R, Agnoletti L, Comini L et al. Oxidative stress during myocardial ischaemia and heart failure. *Eur Heart J* 1998; **19 Suppl B:** B2–11.

38 Thompson DR, Bowman GS, de Bono DP, Hopkins AL, eds. *Cardiac Rehabilitation: Guidelines and Audit Standards.* London: Royal College of Physicians of London, 1997.

39 Dinnes J, Kleijnen J, Leitner M, Thompson DR. Cardiac rehabilitation. *Qual Health Care* 1999; **8:** 65–71.

40 Thompson DR, de Bono DP. How valuable is cardiac rehabilitation and who should get it? *Heart* 1999; **5:** 545–6.

41 Pearson TA, Peters TD. The treatment gap in coronary artery disease and heart failure: community standards and the post-discharge patient. *Am J Cardiol* 1997; **80:** 45–52H.

42 Erhardt L, Cline C. Heart failure clinics: a possible means of improving care. *Heart* 1998; **80:** 428–9.

43 Capewell S, McMurray JJV. 'Chest pain – please admit': is there an alternative? A rapid cardiological assessment service may prevent unnecessary admission. *BMJ* 2000; **320:** 951–2.

44 Cowie MR, Struthers AD, Wood DA et al. Value of natriuretic peptides in assessment of patients with possible new heart failure in primary care. *Lancet* 1997; **350:** 1347–51.

45 McDonagh TA, Cunningham AD, Morrison CE et al. Left ventricular dysfunction, natriuretic peptides, and mortality in an urban population. *Heart* 2001; **86:** 21–6.

46 Simpson RJ, Sueta CA, Boccuzzi SJ, Lulla A, Biggs D et al. Performance assessment model for guideline-recommended pharmacotherapy in the secondary prevention of coronary artery disease and treatment of left ventricular dysfunction. *Am J Cardiol* 1997; **80:** 53–6H.

47 Philbin EF, Andreaou C, Rocco TA, Lynch LJ, Baker SL. Patterns of angiotensin-converting enzyme inhibitor use in congestive cardiac failure in two community hospitals. *Am J Cardiol* 1996; **77:** 832–8.

48 McMurray JJV, Stewart S. Nurse led, multidisciplinary intervention in chronic heart failure. *Heart* 1998; **80:** 430–1.

49 Moser DK. Heart failure management: optimal health care delivery programs. *Ann Rev Nurs Res* 2000; **18:** 91–126.

50 Horowitz JD. Home-based intervention: the next step in treatment of chronic heart failure? *Eur Heart J* 2000; **21:** 1807–9.

51 Stewart, S. Blue L. Key components of specialist nurse-led program in chronic heart failure. In: Stewart S, Blue L, eds. *Improving Outcomes in Chronic Heart Failure.* London: BMJ Books, 2000: 114–18.

52 Stewart S, Horowitz JD. Home-based intervention in congestive heart failure: long-term implications on readmission and survival. *Circulation* 2002; **105:** 2861–6.

53 Rol!nick S, Mason P, Butler C. *Health Behaviour Change: A Guide for Practitioners.* London: Churchill Livingstone, 1999.

54 Miller WR, Rollnick S. *Motivational Interviewing: Preparing People for Change,* 2nd edn. New York: Guilford Press, 2002.

55 Miller NH, Taylor CB. *Lifestyle Management for Patients with Coronary Heart Disease.* Champaign, IL: Human Kinetics, 1995.

56 Becker MH. The Health Belief Model and personal health behavior. *Health Ed Mon* 1974; **2:** 236–508.

57 Prochaska JO, DiClemente CC. Stages and process of self-change of smoking: towards an integrative model of change. *J Consult Clin Psychol* 1983; **51:** 390–5.

58 Dracup K, Baker DW, Dunbar SB, Dacey RA, Brooks NH et al. Management of heart failure. II. Counseling, education, and lifestyle modifications. *JAMA* 1994; **272:** 1442–6.

59 Krumholz HM, Amatruda J, Smith GL et al. Randomized trial of an education and support intervention to prevent readmission of patients with heart failure. *J Am Coll Cardiol* 2002; **39:** 83–9.

60 Jaarsma T, Halfens R, Huijer Abu-Saad H et al. Effects of education and support on self-care and resource utilization in patients with heart failure. *Eur Heart J* 1999; **20:** 673–82.

61 Michalsen A, Konig G, Thimmes W. Preventable causative factors leading to hospital admission with

decompensated heart failure. *Heart* 1998; **80:** 437–41.

62 Bennett S, Milgrom L, Champion V, Hyster G. Beliefs about medication and dietary compliance in people with heart failure: an instrument development study. *Heart Lung* 1997; **26:** 273–9.

63 Bennett SJ, Cordes DK, Westmoreland G, Castro R, Donnelly E. Self-care strategies for symptom management in patients with chronic heart failure. *Nurs Res* 2000; **49:** 139–45.

64 Rockwell JM, Riegel B. Predictors of self-care in persons with heart failure. *Heart Lung* 2001; **30:** 18–25.

65 Riegel B, Carlson B, Glaser D. Development and testing of a clinical tool measuring self-management of heart failure. *Heart Lung* 2000; **29:** 4–15.

66 Artinian NT, Magnan M, Sloan M, Lange MP. Self-care behaviors among patients with heart failure. *Heart Lung* 2002; **31:** 161–72.

67 Carlson B, Riegel B, Moser DK. Self-care abilities of patients with heart failure. *Heart Lung* 2001; **30:** 351–9.

68 Riegel B, Carlson B. Facilitators and barriers to heart failure self-care. *Patient Educ Couns* 2002; **46:** 287–95.

69 Martensson J, Dracup K, Fridlund B. Decisive situations influencing spouses' support of patients with heart failure: a critical incident technique analysis. *Heart Lung* 2001; **30:** 341–50.

70 Neily JB, Toto KH, Gardner EB et al. Potential contributing factors to noncompliance with dietary sodium restriction in patients with heart failure. *Am Heart J* 2002; **143:** 29–33.

71 Jaarsma T. Sexual problems in heart failure patients. *Eur J Cardiovasc Nurs* 2002; **1:** 61–67.

72 Evangelista LS, Berg J, Dracup K. Relationship between psychosocial variables and compliance in patients with heart failure. *Heart Lung* 2001; **30:** 294–301.

73 Stromberg A, Brostrum A, Dahlstrom U, Fridlund B. Factors influencing patient compliance with therapeutic regimens in chronic heart failure: a critical incident technique analysis. *Heart Lung* 1999; **28:** 334–41.

74 Albert NM, Collier S, Sumodi V et al. Nurses' knowledge of heart failure education principles. *Heart Lung* 2002; **31:** 102–12.

75 Stromberg A, Ahlen H, Fridlund B, Dahlstron U. Interactive education on CD-ROM – a new tool in the education of heart failure patients. *Patient Educ Couns* 2002; **46:** 75–81.

76 Koenig HG. Depression in hospitalised older patients with congestive heart failure. *Gen Hosp Psychiat* 1998; **20:** 29–43.

77 Friedman MM, Griffin JA. Relationship of physical symptoms and physical functioning to depression in patients with heart failure. *Heart Lung* 2001; **30:** 98–104.

78 Mahoney JS. An ethnographic approach to understanding the illness experiences of patients with congestive heart failure and their family members. *Heart Lung* 2001; **30:** 429–36.

79 Riedinger MS, Dracup KA, Brecht M-L et al. Quality of life in patients with heart failure: do gender differences exist? *Heart Lung* 2001; **30:** 105–16.

80 Westlake C, Dracup K, Creaser J et al. Correlates of health-related quality of life in patients with heart failure. *Heart Lung* 2002; **31:** 85–93.

81 Berry C, McMurray JJV. A review of quality of life evaluation in patients with congestive heart failure. *Pharmacoeconomics* 1999; **16:** 247–71.

82 Rector TS, Kubo SH, Cohn JN. Patients' self-assessment of their congestive heart failure: content, reliability and validity of a new measure, the Minnesota Living with Heart Failure questionnaire. *Heart Failure* 1987; **3:** 198–209.

83 Sneed NV, Paul S, Michel Y, VanBakel A, Hendrix G. Evaluation of 3 quality of life measurement tools in patients with chronic heart failure. *Heart Lung* 2001; **30:** 332–40.

84 Wenger NK, Froelicher ES, Smith LK et al. Cardiac Rehabilitation. Clinical Practice Guideline No. 17. Rockville, MD: US Department of Health and Human Services Public Health Service, Agency for Health Care Policy and Research and the National Heart, Lung and Blood Institute, 1995.

85 Working Group on Cardiac Rehabilitation and Exercise Physiology and Working Group on Heart Failure of the European Society of Cardiology. Recommendations for exercise training in chronic heart failure patients. *Eur Heart J* 2001; **22:** 125–35.

86 Bowman GS, Thompson DR, Lewin RJP. Why are patients with heart failure not routinely offered cardiac rehabilitation? *Coronary Health Care* 1998; **2:** 187–92.

87 Goodwin BA. Home cardiac rehabilitation for congestive heart failure: a nursing case management appoach. *Rehabil Nurs* 1999; **24:** 143–7.

88 Oka RK, De Marco T, Haskell WL et al. Impact of a home-based walking and resistance training program on quality of life with heart failure. *Am J Cardiol* 2000; **85:** 365–9.

89 Thompson DR. Involvement of the partner in rehabilitation. In: Jobin J, Maltais F, Poirier P, LeBlanc P, Simard C, eds. *Advancing the Frontiers of Cardiopulmonary Rehabilitation*. Champaign, IL: Human Kinetics, 2002: 211–15.

90 Harrison MB, Browne GB, Roberts J et al. Quality of life of individuals with heart failure. A randomised trial of the effectiveness of two models of hospital-to-home transition. *Med Care* 2002; **40:** 271–82.

91 Rich MW, Beckham V, Wittenberg C et al. A multidisciplinary intervention to prevent the readmission of elderly patients with congestive heart failure. *N Engl J Med* 1995; **333:** 1190–5.

92 Stewart S, Pearson S, Luke CG, Horowitz JD. Effects of home-based intervention on unplanned reamissions and out-of-hospital deaths. *J Am Geriatr Soc* 1998; **46:** 174–80.

93 Stewart S, Pearson S, Horowitz JD. Effects of a home-based intervention among patients with congestive heart failure discharged from acute hospital care. *Arch Intern Med* 1998; **158:** 1067–72.

94 Cline CMJ, Israelsson BYA, Willenheimer RB, Broms K, Erhardt LR. Cost effective management programme for heart failure reduces hospitalisation. *Heart* 1998; **80:** 442–6.

95 Jaarsma T, Halfens R, Tan F et al. Self-care and quality of life in patients with advanced heart failure: the effect of a supportive educational intervention. *Heart Lung* 2000; **29:** 319–30.

96 Stewart S, Marley JE, Horowitz JD. Effects of a multidisciplinary, home-based intervention on unplanned readmissions and survival among patients with chronic congestive heart failure: a randomised controlled study. *Lancet* 1999; **354:** 1077–83.

97 Vale MJ, Jelinek MV, Best JD, Santamaria JD. Coaching patients with coronary heart disease to achieve the target cholesterol: a method to bridge the gap between evidence-based medicine and the 'real world' – randomized controlled trial. *J Clin Epidemiol* 2002; **55:** 245–52.

98 Jerant AF, Azari R, Nesbitt TS. Reducing the cost of frequent hospital admissions for congestive heart failure. A randomised trial of a home telecare intervention. *Med Care* 2001; **39:** 1234–45.

99 McKinley S, Moser DK, Dracup K. Treatment-seeking behavior for acute myocardial infarction symptoms in North America and Australia. *Heart Lung* 2000; **29:** 237–47.

100 Marenco JP, Wang PJ, Link MS et al. Improving survival from sudden cardiac arrest: the role of the automated external defibrillator. *JAMA* 2001; **285:** 1193–200.

101 Capucci A, Aschieri D, Piepoli MF et al. Tripling survival from sudden cardiac arrest via early defibrillation without traditional education in cardiopulmonary resuscitation. *Circulation* 2002; **106:** 1065–70.

102 Bernard SA, Gray TW, Jones BM et al. Treatment of comatose survivors of out-of-hospital cardiac arrest with induced hypothermia. *N Engl J Med* 2002; **346:** 557–63.

103 Capewell S, MacIntyre K, Stewart S et al. Age, sex and social trends in out-of-hospital cardiac deaths in Scotland 1986–1995: a retrospective cohort study. *Lancet* 2001; **358:** 1213–17.

104 Perusse L, Bouchard C. Role of genetic factors in childhood obesity and in susceptibility to dietary variations. *Ann Med* 1999; **SI:** 19–25.

105 Leeson CP, Kattenhorn M, Morley R et al. Impact of low birth weight and cardiovascular risk factors on endothelial function in early adult life. *Circulation* 2001; **103:** 1264–8.

6 Clinical assessment and investigation of patients with suspected heart failure

John Byrne, Andrew P Davie and John JV McMurray

Introduction

The clinical assessment and investigation of patients with heart failure is a complex and rapidly evolving area. In part the difficulty arises because of the lack of a satisfactory definition of what 'heart failure' is. Indeed the fact that 'heart failure' is a syndrome (a constellation of symptoms and signs) rather than a strict diagnosis is itself a problem. The syndrome of heart failure has many mimics (e.g. anaemia, obesity, chronic lung disease) and many causes (e.g. valvular, pericardial, epicardial, myocardial and electrical abnormalities, alone or in combination), adding even more confusion. Not surprisingly, therefore, as we will see, clinical symptoms and signs are of limited value and investigations are vital. As will be discussed, new investigative tools, both biochemical and imaging, are currently emerging and are likely to change clinical practice in the next 5–10 years. Excellent guidelines on the diagnosis of heart failure have recently been published.[1,2]

Use of symptoms and signs in clinical diagnosis

The simplest pathophysiological definition of heart failure was provided by Wood: '*a state in which the heart fails to maintain an adequate circulation for the needs of the body despite a satisfactory venous filling pressure*'.[3] This was refined somewhat by Braunwald and Grossman in one of the most widely quoted definitions of heart failure: '*a state in which an abnormality of cardiac function is responsible for failure of the heart to pump blood at a rate commensurate with the requirements of the metabolizing tissues or, to do so, only from an elevated filling pressure*'.[4] Others have emphasized the multi-system nature of the disorder, most notably Packer[5] and Poole-Wilson.[6] Perhaps the most useful, certainly the most pragmatic, definition has been provided by the European Task Force[1] – refer to Table 6.1 for this and the other key definitions. All of these definitions emphasize to varying degrees the importance of

Table 6.1. *Key definitions of heart failure*

Wood, 1968[3]	'*A state in which the heart fails to maintain an adequate circulation for the needs of the body despite a satisfactory venous filling pressure*'
Braunwald and Grossman, 1992[4]	'*A state in which an abnormality of cardiac function is responsible for failure of the heart to pump blood at a rate commensurate with the requirements of the metabolizing tissues or, to do so, only from an elevated filling pressure*'
Packer, 1988[5]	'*A complex clinical syndrome characterized by abnormalities of left ventricular function and neurohormonal regulation which are accompanied by effort intolerance, fluid retention and reduced longevity*'
Poole-Wilson, 1985[6]	'*A clinical syndrome caused by an abnormality of the heart and recognized by a characteristic pattern of haemodynamic, renal, neural and hormonal responses*'
European Task Force on Heart Failure, 2001[1]	'*Symptoms of heart failure at rest or on effort, combined with objective evidence of cardiac dysfunction at rest, together with a response to treatment directed towards heart failure*'

objective evidence of cardiac (usually left ventricular) dysfunction (and more latterly, the importance of a clinical response to treatment). The question arises as to what extent that objective evidence can be provided by clinical assessment (without at least the potentially compelling evidence gained from clinical intervention).

Evaluation of symptoms, signs and other aspects of the medical history

The following sections summarize and review the few studies which have evaluated the usefulness of symptoms and signs in diagnosis. The problem of course is the 'gold standard'. Several of the studies described used the presence of left ventricular systolic dysfunction as the 'gold standard', indicative of definitive heart failure. Of course, there is now the strongly held view that heart failure can occur in patients with preserved systolic function (and maybe a third to a half of patients with heart failure have preserved systolic function).[7,8]

Symptoms of heart failure

The cardinal symptoms of heart failure are breathlessness, ankle swelling and tiredness. Unfortunately these symptoms, even in combination, are very non-specific. Tiredness is probably the commonest and therefore least specific of all symptoms. The majority of patients presenting to their general practitioner complaining of tiredness ('I'm tired all the time, Doctor!') have little objective evidence of any pathophysiological abnormality whatsoever,[9] let alone any cardiac abnormality. Notwithstanding, tiredness is one of the most debilitating symptoms of heart failure itself, and contributes to the extremely disabling nature of the disorder.[10] Symptoms of orthopnoea (breathlessness on lying flat) or paroxysmal nocturnal dyspnoea (waking with sudden-onset breathlessness during the night) might be expected to be more specific than breathlessness on exertion or breathlessness at rest.

The above symptoms have been subjected to objective assessment, and sensitivity, specificity and positive and negative predictive values can be calculated for the purpose of objective comparison (see Table 6.2 for definitions of these terms, Table 6.3 and references[11–15] for results). However, whilst orthopnoea and paroxysmal nocturnal dyspnoea can be seen to be much more specific than dyspnoea on exertion, they are much less sensitive. That is to say, whilst a clear majority (66–100%) of patients *with* confirmed heart failure *are* breathless on exertion (sensitivity), it is probably only a minority (15–52%) of similar patients *without* heart failure who do *not* have the

Table 6.2. Definition of sensitivity, specificity and positive and negative predictive values

	Test positive	Test negative
CHF present	True positive	False negative
CHF absent	False positive	True negative

Sensitivity = true positives / (true positives + false negatives)
= chance of detecting CHF with a positive result

Specificity = true negatives / (true negatives + false positives)
= chance of excluding CHF with a negative result

Positive predictive value = true positives / (true positives + false positives)
= chance that a positive result is representative of CHF being present

Negative predictive value = true negatives / (true negatives + false negatives)
= chance that a negative result is representative of CHF being absent

CHF, congestive heart failure

same symptoms (specificity). Furthermore, whilst a probable majority (40–100%) of patients *without* confirmed heart failure do *not* have orthopnoea or paroxysmal nocturnal dyspnoea (specificity), it is probably only a minority (21–91%) of patients *with* confirmed heart failure who *do* have the same symptoms (sensitivity). It can also be seen that none of these symptoms achieves a significant positive predictive value, although the negative predictive value of breathlessness on exertion is very high. That is to say that, only about one-quarter of patients with any of these symptoms are likely to turn out to have heart failure (2–100%) (positive predictive value), although the vast majority (75–100%) of patients without breathlessness on exertion will turn out not to have heart failure (negative predictive value). In short, these findings underline the sensitivity but lack of specificity or predictive accuracy of *any* particular symptom in heart failure.

Signs of heart failure

The signs of heart failure might be expected to be more helpful in the clinical diagnosis of heart failure, more specific and, perhaps, more predictive. After all, however expert at history-taking, the clinician is still reliant upon

Table 6.3. *Sensitivity (Se), specificity (Sp), positive (+) & negative (−) predictive value of symptoms in diagnosis of congestive heart failure*

		Harlan[11]	Chakko[12]	Stevenson[13]	Echeverria[14]	Davie[15]
Patients (n)		329	52	50	50	259
DoE	Se	66			97	100
	Sp	52			15	17
	+	23			63	18
	−				75	100
Orthopnoea	Se	21	66	91	73	22
	Sp	81	47	100	40	74
	+	2	61	100	65	14
	−		37	64	50	83
PND	Se	33			50	39
	Sp	76			45	80
	+	26			58	27
	−				38	87
AS	Se	23	46	23	23	49
	Sp	80	73	100	70	47
	+	22	79	100	54	15
	−		37	18	38	83

DoE, dyspnoea on exertion; PND, paroxysmal nocturnal dyspnoea; AS, ankle swelling

the patient's subjective and (hopefully) untutored account. When it comes to clinical examination, the clinician's highly refined skills of objective assessment should surely come into play. The signs of heart failure can be divided into three groups of signs of different aspects of the condition: signs of fluid retention (e.g. elevated jugular venous pulsation, pulmonary crackles and ankle oedema); signs of cardiac enlargement (e.g. increased area of cardiac dullness to percussion and displaced apex beat); and signs of cardiac strain (e.g. tachycardia, decreased proportional pulse pressure and third heart sound). These are mostly signs of decompensated heart failure, and whilst the diagnosis of decompensated heart failure may be relatively easy, decompensated heart failure is much less common than heart failure which is more or less compensated. Furthermore, there is a limit to the extent to which any of these signs on their own has any particular, sensitivity, specificity or predictive value for the diagnosis of heart failure (Table 6.4 and references[11–18]).

Signs of fluid retention

Fluid retention in one form or another is regarded as almost pathognomic of heart failure. It is certainly pathognomic of the vicious cycle which characterizes decompensating heart failure (and perhaps that which characterizes the development of symptomatic heart failure in the first place). The definitions we referred to earlier ('a state in which an abnormality of cardiac function is responsible for failure of the heart to pump blood at a rate commensurate with the requirements of the metabolizing tissues or, to do so, only from an elevated filling pressure') make clear how fluid retention is an integral part of this vicious cycle. Failure of the heart to pump blood at a rate commensurate with the requirements of the kidneys results in reduced salt and water clearance and hence fluid retention. Whilst this is initially compensatory (allowing the heart to pump blood from an elevated filling pressure), it is ultimately deleterious, as the failing heart ultimately functions even less efficiently when subjected to prolonged elevation of filling pressures.

Table 6.4. Sensitivity (Se), specificity (Sp), positive (+) and negative (–) predictive value of signs in diagnosis of congestive heart failure

		Harlan[11]	Heckerling[16]	O'Neill[17]	Chakko[12]	Butman[18]	Stevenson[13]	Echeverria[14]	Davie[15]
Patients (n)		329	100	100	52	52	50	50	259
↑P	Se	7							22
	Sp	99							92
	+	6							33
	–								86
↓PPP	Se						91		0
	Sp						8		100
	+						91		
	–						87		84
↑JVP	Se	10			70	57	58	47	17
	Sp	97			79	93	100	65	98
	+	2			85	95	100	67	64
	–				62	47	28	45	86
↑DTP	Se		94						
	Sp		67						
	+								
	–								
→AB	Se			59				60	66
	Sp			76				50	96
	+			59				64	75
	–			77				45	94
S3	Se	31			73	68	98	63	24
	Sp	95			42	73	14	55	99
	+	61			66	86	88	68	77
	–				85	48	50	50	87
Murmur	Se								49
	Sp								67
	+								22
	–								87
Crackles	Se	13			66	24	19	70	29
	Sp	91			84	100	100	35	77
	+	27			87	100	100	62	19
	–				61	35	17	44	85
Wheeze	Se								12
	Sp								82
	+								11
	–								83

Table 6.4. (Continued)

		Harlan[11]	Heckerling[16]	O'Neill[17]	Chakko[12]	Butman[18]	Stevenson[13]	Echeverria[14]	Davie[15]
Patients (n)		329	100	100	52	52	50	50	259
Oedema	Se	10			46		23	40	20
	Sp	93			73		100	70	86
	+	3			79		100	67	21
	–				46		18	44	85

↑P, tachycardia; ↓PPP, decreased proportional pulse pressure; ↑JVP, jugular venous distension; ↑DTP, increased area of cardiac dullness to percussion; →AB, displaced apex beat; S3, triple rhythm

Despite the above considerations, signs of fluid retention are perhaps surprisingly non-specific. Ankle oedema (sensitivity 10–46%, specificity 70–100%, positive predictive value 3–100%, negative predictive value 18–85%) is more likely to be caused by chronic venous insufficiency than by congestive heart failure, especially in the middle-aged woman who also complains of tiredness and perhaps breathlessness on exertion. An elevated jugular venous pulsation (sensitivity 10–70%, specificity 65–100%, positive predictive value 2–100%, negative predictive value 28–86%) is quite a 'hard' sign, but is as likely to be caused by right heart failure secondary to pulmonary hypertension secondary to chronic pulmonary disease ('cor pulmonale' – not at all part of the spectrum of congestive heart failure) as it is by congestive heart failure, especially in the middle-aged or elderly chronic tobacco abuser who complains very justifiably of breathlessness on exertion. Pulmonary crackles (sensitivity 13–70%, specificity 35–100%, positive predictive value 19–100%, negative predictive value 17–85%) ought to be a very specific sign, but somehow turns out not to be, perhaps because the crepitations of pulmonary alveolar oedema are so easily confused with those of chronic pulmonary disease or even those of stasis, especially if the patient does not clear his chest with a good cough. Ascites is an unusual (and late) sign which is difficult to elicit and which needs to be approached with as open a mind as possible as other accumulations of fluid in places where it should not be (similarly late signs of heart failure or worse, such as pleural and pericardial effusion).

Signs of cardiac enlargement

Signs of cardiac enlargement might be expected to be a bit more specific still (refer to Figure 6.1). After all, cardiac enlargement is surely a sine qua non of cardiac failure. That might be so if we accept the broadest possible definition of heart failure (enlarged, for example, to include right heart failure), but not if, as is so often the case, what we are really interested in is heart failure secondary to left ventricular systolic dysfunction. For if we think of the capacity for enlargement of the different cardiac chambers, we find that the left atrium can enlarge enormously (for example, to 20 cm in diameter in severe chronic mitral valve disease). Similarly the right heart, especially the right atrium, can enlarge without imperilling cardiac function unduly. The left ventricle, on the other

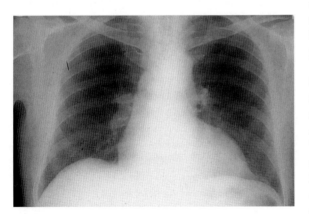

Figure 6.1. Chest X-ray of a patient with chronic heart failure. The patient has been well treated with diuretics and angiotensin-converting enzyme inhibitor. The prominent feature is cardiomegaly, with no evidence of pulmonary oedema. Reproduced with permission from: Heart Failure. Diagnosis and Management. Clark AL, McMurray JJV (eds). London: Martin Dunitz, 2001.

hand, only has to enlarge from around 5 cm in diameter to around 7 cm to be associated with severe left ventricular systolic dysfunction and severe chronic heart failure, and to around 9 cm to be barely compatible with life. It is only because congestive heart failure due to left ventricular systolic dysfunction is associated with congestion, and so with enlargement of left atrium and right heart, that there is any useful association between cardiac size and heart failure at all. The usefulness of these signs is further compromised by the fact that they are rarely used in clinical practice and inter-observer agreement is poor.[16,17,19] Notwithstanding, the evidence suggests that they may be useful clinical tools (increased area of cardiac dullness to percussion: sensitivity 94%, specificity 67%; displaced apex beat: sensitivity 59–66%, specificity 50–96%, positive predictive value 59–75%, negative predictive value 45–94%).

Signs of cardiac strain

Signs of cardiac strain should clearly be very specific markers of heart failure; after all, they purport to detect the very thing we are looking for. Indeed, if the heart is failing, it must be doing so because it is under unacceptable strain (although, if it is under strain, that does not mean it is necessarily failing). However, the main problem with these signs is their subtlety. Apart from tachycardia, which is all too easy to elicit (sensitivity 7–22%, specificity 92–99%, positive predictive value 6–33%, negative predictive value 86%), decreased proportional pulse pressure (proportion of systolic blood pressure over and above diastolic blood pressure) seems to be very difficult to elicit, and third heart sound is very unreliable.[20] One study claimed great sensitivity and predictive value for decreased proportional pulse pressure[13] (sensitivity 91%, specificity 8%, positive predictive value 91%, negative predictive value 87%), whereas another study did not find a single patient with heart failure who had a decreased proportional pulse pressure.[15] The elicitation of a third heart sound is notoriously unreliable and subject to inter-observer variability[20] (sensitivity 24–98%, specificity 14–99%, positive predictive value 61–88%, negative predictive value 48–87%).

None of these symptoms or signs seem to be good at differentiating 'systolic' from 'diastolic' dysfunction.[21–23]

Combinations of symptoms and/or signs

Clinical diagnosis is well recognized to be a process of pattern recognition. It is therefore somewhat unreasonable to suppose that any one symptom or sign would be at all specific, let alone sensitive, for the diagnosis of heart failure due to left ventricular systolic dysfunction. It becomes very much more complicated, and very difficult, to provide an objective assessment of the value, predictive or otherwise, of such combinations of symptoms and signs. Certainly such combinations could be expected to be more specific and predictive, although less sensitive. This has not often been attempted, but when most recently done, it was past medical history of myocardial infarction and displaced apex beat on examination which emerged as the best single predictors of left ventricular systolic dysfunction, and a combination of these two which emerged as a very valuable combined predictor of left ventricular systolic dysfunction.[15] A past medical history of myocardial infarction is in fact much more predictive of significant left ventricular systolic dysfunction than any conventional symptom, despite the fact that a minority of such patients have significant left ventricular systolic dysfunction.

Scoring systems

It is a small step from looking at combinations of symptoms and signs to thinking of scoring systems for the diagnosis of heart failure.[24–29] There have been numerous attempts to devise such scoring systems, even equations for the calculation of left ventricular ejection fraction, but none of these has found common acceptance, perhaps because they are so much more complicated than simple investigations. In fact, most of them have included simple investigations, and are therefore outside of the remit of this chapter. Scoring systems restricted to clinical information, readily volunteered symptoms and readily demonstrated signs, have been mainly the preserve of epidemiologists. There have been three sets of clinical scoring systems in common use, the Framingham criteria, the Duke criteria and the Boston criteria; however, these have mainly been used to define patients as having heart failure for epidemiological purposes. The fact that patients who fulfil these criteria are accepted as having heart failure, by definition, may be useful for epidemiological surveys, but it is hardly likely to be useful in clinical practice, given that we can all think of patients who would fulfil such criteria, whom we would not regard as having heart failure.

A few examples

It may be useful to give a few examples of hypothetical patients, to give some idea of the thought processes involved in the clinical diagnosis of heart failure.

Mr A is 59 years old, a smoker, who had a myocardial infarction and coronary artery bypass grafting 10 years ago. He has noticed increasing breathlessness on exertion recently, which has responded somewhat to prescription of a diuretic. Examination is quite unremarkable. Despite this, the chances of Mr A having heart failure secondary to left ventricular systolic dysfunction are quite high, although the possibility or recurrent ischaemia or lung disease also deserves consideration. Investigation to confirm or deny this clinical impression is mandatory, considering the life-enhancing treatments available.

Mrs B is 56 years old, 10 years' post-menopausal and a smoker, who has had ankle swelling for years. More recently she has complained of weakness, tiredness and breathlessness. The ankle swelling has responded quite well to prescription of a diuretic, although the weakness and tiredness remain. Examination is unremarkable apart from obesity and slight ankle swelling. The chances of Mrs B having heart failure secondary to left ventricular systolic dysfunction are slim, although she certainly merits further investigation, if only to help reassure her.

Miss C is 87 years old, and despite having kept very well all her long life, finds that she has slowed down recently. She is inclined to put her problems down to old age and wonders if she will be able to keep her second-floor flat much longer, given the number of times that she has to stop on the way up her 28 steps to pause for breath. Examination reveals a frail old lady, with obviously elevated jugular venous pulsation and an easily heard systolic murmur with some basal pulmonary crackles. Miss C may very well have heart failure, either due to left ventricular systolic dysfunction or valvular heart disease, and it is quite possible that she may helped a great deal by appropriate medical or even surgical therapy.

Mr D is 69 years old, a heavy smoker who has worked both in the coalfields and in the shipyards. He complains of breathlessness on exertion. Thinking back, it has gone on for some years, but has really become quite a problem recently. Examination reveals obesity and widespread pulmonary wheeze. He could have heart failure secondary to left ventricular systolic dysfunction but is at least as likely to be developing angina of effort, or chronic lung disease.

Summary of signs and symptoms

Our conclusion is that clinical diagnosis of heart failure is very difficult. It is very important to have a high index of suspicion for the possibility of heart failure but it is equally important that clinical suspicion is backed up by objective evidence of cardiac abnormality and preferably by a response to treatment as well. Only in this way will false-negative reassurance and false-positive diagnosis be

avoided. The perils of false-negative reassurance are obvious, the pitfalls of false-positive diagnosis are less so. Apart from the undesirability of providing patients with false information, false-positive diagnosis faces the possible ineffectiveness of treatment, the possible hazards of incorrect treatment and the omission of other potentially efficacious treatments. The truth of the clinical diagnosis (i.e. based only on symptoms and signs) of heart failure is that it should not be attempted. Diagnosis of heart failure should always be backed up by appropriate use of tests. Like much else in clinical cardiology, this is a marked exception to the maxim that 90% of the diagnosis is in the history, 9% in the clinical examination, and only 1% in the results of investigation.

Investigation of patients with suspected heart failure

Because the symptoms and physical signs of cardiac failure are non-specific, and clinical assessment is unreliable, patients in whom the condition is suspected require further investigation.

As has been pointed out, heart failure is a clinical syndrome rather than a diagnosis per se and arises through a number of distinct pathophysiological processes. Attention has tended to focus on patients with left ventricular systolic dysfunction, because they respond well to angiotensin-converting enzyme inhibitor and beta-blocker therapy. However heart failure may also develop because of abnormal ventricular filling (so called 'diastolic dysfunction'), valvular disease, arrhythmias, pericardial disease or metabolic disturbance. This diversity means that there is no easy, all-embracing definition of heart failure, and that no one investigation provides all the answers for each patient. In any case the scope of investigation extends beyond simply confirming the presence of heart failure. For example, evaluation of pathophysiology, aetiology and prognosis may be relevant in determining the most appropriate management. Patients with heart failure who have multivessel coronary artery disease may benefit from revascularization, and surgery is often preferable for patients with valvular disease. Conversely it may be possible to identify patients with severe heart failure awaiting cardiac transplantation, who may respond well to intensified medical therapy.

A further aspect relevant to investigation has emerged recently with the recognition that it is possible to retard or even prevent the development of heart failure. Although chronic heart failure can arise acutely following a major ventricular insult, the usual onset is more insidious, and often preceded by a latent phase of asymptomatic or minimally symptomatic left ventricular dysfunction. Studies show that the natural history of left ventricular dysfunction is one of relentless deterioration, even without additional ventricular damage.[30] However, the rate of progression can be reduced with early recognition and appropriate drug treatment using angiotensin-converting enzyme inhibitors[30] and beta-blockers.[31] The implication is that we need to consider strategies for population screening in order to identify 'at risk' individuals who by definition are unlikely to come to medical attention spontaneously. The potential importance of this problem is illustrated by recent work showing that the prevalence of asymptomatic left ventricular dysfunction is likely to be at least as high as that of overt heart failure itself.[32] The purpose of this section is to review the most important investigations available for patients with heart failure, and also to attempt to offer an insight into some of the latest techniques currently being developed.

Core investigations in heart failure
The electrocardiogram

It is mandatory to record a 12-lead ECG in any patient with suspected heart failure if only to exclude tachy- or bradyarrhythmia. However, the ECG may provide other important clues to the presence of significant cardiac disease. Pathological Q-waves usually indicate previous myocardial infarction, while increased QRS voltage and ST segment changes are characteristic of left ventricular hypertrophy associated with hypertensive heart disease or aortic stenosis (Figure 6.2). The presence of bundle branch block does not invariably indicate the presence of significant cardiac disease, but left bundle branch block can be a marker of ventricular dysfunction, while right bundle branch block may be seen in patients with an atrial septal defect. Conversely a normal 12-lead ECG is unusual in the presence of significant left ventricular dysfunction, and may suggest an alternative diagnosis.[33] In other words, whilst an abnormal ECG is relatively non-specific, a normal ECG has useful negative predictive value, and might have a role in screening patients with suspected heart failure in primary care. In those with an entirely normal ECG initial investigations should probably be directed towards finding other causes for their symptoms, for example pulmonary disease.

The chest X-ray

The chest X-ray has traditionally been one of the core investigations of heart failure, and remains important in patients with acute dyspnoea. Its relative importance in chronic heart failure has diminished with the advent of cardiac ultrasound techniques, but its ready availability ensures that it will continue to be requested in many patients. A number of abnormalities in the cardiac silhouette or in the pulmonary vasculature may provide pointers to cardiac pathology. Cardiomegaly may indicate dilatation of the cardiac chambers, myocardial hypertrophy or pericardial effusion (refer to Figure 6.1). If this is associated with pulmonary oedema or congestion of the upper lobe vessels then heart failure is likely, although the chest X-ray does not provide a reliable estimate of pulmonary capillary pressure,[12] and correlates poorly with other measures of left ventricular function such as echocardiography.[34]

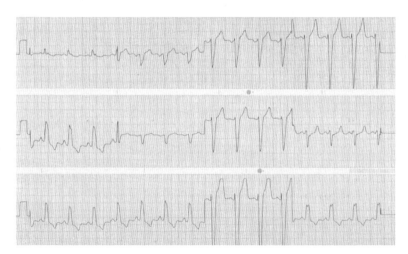

Figure 6.2. *The 12-lead electrocardiogram of a 48-year-old man with a dilated cardiomyopathy (left ventricular ejection fraction 18%). There is a left bundle branch block, and some evidence of left atrial enlargement. Reproduced with permission from: Heart Failure. Diagnosis and Management. Clark AL, McMurray JJV (eds). London: Martin Dunitz, 2001.*

Valvular calcification may be seen in patients with mitral or aortic valve disease, while linear calcification along the pericardial border raises the suspicion of pericardial constriction. Enlargement of the pulmonary arteries may result from shunting of blood through a significant atrial septal defect, and the aortic knuckle may be correspondingly small. Ultimately, however, the most important role of the chest X-ray remains the exclusion of alternative pathology such as pleural effusion, pneumonia, emphysema, tumour or pulmonary fibrosis, all of which may masquerade as heart failure.

Routine blood tests

A number of biochemical and haematological tests may be relevant in the investigation of patients with suspected heart failure. Measurement of serum electrolytes and hepatic function is important before and after initiation of drug treatment for heart failure. Renal impairment at baseline may be due to renovascular disease which is a contraindication to angiotensin-converting enzyme inhibitor therapy. Excessive doses of diuretics may precipitate a deterioration in renal function, and there is also a danger of inducing hypokalaemia or hyponatraemia. Hyponatraemia itself is an ominous feature in patients with established heart failure.[35]

It is important to exclude anaemia as the cause of symptoms in any patient who presents with breathless or fatigue, and similarly both hyper- and hypothyroidism can mimic heart failure. Serum ferritin is performed as a screening test for haemochromatosis in patients with unexplained heart failure, especially if they have diabetes or skin pigmentation, and urinary catecholamine levels provide a method for detecting phaechromocytoma as a rare cause of dilated cardiomyopathy.

The echocardiogram

The echocardiogram is the single most important investigation in patients with heart failure. A meaningful assessment can be obtained in just a few minutes by an experienced operator allowing real time estimation of global and regional left ventricular function, while also identifying gross abnormalities of cardiac anatomy including valvular disease (Figure 6.3). Ultrasound machines are sufficiently portable to allow bed-side assessment in casualty departments, in intensive care settings, in the operating theatre, as well as in the cardiology department. Serial examinations can be performed safely in an individual to document the progression of cardiac disease. The main disadvantage is that image quality is poor in a minority of subjects, espe-

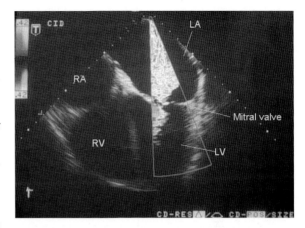

Figure 6.3. *Transoesophageal echocardiogram of a patient whose heart failure was due to mitral regurgitation. The left atrium is closest to the transducer (top). The mitral regurgitation is seen as a colour jet from left ventricle to left atrium. Reproduced with permission from: Heart Failure. Diagnosis and Management. Clark AL, McMurray JJV (eds). London: Martin Dunitz, 2001.*

cially those who are obese or have significant pulmonary disease. Unfortunately these may be the very patients who are most at risk from cardiovascular events.[36]

Echocardiography and ventricular function

Left ventricular function assessment is now the commonest reason for requesting an echocardiogram,[37] and is also the main reason behind the establishment of 'open' or 'direct' access echocardiography services, which allow general practitioners to refer patients with suspected heart failure directly for investigation.[38] The burgeoning popularity of these services is a testament to the widely perceived advantages of the technique. An 'eyeball' assessment of left ventricular contractility takes only a few minutes, and with experience it is possible to provide an accurate estimate of global function which correlates reasonably well with other techniques.[39] Sometimes, however, a more quantitative assessment is required. Fractional shortening is widely reported as a simple index of ventricular contractility (calculated as the ratio of end-systolic and end-diastolic left ventricular diameters measured at the base of the heart). It is reproducible but can be misleading in patients with regional dysynergy, in whom alternative techniques are to be preferred. The left ventricular ejection fraction is the most widely used index of cardiac function and is recognized as an important prognostic indicator in heart failure.[35,40] It can be derived using a number of different echocardiographic techniques, but the

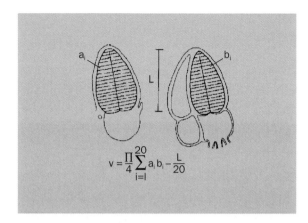

$$v = \frac{\Pi}{4} \sum_{i=1}^{20} a_i b_i - \frac{L}{20}$$

Figure 6.4. *Estimating cardiac volume using Simpson's rule. The volume of 20 discs is summed. The left ventricular ejection fraction (LVEF) is derived from the end-diastolic volume (EDV) and end-systolic volume (ESV: LVEF= (EDV–ESV)/EDV × 100 (%). Reproduced with permission from: Heart Failure. Diagnosis and Management. Clark AL, McMurray JJV (eds). London: Martin Dunitz, 2001.*

modified Simpson's (disc summation) method is probably the most accurate, especially in patients with regional wall motion abnormalities[41] (Figure 6.4). The technique is time-consuming and technically demanding, but many machines now have on-line analysis packages which facilitate measurements. Reproducibility remains an important problem, however, unless excellent image quality can be obtained, and the suitability of this technique for everyday clinical use is questionable. It should be stressed that there is no universal cut-off ejection fraction value which defines left ventricular dysfunction,[42] although values of 35%[43] and 40%[44] have been used as the entry criteria in some clinical trials.

Another clinically useful method for assessing left ventricular contractility is wall motion analysis, which may provide even greater prognostic information than ejection fraction in heart failure.[45] The ventricle is divided up into a number of segments and contractility is assessed individually. The scores are averaged and an overall 'wall motion index' obtained. Recently a nine-segment model has been used successfully to stratify patients surviving myocardial infarction.[46] A wall motion index of 1.2 or less using this model corresponds approximately to a left ventricular ejection fraction of ≤ 35%.

Doppler
Doppler echo techniques have an important role in evaluating patients with heart failure. Colour flow Doppler

readily identifies abnormal valve function or the presence of intracardiac shunts. Quantitative Doppler techniques allow non-invasive measurement of gradients across stenotic valves, estimation of cardiac output, and can be used to obtain an indirect assessment of pulmonary artery pressure. A semiquantitative assessment of valvular regurgitation is also possible, and techniques are still being refined.

Doppler echocardiography can also be used to assess left ventricular diastolic filling using the pattern of early ('E wave') and late ('A wave') inflow through the mitral valve. Abnormal diastolic function is said to be the cause of symptoms in as many as one-third of heart failure patients.[47] The 'E/A ratio' is probably the most frequently quoted index of diastolic function, but is also perhaps the least useful.[48] Reversal of the E/A ratio is often assumed to be synonymous with diastolic dysfunction, but in fact is common with increasing age. Conversely, an apparently normal E/A ratio ('pseudo-normalization') may be seen in patients with marked abnormalities of left ventricular filling. A 'restrictive' filling pattern characterized by a short E-wave deceleration time (less than 100 msec) may be more specific, and develops in patients with severe diastolic dysfunction. It indicates a poor prognosis in heart failure patients.[49] Other measures such as intraventricular relaxation time and pulmonary vein flow patterns may also be useful, but most would agree that both the assessment and management of diastolic dysfunction is less well characterized than that of systolic dysfunction.[50] The complex issue of evaluating diastolic function has been reviewed in detail elsewhere.[51–55]

Low-dose dobutamine echocardiography
Dobutamine stress echocardiography is now well-established as an alternative to nuclear techniques for assessing myocardial ischaemia, but infusion of lower doses of dobutamine (typically 5–10 μg/kg/minute) allows assessment of myocardial viability in patients with advanced left ventricular dysfunction.[56] In many cases such ventricular impairment is the result of irreversible myocardial necrosis and scarring. In others, however, there may be areas of viable, but non-contractile myocardium, known as 'hibernating myocardium'. This is thought to occur as a response to chronic ischaemia, or recurrent episodes of ischaemia. The key importance of recognizing the presence of hibernating myocardium is that it can recover contractile function if it is revascularized.[57–59] The gold standard for identifying hibernating myocardium is probably positron emission tomography, but its availability is too

limited for it to be clinically useful.[60,61] Low-dose dobutamine echocardiography provides an alternative approach. Areas of hibernating tissue appear akinetic initially, but begin to contract or thicken as dobutamine is infused, though at higher doses function may again be lost as the tissue becomes more ischaemic. This biphasic response is highly indicative of recovery after revascularization.[62] Hibernating myocardium should be differentiated from 'stunned myocardium' which has superficial similarities. The key difference is that stunning occurs following a single, transient episode of ischaemia, and myocardial function recovers spontaneously.

Recent developments in echocardiography

Other techniques promise to extend the role of echocardiography in heart failure still further.[63] Contrast echocardiography employs intravenous contrast agents which cross the pulmonary vascular bed and enter the systemic circulation. Most of these agents contain microbubbles or spheres which reflect ultrasound energy, opacifying the blood pool and so improving endocardial boundary definition. In addition, ultrasound causes these microspheres to resonate at specific harmonic frequencies which can be selectively amplified ('second harmonic imaging') to improve signal-to-noise ratio. Contrast echo should make it possible to obtain a quantitative assessment of cardiac function in many patients in whom images were previously considered inadequate. New image-processing techniques may even permit evaluation of myocardial perfusion using these agents, thus providing a direct assessment of coronary patency, and perhaps tissue viability.

Transoesophageal echocardiography

Transoesophageal echocardiography is occasionally valuable in the assessment of patients with heart failure if transthoracic echo images are inadequate.[64] It also allows detailed evaluation of structures which may not be seen particularly well using transthoracic imaging, including prosthetic heart valves, the intra-atrial septum and the pulmonary veins.

Ancillary investigations in heart failure

Cardiac catheterization

Cardiac catheterization is rarely if ever required to make the diagnosis of chronic heart failure. However, it has an important part to play in elucidating the aetiology and pathophysiology of heart failure, and it may be valuable in guiding management under certain circumstances.

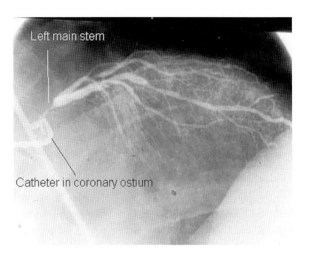

Figure 6.5. *Left coronary artery demonstrated during angiography. There is a tight left main stem stenosis. Severe atheroma throughout the left coronary artery. Reproduced with permission from: Heart Failure. Diagnosis and Management. Clark AL, McMurray JJV (eds). London: Martin Dunitz, 2001.*

More than one-half of patients with left ventricular dysfunction will have underlying coronary artery disease (Figure 6.5). In some of these patients its presence is suspected because anginal symptoms coexist with heart failure, or because there is a documented history of myocardial infarction. In others it is detected by stress testing using conventional treadmill or bicycle exercise testing, radionuclide perfusion imaging, or stress echocardiography. In selected patients found to have triple vessel disease, or left main stem stenosis, the prognosis may be improved by successful bypass surgery. Historically there has been a reluctance to consider conventional revascularization in patients with heart failure and severe ventricular impairment because of the perceived high operative mortality, but this should no longer be the case.

Cardiac catheterization may also provide a useful guide to medical therapy, particularly since physical signs are such an unreliable guide to haemodynamic status.[13] Pulmonary artery catheterization using a Swan–Ganz catheter is already widely used to optimize filling pressures in patients with acute heart failure and cardiogenic shock. However, it can also be valuable in chronic heart failure, although a certain amount of caution is required in the interpretation of the results. It is important to remember that a normal right heart study does not exclude the diagnosis of heart failure. Pharmacological treatment may normalize filling pressures even in patients with severe heart failure, and indeed this is the aim of 'tailored vasodilator therapy' in which the dosages of diuretics and vasodilators are titrated to achieve predefined haemodynamic targets. This aggressive approach has been shown to improve symptomatic status in patients with endstage heart failure,[65] even to the extent of allowing patients to be taken off the waiting-list for cardiac transplantation.

Other procedures which can be performed at the time of cardiac catheterization include myocardial biopsy in cases where primary myocardial disease (e.g. myocarditis) or infiltrative disease (e.g. amyloid) is suspected. Renal angiography may also be considered, particularly in patients with coexistent hypertension, azotaemia, or peripheral vascular disease, in whom the prevalence of atheromatous renovascular disease is higher.[66] Renal artery stenosis may be a contraindication to angiotensin-converting enzyme inhibitor therapy if it is bilateral, or if the patient has a single functioning kidney. Renal artery stenosis itself may precipitate heart failure, both acute ('flash pulmonary oedema'), and chronic.[67] It may be amenable to percutaneous intervention, although the long-term clinical results have been variable, and the technique is not without hazards.[68]

Nuclear techniques
Blood pool imaging
Nuclear techniques can be useful in assessing ventricular function especially when echocardiographic images are inadequate or results seem inconsistent. The left ventricular ejection fraction can be obtained using radionuclide ventriculography (also known as multi-gated acquisition or 'MUGA' scans) in most patients, and regional wall motion can also be evaluated. It offers good reproducibility, and is largely free of the imaging problems faced with echocardiography.

However, there are drawbacks. Gating can be difficult in patients with arrhythmias, and a significant dose of ionizing radiation is administered, limiting the number of studies which can be performed on an individual. Facilities for nuclear cardiology are not as widely available as for echocardiography, and the technique is less convenient to perform. Finally, there is a wide variation in the normal range quoted in different institutions making comparison of results between centres difficult.[69]

Myocardial perfusion imaging
Coronary artery disease is present in the majority of patients who develop heart failure, and bypass surgery improves the prognosis of those with multivessel coronary

disease and ventricular dysfunction. Myocardial perfusion imaging (most commonly using thallium) allows myocardial ischaemia to be recognized in patients with heart failure, and may suggest the need for angiography and revascularization. The technique is more sensitive and specific than treadmill exercise testing, and probably of equivalent predictive accuracy to stress echo techniques. Myocardial perfusion imaging can also be used to assess myocardial viability in patients with severe ventricular dysfunction being considered for conventional revascularization (Figure 6.6).[70] It appears to have comparable accuracy to low-dose dobutamine echocardiography for predicting functional recovery following bypass surgery.[71]

Exercise testing
Simple treadmill or bicycle exercise provides important information in patients with angina or myocardial infarction, but is not particularly useful for actually diagnosing heart failure. However, it may demonstrate evidence of underlying cardiac ischaemia, and the addition of cardiopulmonary testing allows measurement of gas exchange (most commonly peak oxygen consumption or 'VO_2max'), which is widely used as a measure of disease severity and prognosis,[35,40] and increasingly as a guide to the timing of cardiac transplantation.[72] A fall in arterial oxygen saturation during exercise is unusual in heart failure, and points to pulmonary disease as a possible cause of symptoms.[73]

Ambulatory electrocardiogram
A Holter recording, usually carried out over 24 or 48 hours, does not in itself aid the diagnosis of heart failure, but may identify significant tachy- or bradyarrhythmias, which may be amenable to treatment. Patients with paroxysmal atrial fibrillation, for example, might be considered for anticoagulant therapy, while the presence of non-sustained ventricular tachycardia may be regarded as an indication for a ventricular stimulation study, with a view to implantation of a cardioverter-defibrillator.

Magnetic resonance imaging
Magnetic resonance imaging shows great promise for the future.[74] Previously, restricted availability, prolonged imaging protocols, and poor patient tolerability had limited its applicability. Recently, however, improvements in technology have dramatically reduced imaging times while improving image quality. The current generation of scanners are capable of real-time cardiac imaging, producing accurate, reproducible measurements of cardiac volumes, cardiac function, and muscle mass. Magnetic

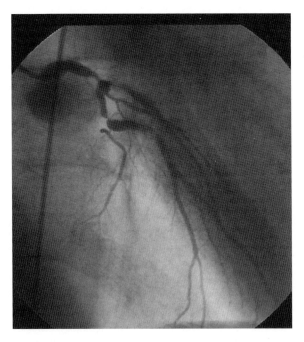 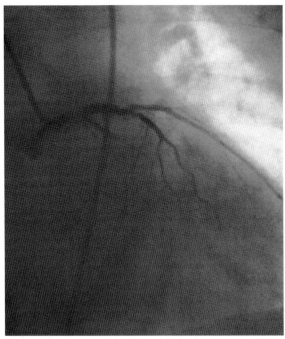

Figure 6.6. *High-grade lesions in the proximal left coronary artery, which caused repetitive stunning and then hibernation. Akinesia existed throughout the anterolateral surface but without Q-waves or a history of myocardial infarction. Reproduced with permission from: Heart Failure. Pathogenesis and Treatment. Narula J (ed). London: Martin Dunitz, 2001.*

resonance coronary angiography is not far away as a practical clinical tool, while magnetic resonance renal angiography is already becoming the method of choice for assessing renal vasculature. It is not unrealistic to foresee a time when it will be possible to assess the body's entire vascular tree quickly in a single, non-invasive study. Perhaps even more excitingly magnetic resonance will be able to combine this with an assessment of myocardial perfusion and viability.[75]

Computed tomography

Computed tomography has a relatively minor role in the investigation of patients with heart failure, but again allows accurate assessment of chamber dimensions. It is also a good technique for demonstrating disease of the pericardium and, in particular, pericardial constriction.

Novel investigations in heart failure
Neurohumoral markers

For many years there has been interest in the role of neurohumoral factors in the pathogenesis of heart failure,[76] and this interest intensified with the realization that there might be a role for some of these neurohormones in the diagnosis,

assessment, and monitoring of heart failure and related conditions.[77] The natriuretic peptides appear to have the greatest potential for clinical use. There are three members of the family of natriuretic peptides altogether, but atrial natriuretic peptide (ANP), and brain or B-type natriuretic peptide (BNP) have been studied most. As the name suggests, ANP is secreted primarily from the atria, whereas BNP is actually predominantly ventricularly derived. Both are synthesized as 'prohormones', and cleaved into an active C-terminal moiety, and a relatively inactive N-terminal fragment (NT-ANP and NT-BNP, respectively). The N-terminal fragments are cleared more slowly from the circulation than the active C-peptides, and might therefore be expected to provide a better reflection of cardiac status.

Both CT-BNP and NT-BNP seem to be the most promising candidates for routine diagnostic use. They are stable in whole blood for several days even at room temperature, which facilitates handling and processing.[78–85] They are superior to other neurohormones for diagnosing left ventricular dysfunction and predicting prognosis in heart failure, and after myocardial infarction. They have been used to establish if there is a cardiac cause of breathlessness in patients in the community, and in patients presenting acutely to hospital. They may also have an important role in screening the wider population in order to identify patients with asymptomatic left ventricular dysfunction who may benefit from the early use of angiotensin-converting enzyme inhibitors. Finally, there is preliminary evidence that they might have a part to play in guiding drug therapy, and monitoring the response to treatment.[86]

Autonomic function assessment

Heart failure is associated with abnormalities of autonomic activity which may be of value in predicting prognosis. As well as an increase in sympathetic nervous system activity there is decreased parasympathetic tone. This may be evident even in the early stages of heart failure, and is reflected in reduced heart rate variability and impaired baroreflex sensitivity (measures of tonic and reflex parasympathetic activity, respectively). The everyday clinical importance of techniques which measure these variables is as yet uncertain.

Summary of investigation

Although a growing number of tools are at the disposal of the physician investigating and managing patients with suspected heart failure, the key is still thorough clinical evaluation combined with simple baseline investigations. The negative predictive value of a normal 12-lead ECG should be more widely appreciated, since it may allow more selective referral for cardiac investigation. Beyond this, echocardiography still provides the cornerstone of investigation, providing as it does a comprehensive, non-invasive assessment of global cardiac function. For the majority of patients this is sufficient to confirm the diagnosis, but if doubt remains there is a range of other techniques available.

The challenge which faces us now is to refine our approach so that patients can be recognized earlier in the course of their disease. If appropriate, effective treatment can be offered more quickly, we may delay or even prevent the development of overt heart failure. This is no idle dream. In the near future, humoral markers may be used to screen for the presence of left ventricular dysfunction in the community, while magnetic resonance imaging will offer a more precise evaluation of all aspects of cardiac pathophysiology, perhaps replacing echocardiography, nuclear techniques, and even angiography. The future of heart failure investigation looks exciting indeed.

References

1 Remme WJ, Swedberg K. Guidelines for the diagnosis and treatment of chronic heart failure. *Eur Heart J* 2001; **22:** 1527–60.

2 Hunt SA, Baker DW, Chin MH et al. ACC/AHA guidelines for the evaluation and management of chronic heart failure in the adult: Executive summary, a report of the American College of Cardiology/American Heart Association Task Force on Practice Guidelines (committee to revise the 1995 guidelines for the evaluation and management of heart failure); developed in collaboration with the International Society for Heart and Lung Transplantation, endorsed by the Heart Failure Society of America. *Circulation* 2001; **104:** 2996–3007.

3 Wood P. *Diseases of the Heart and Circulation*. London: Chapman and Hall, 1968.

4 Braunwald E, Grossman W. Clinical aspects of heart failure. In: Braunwald E, ed. *Heart Disease*, 4th edn. New York: WB Saunders, 1992: 444.

5 Packer M. Survival in patients with chronic heart failure and its potential modification by drug therapy. In: Cohn J, ed. *Drug Treatment of Heart Failure*, 2nd edn. Secaucus, NJ: ATC International, 1988: 273.

6 Poole-Wilson PA. Heart Failure. *Med Int* 1985; 866–71.

7 Vasan RS, Benjamin EJ, Levy D. Prevalence, clinical features and prognosis of diastolic heart failure: an epidemiologic perspective. *J Am Coll Cardiol* 1995; **26:** 1565–74.

8 Vasan RS, Larson MG, Benjamin EJ et al. Congestive heart failure in subjects with normal versus reduced left ventricular ejection fraction: prevalence and mortality in a population-based cohort. *J Am Coll Cardiol* 1999; 1948–55.

9 Ridsdale L, Evans A, Jerrett W et al. Patients with fatigue in general practice: a prospective study. *BMJ* 1993; **307:** 103–6.

10 Stewart AL, Greenfield S, Hays RD et al. Functional status and well-being of patients with chronic conditions. Results from the Medical Outcomes Study. *JAMA* 1989; **262:** 907–13.

11 Harlan WR, Olberman A, Grimm R, Rosati RA. Chronic congestive heart failure in coronary artery disease: clinical criteria. *Ann Intern Med* 1977; **86:** 133–8.

12 Chakko S, Woska D, Martinez H et al. Clinical, radiographic, and hemodynamic correlations in chronic congestive heart failure: conflicting results may lead to inappropriate care. *Am J Med* 1991; **90:** 353–9.

13 Stevenson LW, Perloff JK. The limited reliability of physical signs for estimating haemodynamics in chronic heart failure. *JAMA* 1989; **261:** 884–8.

14 Echevarria HH, Bilsker MS, Myerburg RJ, Kessler KM. Congestive heart failure: echocardiographic insights. *Am J Med* 1983; **75:** 750–5.

15 Davie AP, Francis CM, Caruana L, Sutherland GR, McMurray JJV. Assessing diagnosis in heart failure: which features are any use? *Q J Med* 1997; **90:** 335–9.

16 Heckerling PS, Wiener SL, Moses VK et al. Accuracy of precordial percussion in detecting cardiomegaly. *Am J Med* 1991; **91:** 328–34.

17 O'Neil TW, Barry M, Smith M, Graham IM. Diagnostic value of the apex beat. *Lancet* 1989; **1:** 410–11.

18 Butman SM, Ewy GA, Standen JR, Kern KB, Hahn E. Bedside cardiovascular examination in patients with severe chronic heart failure: importance of rest or inducible jugular venous distension. *J Am Coll Cardiol* 1993; **22:** 968–74.

19 Dans AL, Bossone EF, Guyatt GH, Fallen EL. Evaluation of the reproducibility and accuracy of apex beat measurement in the detection of echocardiographic left ventricular dilatation. *Can J Cardiol* 1994; **11:** 493–7.

20 Ishmail AA, Wing S, Ferguson J et al. Interobserver agreement by auscultation in the presence of a third heart sound in patients with congestive heart failure. *Chest* 1987; **91:** 870–3.

21 Ghali JK, Kadakia S, Cooper RS, Liao YL. Bedside diagnosis of preserved versus impaired left ventricular systolic function in heart failure. *Am J Cardiol* 1991; **67:** 1002–6.

22 Thomas JT, Kelly RF, Thomas SJ et al. Utility of history, physical examination, electrocardiogram, and chest radiograph for differentiating normal from decreased systolic function in patients with heart failure. *Am J Med* 2002; **112:** 437–45.

23 Cheitlin MD. Can clinical evaluation differentiate diastolic from systolic heart failure? If so, is it important? *Am J Med* 2002; **112:** 496–7.

24 Marantz PR, Tobin JN, Wassertheil-Smoller S et al. The relationship between left ventricular systolic function and congestive heart failure diagnosed by clinical criteria. *Circulation* 1988; **77:** 607–12.

25 Remes J, Miettinen H, Reunanen A et al. Validity of clinical diagnosis of heart failure in primary health care. *Eur Heart J* 1991; **12:** 315–21.

26 Carlson KJ, Lee DC-S, Goroll AH et al. An analysis of physicians' reasons for prescribing long-term digitalis therapy in outpatients. *J Chron Dis* 1985; **38:** 733–9.

27 Mattleman SJ, Hakki A-H, Iskandrian AS et al. Reliability of bedside evaluation in determining left ventricular function: correlation with left ventricular ejection fraction determined by radionuclide ventriculography. *J Am Coll Cardiol* 1983; **1:** 417–20.

28 Cease KB, Nicklas JM. Prediction of left ventricular ejection fraction using simple quantitative clinical information. *Am J Med* 1986; **81:** 429–36.

29 Eagle KA, Quertermous T, Singer DE et al. Left ventricular ejection fraction: physician estimates compared with gated blood pool scan measurements. *Arch Intern Med* 1988; **148:** 882–5.

30 Konstam MA, Kronenberg MW, Rousseau MF, Udelson JE, Melin J et al. Effects of the angiotensin converting enzyme inhibitor enalapril on the long-term progression of left ventricular dilatation in patients with asymptomatic systolic dysfunction. SOLVD (Studies of Left Ventricular Dysfunction) Investigators. *Circulation* 1993; **88:** 2277–83.

31 Colucci WS, Packer M, Bristow MR, Gilbert EM, Cohn JN et al. Carvedilol inhibits clinical progression in patients with mild symptoms of heart failure. US Carvedilol Heart Failure Study Group. *Circulation* 1996; **94:** 2800–6.

32 Petrie M, McMurray J. Changes in notions about heart failure. *Lancet* 2001; **358:** 432–4.

33 Davie AP, Francis CM, Love MP, Caruana L, Starkey IR et al. Value of the electrocardiogram in identifying heart failure due to left ventricular systolic dysfunction. *BMJ* 1996; **312:** 222.

34 Clark AL, Coats AJ. Unreliability of cardiothoracic ratio as a marker of left ventricular impairment: comparison with radionuclide ventriculography and echocardiography. *Postgrad Med J* 2000; **76:** 289–91.

35 Parameshwar J, Keegan J, Sparrow J, Sutton GC, Poole-Wilson PA. Predictors of prognosis in severe chronic heart failure. *Am Heart J* 1992; **123:** 421–6.

36 Kober L, Torp-Pedersen C. Clinical characteristics and mortality of patients screened for entry into the Trandolapril Cardiac Evaluation (TRACE) study. *Am J Cardiol* 1995; **76:** 1–5.

37 Gillespie ND, Struthers AD, Pringle SD. Changing echocardiography request patterns between 1988 and 1993. *Health Bulletin* 1996; **54:** 395–401.

38 Francis CM, Caruana L, Kearney P, Love M, Sutherland GR et al. Open access echocardiography in management of heart failure in the community. *BMJ* 1995; **310:** 634–6.

39 Willenheimer RB, Israelsson BA, Cline CMJ, Erhardt LR. Simplified echocardiography in the diagnosis of heart failure. *Scand Cardiovasc J* 1997; **31:** 8–16.

40 Cohn JN, Johnson GR, Shabetai R, Loeb H, Tristani F et al. Ejection fraction, peak exercise oxygen consumption, cardiothoracic ratio, ventricular arrhythmias, and plasma norepinephrine as determinants of prognosis in heart failure. The V-HeFT VA Cooperative Studies Group. *Circulation* 1993; **87:** VI5–16.

41 Schiller NB, Shah PM, Crawford M, DeMaria A, Devereux R et al. Recommendations for quantitation of the left ventricle by two-dimensional echocardiography. American Society of Echocardiography Committee on Standards, Subcommittee on Quantitation of Two-Dimensional Echocardiograms. *J Am Soc Echocardiog* 1989; **2:** 358–67.

42 Ray SG, Metcalfe MJ, Oldroyd KG, Pye M, Martin W et al. Do radionuclide and echocardiographic techniques give a universal cut off value for left ventricular ejection

fraction that can be used to select patients for treatment with ACE inhibitors after myocardial infarction? *Br Heart J* 1995; **73**: 466–9.

43 The SOLVD Investigators. Effect of enalapril on survival in patients with reduced left ventricular ejection fractions and congestive heart failure. *N Eng J Med* 1991; **325**: 293–302.

44 Pfeffer MA, Braunwald E, Moye LA, Basta L, Brown EJ Jr et al. Effect of captopril on mortality and morbidity in patients with left ventricular dysfunction after myocardial infarction. Results of the survival and ventricular enlargement trial. *N Engl J Med* 1992; **327**: 669–77.

45 Madsen BK, Videbaek R, Stokholm H, Mortensen LS, Hansen JF. Prognostic value of echocardiography in 190 patients with chronic congestive heart failure. A comparison with New York Heart Association functional classes and radionuclide ventriculography. *Cardiology* 1996; **87**: 250–6.

46 Kober L, Torp-Pedersen C, Carlsen J, Videbaek R, Egeblad H. An echocardiographic method for selecting high risk patients shortly after acute myocardial infarction, for inclusion in multi-centre studies (as used in the TRACE study). *Eur Heart J* 1994; **15**: 1616–20.

47 Cohn JN, Johnson G. Heart failure with normal ejection fraction. The V-HeFT Study. Veterans Administration Cooperative Study Group. *Circulation* 1990; **81**: III48–53.

48 Davie AP, Francis CM, Caruana L, Sutherland GR, McMurray JJ. The prevalence of left ventricular diastolic filling abnormalities in patients with suspected heart failure. *Eur Heart J* 1997; **18**: 981–4.

49 Giannuzzi P, Temporelli PL, Bosimini E, Silva P, Imparato A et al. Independent and incremental prognostic value of Doppler-derived mitral deceleration time of early filling in both symptomatic and asymptomatic patients with left ventricular dysfunction. *J Am Coll Cardiol* 1996; **28**: 383–90.

50 Vasan RS, Benjamin EJ, Levy D. Congestive heart failure with normal left ventricular systolic function. Clinical approaches to the diagnosis and treatment of diastolic heart failure. *Arch Intern Med* 1996; **156**: 146–57.

51 Vasan RS, Levy D. Defining diastolic heart failure: a call for standarized diagnostic criteria. *Circulation* 2000; **101**: 2118–21.

52 Zile MR, Gaasch WH, Carroll JD et al. Heart failure with a normal ejection fraction: is measurement of diastolic function necessary to make the diagnosis of diastolic heart failure? *Circulation* 2001; **104**: 779–82.

53 Zile MR, Brutsaert DL. New concepts in diastolic dysfunction and diastolic heart failure. I: Diagnosis, prognosis, and measurements of diastolic function. *Circulation* 2002; **105**: 1387–93.

54 Zile MR, Brutsaert DL. New concepts in diastolic dysfunction heart failure. II: Causal mechanisms and treatment. *Circulation* 2002; **105**: 1503–8.

55 (No authors listed). How to diagnose diastolic heart failure. European Study Group on Diastolic Heart Failure. *Eur Heart J* 1998; **19**: 990–1003.

56 La Canna G, Alfieri O, Giubbini R, Gargano M, Ferrari R, Visioli O. Echocardiography during infusion of dobutamine for identification of reversible dysfunction in patients with chronic coronary artery disease. *J Am Coll Cardiol* 1994; **23**: 617–26.

57 Rahimtoola SH. The hibernating myocardium. *Am Heart J* 1989; **117**: 211–21.

58 Wijns W, Vatner SF, Camici PG. Hibernating myocardium. *N Engl J Med* 1998; **339**: 173–81.

59 Bax JJ, Poldermans D, Elhendy A, Cornel JH, Boersma E et al. Improvement of left ventricular ejection fraction, heart failure symptoms and prognosis after revascularization in patients with chronic coronary artery disease and viable myocardium detected by dobutamine stress echocardiography. *J Am Coll Cardiol* 1999; **34**: 163–9.

60 Di Carli MF, Asgarzadie F, Schelbert HR, Brunken RC, Laks H et al. Quantitative relation between myocardial viability and improvement in heart failure symptoms after revascularization in patients with ischemic cardiomyopathy. *Circulation* 1995; **92**: 3436–44.

61 Pagano D, Bonser RS, Townend JN, Ordoubadi F, Lorenzoni R, Camici PG. Predictive value of dobutamine echocardiography and positron emission tomography in identifying hibernating myocardium in patients with postischaemic heart failure. *Heart* 1998; **79**: 281–8.

62 Cornel JH, Bax JJ, Elhendy A, Maat AP, Kimman GJ et al. Biphasic response to dobutamine predicts improvement of global left ventricular function after surgical revascularization in patients with stable coronary artery disease: implications of time course of recovery on diagnostic accuracy. *J Am Coll Cardiol* 1998; **31**: 1002–10.

63 Jarnert C, Mejhert M, Ring M, Persson H, Edner M. Doppler tissue imaging in congestive heart failure patients due to diastolic or systolic dysfunction: a comparison with Doppler echocardiography and the atrio-ventricular plane displacement technique. *Eur J Heart Fail* 2000; **2**: 151–60.

64 Vitarelli A, Gheorghiade M. Transthoracic and transesophageal echocardiography in the hemodynamic assessment of patients with congestive heart failure. *Am J Cardiol* 2000; **86**: 36G–40G.

65 Steimle AE, Stevenson LW, Chelimsky-Fallick C, Fonarow GC, Hamilton MA et al. Sustained hemodynamic efficacy of therapy tailored to reduce filling pressures in survivors with advanced heart failure. *Circulation* 1997; **96**: 1165–72.

66 Greco BA, Breyer JA. The natural history of renal artery stenosis: who should be evaluated for suspected ischemic nephropathy? *Semin Nephrol* 1996; **16**: 2–11.

67 Missouris CG, Belli AM, MacGregor GA. 'Apparent' heart failure: a syndrome caused by renal artery stenoses. *Heart* 2000; **83**: 152–5.

68 Weibull H, Bergqvist D, Jonsson K, Carlsson S, Takolander R. Analysis of complications after percutaneous transluminal angioplasty of renal artery stenoses. *Eur J Vasc Surg* 1987; **1**: 77–84.

69 Underwood R, Gibson C, Tweddel A, Flint J. A survey of nuclear cardiological practice in Great Britain. The British Nuclear Cardiology Group. *Br Heart J* 1992; **67:** 273–7.

70 Ragosta M, Beller GA, Watson DD, Kaul S, Gimple LW. Quantitative planar rest–redistribution 201Tl imaging in detection of myocardial viability and prediction of improvement in left ventricular function after coronary bypass surgery in patients with severely depressed left ventricular function. *Circulation* 1993; **87:** 1630–41.

71 Vanoverschelde JL, D'Hondt AM, Marwick T, Gerber BL, De Kock M et al. Head-to-head comparison of exercise–redistribution–reinjection thallium single-photon emission computed tomography and low dose dobutamine echocardiography for prediction of reversibility of chronic left ventricular ischemic dysfunction. *J Am Coll Cardiol* 1996; **28:** 432–42.

72 Mancini DM, Eisen H, Kussmaul W, Mull R, Edmunds LH Jr, Wilson JR. Value of peak exercise oxygen consumption for optimal timing of cardiac transplantation in ambulatory patients with heart failure. *Circulation* 1991; **83:** 778–86.

73 Clark AL, Coats AJ. Usefulness of arterial blood gas estimations during exercise in patients with chronic heart failure. *Br Heart J* 1994; **71:** 528–30.

74 Prasad S, Pennell DJ. Magnetic resonance imaging in the assessment of patients with heart failure. *J Nucl Cardiol* 2002; **9(Suppl):** 60S–70S.

75 Sensky PR, Jivan A, Hudson NM, Keal RP, Morgan B et al. Coronary artery disease: combined stress MR imaging protocol-one-stop evaluation of myocardial perfusion and function. *Radiology* 2000; **215:** 608–14.

76 Packer M. The neurohormonal hypothesis: a theory to explain the mechanism of disease progression in heart failure. *J Am Coll Cardiol* 1992; **20:** 248–54.

77 Francis GS, Cohn JN, Johnson G, Rector TS, Goldman S, Simon A. Plasma norepinephrine, plasma renin activity, and congestive heart failure. Relations to survival and the effects of therapy in V-HeFT II. The V-HeFT VA Cooperative Studies Group. *Circulation* 1993; **87:** VI40–8.

78 Murdoch DR, Byrne J, Morton JJ, McDonagh TA, Robb SD et al. Brain natriuretic peptide is stable in whole blood and can be measured using a simple rapid assay: implications for clinical practice. *Heart* 1997; **78:** 594–7.

79 Smith H, Pickering RM, Struthers A, Simpson I, Mant D. Biochemical diagnosis of ventricular dysfunction in elderly patients in general practice: observational study. *BMJ* 2000; **320:** 906–8.

80 Krishnaswamy P, Lubien E, Clopton P et al. Utility of B-natriuretic peptide levels in identifying patients with left ventricular systolic or diastolic dysfunction. *Am J Med* 2001; **111:** 274–9.

81 Lubien E, DeMaria A, Krishnaswamy P et al. Utility of B-natriuretic peptide in detecting diastolic dysfunction: comparison with Doppler velocity recordings. *Circulation* 2002; **105:** 595–601.

82 Morrison LK, Harrison A, Krishnaswamy P et al. Utility of a rapid B-natriuretic peptide assay in differentiating congestive heart failure from lung disease in patients presenting with dyspnea. *J Am Coll Cardiol* 2002; **39:** 202–9.

83 McCullough PA, Nowak RM, McCord J et al. B-type natriuretic peptide and clinical judgment in emergency diagnosis of heart failure: analysis from Breathing Not Properly (BNP) Multinational Study. *Circulation* 2002; **106:** 416–22.

84 Maisel AS, Krishnaswamy P, Nowak RM et al. Rapid measurement of B-type natriuretic peptide in the emergency diagnosis of heart failure. *N Engl J Med* 2002; **347:** 161–7.

85 Hobbs FD, Davis RC, Roalfe AK et al. Reliability of N-terminal pro-brain natriuretic peptide assay in diagnosis of heart failure: cohort study in representative and high risk community populations. *BMJ* 2002; **324:** 1498.

86 Troughton RW, Frampton CM, Yandle TG et al. Treatment of heart failure guided by plasma aminoterminal brain natriuretic peptide (N-BNP) concentrations. *Lancet* 2000; **355:** 1126–30.

7 The management of acute cardiogenic pulmonary oedema

John Beltrame and John D Horowitz

Acute pulmonary oedema is a life-threatening condition due to the rapid accumulation of fluid within the pulmonary alveoli. It is a common condition which most health care workers will have witnessed yet its optimal therapy is largely based upon empiric experience rather than evidence-based medicine. In this chapter the acute management of patients presenting with acute pulmonary oedema secondary to a cardiac disorder will be discussed. Following a brief revision of the underlying pathophysiological mechanisms and aetiology of acute pulmonary oedema, a practical guide to the management of this disorder will be outlined and the evidence supporting each particular therapy summarized.

Pathophysiological considerations

To understand the management of acute pulmonary oedema it is essential to grasp the aetiology and underlying pathophysiology of this disorder. Chapter 3 describes the pathophysiological principles of acute pulmonary oedema in detail that are briefly revised below.

Only half a micron separates capillary blood from the air in the lung. From the Frank–Starling law of fluid dynamics (see Chapter 3), there is net flow of fluid into the pulmonary extravascular space. This interstitial fluid is normally approximately 200–300 ml; however, should it increase by a further 100 ml, the results are cataclysmic. To prevent accumulation of interstitial fluid pulmonary lymphatics drain excess fluid resulting in an estimated normal lymph flow of 20 ml/hour.[1]

Pathophysiologically acute pulmonary oedema may occur if (1) the pulmonary capillary hydrostatic pressure increases resulting in increased fluid extravasation into the interstitium beyond that cleared by homeostatic lymph drainage mechanisms; (2) plasma oncotic pressure falls thus reducing transudation forces for fluid return to the capillary; (3) alveolar–capillary membrane disruption thereby increasing capillary permeability and allowing

excess fluid accumulation; and (4) impaired lymphatic drainage resulting in excess interstitial fluid.

The potential aetiological disorders contributing to acute pulmonary oedema and their associated pathophysiological mechanisms are summarized in Table 7.1. The most common mechanism is an increased pulmonary capillary hydrostatic pressure resulting from a cardiac disorder associated with raised left atrial pressures. This form of pulmonary oedema is referred to as 'acute cardiogenic pulmonary oedema' and therapies are directed towards reducing the raised capillary hydrostatic pressure.

In contrast, 'acute non-cardiogenic pulmonary oedema' (often referred to adult respiratory distress syndrome or ARDS) is usually due to disruption of the alveolar–capillary membrane resulting in the leakage of fluid into the interstitium. Thus, therapies involve treating the underlying aetiology whilst providing respiratory support until the alveolar–capillary membrane has healed. Alternatively this form of pulmonary oedema may arise from lymphatic obstruction, which is again managed by supportive therapy.

The above pathogenetic description of the causes of acute pulmonary oedema is an oversimplification since this disorder often involves several pathophysiological processes. For example, in acute cardiogenic pulmonary oedema, three distinct stages have been described.[2] Firstly, there is increased interstitial fluid as a result of the increased pulmonary capillary hydrostatic pressure, producing fluid-distended peribronchial tissues and lymphatics (stage 1). With further fluid accumulation, the more compliant tissues such as alveolar septa, bronchioles, arterioles and venules are distended (stage 2). Finally, fluid begins to enter the alveolar space (stage 3), either as a result of leakage through the less resistant bronchiolar epithelium and overflowing into the alveoli, or due to the disruption of alveolar membrane tight junctions. Alveolar flooding finally occurs when the increasing surface tension reaches a critical point in which the oedematous alveolus shrinks and thus the airspace is replaced with fluid and macromolecules.

Table 7.1. Aetiologies of acute pulmonary oedema

Cardiogenic (cardiac disorder resulting in raised pulmonary hydrostatic pressure)

    1. Acute left ventricular failure (systolic and/or diastolic dysfunction)

    2. Severe mitral stenosis

Non-cardiogenic

    1. Alveolar–capillary membrane permeability dysfunction (adult respiratory distress syndrome)

        (a) Infection – septicaemia, pneumonia

        (b) Aspiration – gastric contents, near-drowning

        (c) Inhalation – smoke, corrosive gases

        (d) Trauma – head injury, fat embolism, non-thoracic trauma

        (e) Haematologic – disseminated intravascular coagulation, post cardiopulmonary bypass

        (f) Metabolic – acute pancreatitis, renal failure, hepatic failure

    2. Impaired lymphatic drainage

        (a) Lymphangitis carcinomatosis

        (b) Post lung transplant

    3. Unclear mechanisms

        (a) Neurogenic pulmonary oedema

        (b) Narcotic overdose

        (c) High altitude pulmonary oedema

        (d) Eclampsia

        (e) Post cardioversion

A practical management strategy

Health care workers who have witnessed an episode of acute pulmonary oedema will attest to the severe distress of the affected patient's experience and therefore the urgency in administering therapy. Thus, unlike many medical conditions, emergency therapeutic measures must be rapidly instituted before the patient can be fully evaluated. Hence the treatment of acute cardiogenic pulmonary oedema can be considered to involve the following phases:

1. Immediate emergency resuscitation of hypoxaemia.
2. Urgent evaluation of the differential diagnosis.
3. Initial pharmacological therapy.
4. Aetiology-directed therapies.

Although these are listed as distinct phases for simplicity, they reflect a continuum with different phases often being addressed simultaneously by the experienced clinician.

Immediate emergency resuscitation

The characteristic clinical appearance of a patient with acute pulmonary oedema is of a patient sitting on the side of the bed with profuse sweating, severe dyspnoea with air hunger and possibly expectorating pink frothy sputum. Indeed it appears they are 'drowning in their own fluid'. The importance of sitting upright is to optimize the gravity-dependent pulmonary capillary flow distribution in order to minimize the lung zones affected by the raised intravascular pressure or leaking alveolar–capillary membrane.

Following the traditional 'ABC' resuscitation principles, it is usually evident that the 'Airway' is not compromised and that the distressed 'Breathing' requires immediate high flow oxygen administration to begin correction of the associated hypoxaemia. A rapid assessment must then be made regarding the patient's level of respiratory fatigue. If the patient is struggling to maintain respiratory effort (e.g. reduced respiratory rate and/or inspiratory volume) then mechanical ventilation may be required immediately. However, if the level of fatigue is reasonable, less invasive therapies may be employed initially.

The 'Circulation' must also be assessed including the pulse rate, cardiac rhythm and blood pressure. Intravenous access should also be rapidly established and a baseline arterial blood gas taken as soon as practical.

Table 7.2. Causes of acute severe dyspnoea

Acute pulmonary oedema: Cardiogenic
Non-cardiogenic
Acute exacerbation of chronic obstructive airways disease
Acute massive pulmonary embolism
Pneumothorax
Foreign body aspiration
Hyperventilation syndrome

Urgent evaluation of the differential diagnosis

Differential diagnosis of acute dyspnoea

After commencing resuscitative measures a rapid assessment as to the cause of the acute dyspnoea must be made. Table 7.2 summarizes important causes of acute dyspnoea. Whilst this chapter focuses upon acute cardiogenic pulmonary oedema other causes must also be considered. Most of these disorders can be readily distinguished from acute pulmonary oedema by clinical examination and basic investigations. However, the different forms of acute pulmonary oedema and exacerbation of chronic obstructive airways are often more difficult to delineate.

Delineating features for acute pulmonary oedema

Table 7.3 summarizes the clinical features which aid in differentiating between chronic obstructive airways disease exacerbation, acute cardiogenic and non-cardiogenic pulmonary oedema. The patient with an exacerbation of chronic obstructive airways disease will usually have a history of this disorder and presents with a progressive deterioration in dyspnoea over several days following an antecedent respiratory tract infection. The clinical manifestation of their chronic disease is usually evident and signs of a pneumonic process may be detected. The chest X-ray is particularly useful in excluding this cause from acute pulmonary oedema.

The patient presenting with acute cardiogenic pulmonary oedema generally has a history of a cardiac disorder and frequently prior admissions with acute pulmonary oedema. They typically present in the early hours of the morning reflecting a circadian variation similar to other cardiac disorders.[3] Clinical examination and investigation of these patients will reveal features of the underlying cardiac disorder (e.g. heart failure or valvular heart disease)

or the initiating event (e.g. acute myocardial infarction on ECG and/or cardiac enzymes).

In contrast to above, patients with acute non-cardiogenic pulmonary oedema may not have any significant past medical history. However, they often initially present with the precipitating insult (e.g. trauma, surgery, etc.) 24–48 hours prior to the onset of acute pulmonary oedema. Hence, these patients are often severely compromised and admitted to the intensive care unit as a result of the initiating insult.

Whilst the diagnosis of acute cardiogenic pulmonary oedema can often be made on clinical grounds it may be difficult in some patients, particularly those with multiple medical problems, e.g. the patient with chronic obstructive airways disease presenting with acute cardiogenic pulmonary oedema secondary to myocardial ischaemia. In these patients, invasive haemodynamic monitoring with the measurement of pulmonary capillary wedge pressure is particularly useful. If the mean pulmonary capillary wedge pressure is elevated (typically above 18 mmHg), then the pulmonary oedema is of cardiogenic origin and reflects an underlying raised hydrostatic pressure.

The extent of the difficulty in differentiating acute cardiogenic pulmonary oedema from other causes is illustrated by a recent study completed by Beltrame et al.[29] In this study, experienced emergency care physicians recruited patients with suspected acute cardiogenic pulmonary oedema. However, subsequent investigations demonstrated alternative causes for the acute dyspnoea presentation in 6% of the patients (obstructive airways disease exacerbation in 3% and 3% with acute non-cardiogenic pulmonary oedema). In another investigation where paramedics recruited acute cardiogenic pulmonary oedema patients, 23% were subsequently found to have alternative diagnoses with most having obstructive airways disease.[4] Hence, even in structured clinical studies where patients are specifically selected for presumed acute cardiogenic pulmonary oedema, there is difficulty in making the diagnosis.

Initial pharmacological therapy of acute cardiogenic pulmonary oedema

Once the diagnosis of acute cardiogenic pulmonary oedema is apparent it is imperative that pharmacological therapy be instituted promptly. Initial therapy would include sublingual nitrates provided that the systolic blood pressure is greater than 100 mmHg. This easily administered therapy is not only beneficial but also has a rapid onset of action and is relatively safe. Blood

Table 7.3. Differential diagnosis of acute pulmonary oedema

FEATURE	ACUTE PULMONARY OEDEMA		EXACERBATION
	Cardiogenic	Non-Cardiogenic	of COAD
History			
Past history	Ischaemic heart disease	Nil specific	COAD
	Chronic heart failure		
	Valvular heart disease		
Medications	Cardiac medications (e.g. diuretics)	Precipitants: nitrofurantoin	Bronchodilator puffers
Onset	Often as PND	Often 24–48 hours after insult	Progressive onset hours–days
Precipitant	Myocardial infarct	Trauma/surgery	Chest infection
	New/uncontrolled atrial fibrillation	Organ failure	
Clinical Examination			
Periphery	Cool (peripheral shut-down)	Warm (hyperdynamic circulation)	Cyanosed
	Profuse sweating	May be febrile	
JVP	Elevated if biventricular failure	Often not elevated	May be elevated (cor pulmonale)
Praecordium	Previous cardiac surgery	Trauma	Hyperinflated chest
	Cardiomegaly often present	Cardiomegaly usually absent	Cardiomegaly absent
	3rd and 4th heart sounds present	Added heart sounds usually absent	Soft heart sounds
	Murmurs may be present	Murmurs often absent	
Lung fields	Diffuse moist crepitations	Dry crepitations	Poor air entry/wheeze
Investigations			
ECG	Ischaemic/infarct changes	Usually normal	Tall P wave, low voltage, right axis
Chest X-ray	Perihilar distribution	Peripheral distribution	Hyperinflated/consolidation
Cardiac enzymes	May be elevated	Usually normal	Usually normal
PcWP	Elevated	Usually normal	Usually normal

COAD, chronic obstructive airways disease; JVP, jugular venous pulse; PND, paroxysmal nocturnal dyspnoea; PcWP, pulmonary capillary wedge pressure

pressure should continue to be monitored and further sublingual nitrates withheld should nitrate-associated hypotension occur.

Once intravenous access is established, intravenous nitrates should be commenced with continued blood pressure monitoring. Intravenous frusemide and/or morphine should also be administered provided the patient has no contraindication (particularly with the use of morphine in obstructive airways disease).

This initial pharmacological therapy of nitrates/diuretics and morphine should be administered under close supervi-sion with regular clinical observations, cardiac and oxygen saturation monitoring. Clinical reassessment of the patient should occur at 30 and 60 minutes after initiating therapy with arterial blood gases being performed if necessary. Based upon our previous experience, the clinical signs should begin to improve within 30 minutes of therapy and continue to improve with time. Incremental pharmacolog-ical or mechanical therapy may be required depending upon the patient's clinical status, with mechanical sup-portive therapies being essential if the patient develops res-piratory fatigue.

Aetiology-directed therapy of acute cardiogenic pulmonary oedema

Good clinical practice requires not only the diagnosis of acute cardiogenic pulmonary oedema but also recognition of its underlying aetiology. If not evident initially, efforts should be directed towards identifying the underlying cause whilst awaiting the clinical response to the above initial therapy. Thereafter specific therapies directed towards ameliorating these aetiologies can be initiated.

Acute cardiogenic pulmonary oedema aetiology

Identifying the aetiology of acute cardiogenic pulmonary oedema involves evaluating both the underlying cardiac pathology and the responsible precipitating factor (Table 7.4). Left ventricular systolic dysfunction is the most common underlying cardiac pathology responsible for acute pulmonary oedema. This is usually a chronic state with acute heart failure occurring following a decompensating precipitant; however, a large ischaemic zone/infarct may also be responsible. Left ventricular diastolic dysfunction may further compromise a ventricle with impaired systolic function or may be the major mechanism responsible for the acute pulmonary oedema. Isolated acute dias-

tolic heart failure may often be found in patients with systolic hypertension on admission.[5]

Identification of the precipitant responsible for the acute presentation is also important. In a retrospective study of patients presenting with acute cardiogenic pulmonary oedema, Goldberger et al[6] found that progressively deteriorating left ventricular function (25% of patients) and acute myocardial infarction (26% of patients; transmural infarcts in 10%, subendocardial in 16%) were the most common precipitants. Others included coronary insufficiency (21%), arrhythmias (8%) and non-compliance (7%).

Specific aetiology-directed therapies of acute cardiogenic pulmonary oedema

Specific emergency therapies for the precipitating cause include routine acute myocardial infarction management strategies and control of the ventricular response rate in atrial fibrillation with digoxin. Specific therapies for the underlying cardiac pathology include (a) preload reduction with nitrates and diuretics for systolic heart failure and mitral stenosis; (b) anti-ischaemic agents and revascularization for ischaemia-associated diastolic heart failure; and (c) intra-aortic balloon pump counterpulsation and

---

Table 7.4. Acute cardiogenic pulmonary oedema aetiology

Underlying cardiac pathology	
Left ventricular systolic dysfunction	– Prior myocardial infarction
	– Left ventricular aneurysm
	– Stunned/hibernating myocardium
	– Cardiomyopathy
	– Chronic mitral regurgitation
Left ventricular diastolic dysfunction	– Hypertensive heart disease
	– Hypertrophic cardiomyopathy
	– Aortic stenosis
Normal left ventricular function	– Mitral stenosis

Precipitant
Deteriorating cardiac failure
Myocardial ischaemia/infarction
Uncontrolled atrial fibrillation
Fluid overload
Medication non-compliance

inotropic support for severe systolic dysfunction associated with a poor cardiac output. The long-term management of these patients will also involve treatment directed towards the underlying aetiology.

The evidence for acute pulmonary oedema therapies

Clinical studies of acute cardiogenic pulmonary oedema are difficult to conduct because of the emergency life-threatening nature of the condition and thus it is not surprising that there are no placebo-controlled studies. Early investigations were observational in nature and are the basis upon which many of our current therapies are rationalized. More recently, comparative therapeutic studies have been undertaken to further define optimal therapy.

Pharmacological therapies

Clinical studies investigating pharmacological therapies of acute cardiogenic pulmonary oedema are diverse in (a) the clinical spectrum of the recruited patients; (b) the study design; and (c) the endpoints investigated. The spectrum of patients investigated includes those with acute fulminant pulmonary oedema recruited by paramedics en route to hospital, to patients with acute myocardial infarction admitted to the coronary care unit who had stable observations but a raised pulmonary capillary wedge pressure. The study designs vary from case reports and observational studies to controlled comparative studies of therapeutic alternatives. The endpoints studied include invasive haemodynamic parameters such as the pulmonary capillary wedge pressure, clinical markers such as urine output, and cardiorespiratory event studies such as the need for mechanical respiratory support.

Haemodynamic studies

Before embarking on a discussion of the haemodynamic trials of acute cardiogenic pulmonary oedema, further comment is required regarding the methodology utilized. A number of the important haemodynamic studies were conducted in the prethrombolytic era on acute myocardial infarction patients who were recruited after receiving opioid therapy and documented elevated pulmonary capillary wedge pressure (usually >18 mmHg). The conclusions from these haemodynamic investigations may be limited when considering the management of an acute fulminant pulmonary oedema patient arriving at the hospital since the study patients (a) all had acute myocardial infarction;

(b) all received baseline opioid therapy; (c) the dyspnoea had to be sufficiently controlled to allow insertion of a pulmonary arterial catheter; and (d) the time delay from onset of symptoms to obtaining haemodynamic parameters. Despite these limitations, these studies are the major source of haemodynamic data assessing pharmacological therapeutic strategies for 'acute cardiogenic pulmonary oedema'.

Investigations assessing pulmonary capillary wedge pressure changes in patients with acute pulmonary oedema associated with myocardial infarction have demonstrated a fall in filling pressure with (a) diuretics (frusemide[7–9]); (b) nitrates (sublingual glyceryl tritrate,[10] transdermal nitrates,[11] isosorbide dinitrate,[8,12,13] and isosorbide mononitrate[14]); (c) inotropes (amrinone,[15,16] prenalterol[17]); and (d) arterial vasodilators (doxazosin,[18] α-antagonists,[19] hydralazine,[12,17] nifedipine[20] and enaliprat[18]). Digoxin[21,22] does not produce beneficial haemodynamic effects and the effects of dobutamine are equivocal.[16,21,22] Morphine has been shown to have favourable haemodynamics in animal pulmonary oedema models;[23] however, it has not been assessed in the clinical setting. Vismara et al measured dorsal hand vein pressure responses to intravenous morphine in acute pulmonary oedema patients and observed only a mild change in venous tone thus adding further speculation as to morphine's benefit in this disorder.[24]

With haemodynamic benefits demonstrated for a number of agents, comparative studies have been undertaken to determine the optimal therapy. Verma et al[17] compared the haemodynamic responses to intravenous frusemide, isosorbide dinitrate, hydralazine and prenalterol in patients with acute myocardial infarction and raised pulmonary capillary wedge pressure. They concluded that the optimal haemodynamic strategy was ranked as follows: (a) nitrate-induced venodilation provided the optimal reduction in left ventricular filling pressure/work; (b) frusemide produced a reduced filling pressure/work but initially produced a detrimental transient vasoconstrictor effect; (c) hydralazine's arterial vasodilating effect reduced filling pressures but this was offset by reflex tachycardia; and (d) prenalterol's positive inotropic properties did not improve filling pressure but produced tachycardia and increased left ventricular afterload.

Several studies have compared the haemodynamic benefits of combination therapy in acute pulmonary oedema. Nelson et al[25] compared intravenous isosorbide dinitrate ± frusemide with hydralazine ± frusemide. Frusemide combined with nitrates produced a small incremental benefit to nitrates alone and combined hydralazine/frusemide therapy was equivalent to nitrates alone. Verma et al found monotherapy with intravenous doxazosin or enalaprilat was haemodynamically similar to the combination of intravenous isosorbide dinitrate and hydralazine except that the latter had hydralazine-associated tachycardia.[18]

The conclusion from the above studies is that nitrates and frusemide have the optimal haemodynamic profile for acute cardiogenic pulmonary oedema associated with acute myocardial infarction and that the combination appears to be slightly more favourable than nitrate monotherapy. However, these conclusions are limited considering the difficulties described above with the population studied.

Clinical marker studies

A small number of studies have utilized less invasive clinical endpoints to assess the response to therapies in acute cardiogenic pulmonary oedema, thereby allowing earlier recruitment of a broader population sample. The parameters assessed include respiratory rate, pulse rate, blood pressure, dyspnoea scores, urine output and arterial blood gas results.

Utilizing urine output as an endpoint, Lesch et al demonstrated that intravenous ethacrynic acid was more effective than the intramuscularly administered mercurial diuretic, mercaptomerin.[26] Subsequently, ethacrynic acid became the mainstay diuretic therapy for acute pulmonary oedema until it was replaced by the less toxic frusemide. The diuresis induced by frusemide is evident approximately 15–30 minutes following intravenous administration. However, the haemodynamic benefits are seen much earlier,[27] suggesting that frusemide's venodilating properties may account for these early effects.[28]

Arterial blood gas is frequently utilized in clinical practice to assess the patient's response to therapy in acute pulmonary oedema. Recently we performed serial clinical and blood gas measurements in patients with acute cardiogenic pulmonary oedema not associated with acute transmural myocardial infarction, in order to compare combined intravenous morphine/frusemide therapy with intravenous nitrates.[29] Both treatments had improved arterial oxygenation by 60 minutes although this was only statistically significant for the nitrate therapy. Furthermore, other clinical indices such as extent of dyspnoea and crepitations, respiratory rate, pulse rate and systolic blood pressure had improved within an hour of therapy with no differences observed between the randomized treatments. Hence,

these therapies are equieffective in the management of acute cardiogenic pulmonary oedema not associated with acute transmural myocardial infarction.

Hoffman and Reynolds[4] compared intravenous morphine, frusemide and nitroglycerin alone and in combination, on patients with suspected prehospital acute cardiogenic pulmonary oedema. They qualitatively defined clinical improvement or deterioration based upon a 20% change in respiratory rate and/or heart rate from baseline values. They concluded that nitrate therapy resulted in clinical improvement more frequently than the other therapies and morphine was most often associated with a deleterious effect. However, as mentioned previously, their conclusions are tainted as 23% of patients did not have pulmonary oedema (many of whom had obstructive airways disease).

Cardiorespiratory event studies

The merits of nitrate therapy compared with diuretic therapy have been further examined in a prehospital acute cardiogenic pulmonary oedema study where death, myocardial infarction and need for mechanical ventilation in the first 12 hours were the major endpoints.[30] This study randomized 110 patients to either high-dose nitrate therapy or high-dose diuretic therapy after all patients received baseline frusemide/morphine therapy. Whilst the study observed less frequent myocardial infarction and need for intubation in patients on high-dose nitrate therapy, the findings may be difficult to generalize since acute myocardial infarction patients were not excluded.[31]

Conclusions

Based upon the haemodynamic, clinical and event studies, nitrate therapy is clearly the most fundamental therapy for acute cardiogenic pulmonary oedema. Frusemide and morphine may provide a modest incremental benefit; however, clinicians should beware of their potential detrimental effects. Other therapies such as arterial vasodilators, inotropes, digoxin and aminophylline generally have less clear roles; however, they may be useful in particular subsets of acute cardiogenic pulmonary oedema patients (e.g. digoxin in uncontrolled atrial fibrillation).

Mechanical therapies
Intubation and mechanical ventilation

Mechanical ventilatory support for acute cardiogenic pulmonary oedema is considered mandatory in patients who are moribund at presentation or who fail to respond adequately to medical therapy. Thus, not surprisingly, there is little objective trial evidence as to the benefits of this therapy. Physiologically, ventilatory support not only oxygenates the patient but also reduces cardiac workload thereby providing the assistance required for the failing myocardium to recover. Further assistance is provided by positive end-expiratory pressure and adjunct pharmacological therapy.

The frequency of mechanical ventilation in acute cardiogenic pulmonary oedema varies between 5% and 60%. While this in part exhibits the severity of the pulmonary oedema in the recruited patients, it also reflects the subjective nature of the clinical decision to ventilate. Griner reported the frequency of intubation in acute pulmonary oedema patients before and after the opening of an intensive care unit.[32] Although 6-month mortality was similar, there was a doubling of intubation rates after the establishment of the intensive care unit suggesting a lower clinical decision threshold to intubate.

Continuous positive airway pressure

Several studies have demonstrated the therapeutic benefit of continuous positive airway pressure administered by face mask (CPAP) in patients with acute cardiogenic pulmonary oedema.[33–35] Bersten et al[33] randomized 39 consecutive acute cardiogenic pulmonary oedema patients to high-flow oxygen therapy or CPAP. Patients receiving CPAP therapy not only showed an earlier improvement in respiratory rate and oxygenation but also none required mechanical ventilation whereas 35% of those receiving high-flow oxygen needed intubation.

Other therapies

A variety of other mechanical therapies have been employed in the management of acute cardiogenic pulmonary oedema, which warrant brief discussion. Time-honoured therapies include venesection and rotating tourniquets. These treatments are thought to be effective by reducing preload although their efficacy has been questioned.[36]

The intra-aortic balloon pump is often utilized in patients with acute pulmonary oedema and cardiogenic shock. Its routine use in acute pulmonary oedema in the absence of cardiogenic shock is not warranted considering the invasive nature of the intervention. However, it is essential in patients who have fulminant pulmonary oedema secondary to extensive myocardial ischaemia which requires urgent revascularization.

Conclusions

The management of acute cardiogenic pulmonary oedema is a cardiac emergency requiring urgent implementation of resuscitative procedures ('ABC') followed by early initiation of pharmacological therapy (nitrates, diuretics, and/or morphine) and/or mechanical therapies if required. Management also requires the rapid evaluation of the underlying cause with therapy directed towards the specific underlying problem.

Although evidence for a variety of therapies of acute cardiogenic pulmonary oedema have been investigated, many questions remain unanswered. Thus further studies of this life-threatening condition are required if treatment strategies are to improve.

References

1. West JB. *Pulmonary Pathophysiology – The Essentials*. Baltimore: Williams & Wilkins, 1977: 227.
2. Prichard JS. Pulmonary Edema. In: Weatherall DJ, Ledingham JGG, Warrell DA, eds. *Oxford Textbook of Medicine*. Oxford: Oxford Medical Publications, 1996: 2504.
3. Barash D, Silverman R, Gennis P, Budner N, Matos M, Gallagher E. Circadian variation in the frequency of myocardial infarction and death associated with acute pulmonary edema. *J Emerg Med* 1989; **7:** 119–21.
4. Hoffman JR, Reynolds S. Comparison of nitroglycerin, morphine and furosemide in treatment of presumed pre-hospital pulmonary edema. *Chest* 1987; **92:** 586–93.
5. Gandhi SK, Powers JC, Nomeir AM et al. The pathogenesis of acute pulmonary edema associated with hypertension. *N Engl J Med* 2001; **344:** 17–22.
6. Goldberger J, Peled H, Stroh J, Cohen M, Frishman W. Prognostic factors in acute pulmonary edema. *Arch Intern Med* 1986; **146:** 489–93.
7. Kiely J, Kelly D, Taylor D, Pitt B. The role of furosemide in the treatment of left ventricular dysfunction associated with acute myocardial infarction. *Circulation* 1973; **48:** 581–7.
8. Nelson G, Silke B, Ahuja R, Hussain M, Taylor S. Haemodynamic advantages of isosorbide dinitrate over frusemide in acute heart-failure following myocardial infarction. *Lancet* 1983; **1:** 730–3.
9. Biddle T, Yu P. Effect of furosemide on hemodynamics and lung water in acute pulmonary edema secondary to myocardial infarction. *Am J Cardiol* 1979; **43:** 86–90.
10. Bussmann WD, Schupp D. Effect of sublingual nitroglycerin in emergency treatment of severe pulmonary edema. *Am J Cardiol* 1978; **41:** 931–6.

11. Verma SP, Silke B, Reynolds GW et al. Haemodynamic dose–response effects of a transdermal nitrate delivery system in acute myocardial infarction with and without left heart failure. *J Cardiovasc Pharmacol* 1988; **11:** 151–7.

12. Nelson GI, Ahuja RC, Silke B, Hussain M, Taylor SH. Arteriolar or venous dilatation in left ventricular failure following acute myocardial infarction: a haemodynamic trial of hydralazine and isosorbide dinitrate. *J Cardiovasc Pharmacol* 1983; **5:** 574–9.

13. Rabinowitz B, Tamari I, Elazar E, Neufeld HN. Intravenous isosorbide dinitrate in patients with refractory pump failure and acute myocardial infarction. *Circulation* 1982; **65:** 771–8.

14. Rabinowitz B, Katz A, Shotan A, Chouraqui P, Neufeld HN. Haemodynamic effects of intravenous isosorbide-5-mononitrate in acute and chronic left heart failure of ischaemic aetiology. *Eur Heart J* 1988; **9:** 175–80.

15. Taylor SH, Verma SP, Hussain M et al. Intravenous amrinone in left ventricular failure complicated by acute myocardial infarction. *Am J Cardiol* 1985; **56:** 29B–32B.

16. Silke B, Verma SP, Midtbo KA, Reynolds G, Taylor SH. Comparative haemodynamic dose-response effects of dobutamine and amrinone in left ventricular failure complicating acute myocardial infarction. *J Cardiovasc Pharmacol* 1987; **9:** 19–25.

17. Verma SP, Silke B, Hussain M et al. First-line treatment of left ventricular failure complicating acute myocardial infarction: a randomised evaluation of immediate effects of diuretic, venodilator, arteriodilator, and positive inotropic drugs on left ventricular function. *J Cardiovasc Pharmacol* 1987; **10:** 38–46.

18. Verma SP, Silke B, Reynolds GW, Kelly JG, Richmond A, Taylor SH. Vasodilator therapy for acute heart failure: haemodynamic comparison of hydralazine/isosorbide, alpha-adrenoceptor blockade, and angiotensin-converting enzyme inhibition. *J Cardiovasc Pharmacol* 1992; **20:** 274–81.

19. Silke B, Nelson GI, Verma SP et al. Haemodynamic dose-response effects of intravenous indoramin in acute heart failure complicating myocardial infarction. *J Cardiovasc Pharmacol* 1986; **8:** S102–6.

20. Polese A, Fiorentini C, Olivari MT, Guazzi MD. Clinical use of a calcium antagonistic agent (Nifedipine) in acute pulmonary edema. *Am J Med* 1979; **66:** 825–30.

21. Verma SP, Silke B, Reynolds GW, Richmond A, Taylor SH. Modulation of inotropic therapy by venodilation in acute heart failure: a randomised comparison of four inotropic agents, alone and combined with isosorbide dinitrate. *J Cardiovasc Pharmacol* 1992; **19:** 24–33.

22. Goldstein RA, Passamani ER, Roberts R. A comparison of digoxin and dobutamine in patients with acute infarction and cardiac failure. *N Engl J Med* 1980; **303:** 846–50.

23. Vasko JS, Henney RP, Oldham HN, Brawley RK, Morrow AG. Mechanisms of action of morphine in the treatment of experimental pulmonary edema. *Am J Cardiol* 1966; **18:** 876–83.

24. Vismara L, Leaman D, Zelis R. The effects of morphine on venous tone in patients with acute pulmonary edema. *Circulation* 1976; **54:** 335–7.

25. Nelson GI, Silke B, Forsyth DR, Verma SP, Hussain M, Taylor SH. Hemodynamic comparison of primary venous or arteriolar dilatation and the subsequent effect of furosemide in left ventricular failure after acute myocardial infarction. *Am J Cardiol* 1983; **52:** 1036–40.

26. Lesch M, Caranasos G, Mulholland J. Controlled study comparing ethacrynic acid to mercaptomerin in the treatment of acute pulmonary edema. *N Engl J Med* 1968; **279:** 115–22.

27. Taylor SH. Diuretics in postinfarction heart failure. *Cardiovasc Drugs Ther* 1993; **7:** 885–9.

28. Mukherjee SK, Katz MA, Michael UF, Ogden DA. Mechanisms of hemodynamic actions of furosemide: differentiation of vascular and renal effects on blood pressure in functionally anephric hypertensive patients. *AHJ* 1981; **101:** 313–8.

29. Beltrame JF, Zeitz CJ, Unger SA et al. Nitrate therapy is an alternative to furosemide/morphine therapy in the management of acute cardiogenic pulmonary edema. *J Cardiac Fail* 1998; **4:** 271–9.

30. Cotter G, Metzkor E, Kaluski E et al. Randomised trial of high-dose isosorbide dinitrate plus low-dose furosemide versus high-dose furosemide plus low-dose isosorbide dinitrate in severe pulmonary oedema. *Lancet* 1998; **351:** 389–93.

31. Beltrame JF, Zeitz CJ, Moran JL, Horowitz JD. Nitrates for myocardial infarction. *Lancet* 1998; **351:** 1731–2; discussion 1732–3.

32. Griner PF. Treatment of acute pulmonary edema. *Ann Int Med* 1972; **77:** 501–6.

33. Bersten A, Holt A, Vedig A, Skowronski G, Baggoley C. Treatment of severe cardiogenic pulmonary oedema with continuous positive airway pressure delivered by face mask. *N Engl J Med* 1991; **325:** 1825–30.

34. Rasanen J, Heikkila J, Downs J, Nikki P, Vaisanen I, Viitanen A. Continuous positive airway pressure by face mask in acute cardiogenic pulmonary edema. *Am J Cardiol* 1985; **55:** 296–300.

35. Vaisanen I, Rasanen J. Continuous positive airway pressure and supplemental oxygen in the treatment of cardiogenic pulmonary edema. *Chest* 1987; **92:** 481–5.

36. Bertel O, Steiner A. Rotating tourniquets do not work in acute congestive heart failure and pulmonary oedema [letter]. *Lancet* 1980; **1:** 762.

8 Pharmacological treatment of chronic heart failure

Robert N Doughty

Introduction

Patients with heart failure experience symptoms of shortness of breath, fluid retention, exercise intolerance and fatigue. In addition, heart failure frequently results in hospital admission and premature death. In recent decades there have been considerable advances in the pharmacological management of patients with the clinical syndrome of heart failure. Despite the proven benefits of these drugs, the uptake into clinical practice for many patients with heart failure is often slow. Aims of treatment for patients with heart failure include relief of symptoms of shortness of breath, improved exercise capacity and quality of life, improved left ventricular function, decreased hospital admissions and improved survival. While all of these aims are important some may have relative greater importance at certain stages of the disease or in different patient groups. For example, improved quality of life may be of utmost importance for an elderly patient with multiple comorbidities, while improved survival may have lesser importance to this individual patient.

Numerous clinical practice guidelines for the management of patients with heart failure are available, many of which are in formats easy to download from the internet. The aim of this chapter is to provide a practical approach to the current evidence-based pharmacological treatment for patients with heart failure. It is not intended to provide a comprehensive in-depth review of each class of drug, rather to provide practical information on the use of each drug in patients with chronic heart failure. Before the specific therapies are reviewed several points should be considered.

Impaired vs preserved left ventricular systolic function

In general, the clinical trials of pharmacological agents for heart failure have selected patients with heart failure and impaired left ventricular (LV) systolic function (low LV ejection fraction). However, the clinical syndrome of heart failure can occur in patients with preserved or only mildly impaired LV systolic function, so called 'diastolic heart failure'. It appears that this may occur more frequently in the elderly and in those with a history of hypertension.[1–3] The evidence base for the treatment recommendations in most heart failure guidelines thus refers specifically to those patients with heart failure and impaired LV systolic function. Little evidence is currently available for the treatment of heart failure with preserved LV systolic function, although clinical trials are ongoing in this area (see later).

Clinical trials vs the 'real world' of heart failure

Clinical trials have often enrolled selected groups of patients who may not be representative of patients with heart failure in clinical practice. For example, clinical trial patients are often young, have heart failure alone with few comorbidities, have simple drug regimes and optimal compliance. However, many patients with heart failure in the community are older, have multiple comorbidities, are receiving multiple drugs and have variable compliance. Thus, as such, the clinical trials may not be directly generalizable to the 'average' patient with heart failure in the community. Having said this, we must be guided by the current evidence for treatment and extrapolate these data sensibly to apply to the non-trial setting, until such time as further clinical trial data are available.

Pharmacological treatment for heart failure

Diuretics

Symptoms of shortness of breath and fluid retention are common in patients with heart failure. Diuretics are essential therapy to help control these symptoms. However, most diuretics, with the exception of spironolactone,[4] have not been subjected to long-term clinical trials and thus the effects on survival are uncertain. While diuretics do

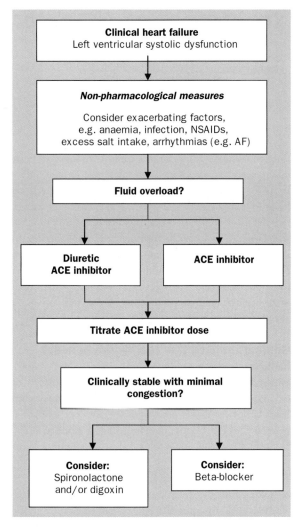

Figure 8.1. *Treatment algorithm for initial management of heart failure. Refer to sections regarding details for specific drugs; this algorithm suggests a simplified approach to initial treatment and further treatment and/or investigations may be required for many patients. Modified with permission from the New Zealand Guideline for the Management of Heart Failure – Treatment Algorithm. Heart Foundation of New Zealand, 2001.*

achieve relief of symptoms associated with fluid retention, the addition of diuretics may actually contribute to the neurohormonal activation in patients with mild heart failure. Data from the SOLVD trial[5] have demonstrated that activation of the renin–angiotensin–aldosterone system was potentiated when patients were commenced on

diuretics. Thus, diuretics should not be used as mono-therapy for patients with heart failure.

Expected benefits of diuretics

Initiation of diuretic therapy should be associated with improvement in symptoms of shortness of breath and decrease in oedema. The patient can monitor their progress by simple recording of daily weight. There is an important overlap between drug therapy for heart failure and non-pharmacological therapy, which will include education regarding the expected effects of any drugs used and ways in which the patient can monitor their own condition.

Recommended diuretics and dosages

Diuretics should be started for patients with symptoms and signs of fluid retention. While a thiazide may suffice for mild symptoms, in practice, many patients with heart failure require a more potent loop diuretic such as frusemide. The diuretic can usually be started a low dose, e.g. frusemide 40 mg daily. Early review within a few days is often required to help gauge the patient's response to treatment and allow subsequent dose adjustment.

Adverse effects of diuretics

Hypokalaemia is a common problem with diuretics. However, this effect is lessened for heart failure patients as an angiotensin-converting enzyme (ACE) inhibitor should be started at the same time (see below). Hypotension and worsening renal function may occur with over-diuresis but can often be minimized by early clinical review. From the patients perspective, one of the most troublesome effects of diuretics is the exacerbation of gout.

Angiotensin-converting enzyme inhibitors

The ACE inhibitors have been shown to improve symp-toms, exercise capacity, LV function and survival in a wide range of patients with heart failure and asymptomatic LV systolic dysfunction.[6–8] ACE inhibitors are thus established as first line agents, along with diuretics, for the treatment of patients with heart failure (Table 8.1).

Expected benefits of angiotensin-converting enzyme inhibitors

ACE inhibitors in combination with diuretics can improve the symptoms and signs of heart failure. However, as ACE inhibitors have been shown to decrease hospital admis-sions and improve survival they should be used even if

Table 8.1.

ACE inhibitor therapy

Check
- For risk factors for first-dose hypotension
- Renal function at baseline and after 1 and 4 weeks

Initiation/titration
- Start at low dose, e.g. enalapril 2.5 mg daily or twice daily*
- Titrate to maximum tolerated dose over 2–4 weeks, e.g. enalapril 10–20 mg twice daily
- Use in combination with diuretic if symptoms/signs of congestion

Possible adverse effects
- Hypotension
- Worsening renal function
- Hyperkalaemia
- Cough (see text re management of cough)

Beta-blockers

Check
- For contraindications to beta-blocker, e.g. asthma or heart block (in the absence of a permanent pacemaker)

Initiation/titration
- Start at low dose, e.g. metoprolol CR 47.5 mg $\frac{1}{4}$ tablet or carvedilol 3.125–6.25 mg
- Give under supervision in outpatient setting, observe patient for 2 hours (BP/HR)
- Fortnightly visits to titrate dose of beta-blocker. Check specifically for signs of worsening congestion, hypotension or bradycardia at each visit
- Withhold the morning dose on the day of the visit, observe patient for 2 hours after each dose increment
- Doubling of the dose every 2 weeks is a reasonable titration regime. However, titration can occur slowly and sometimes may take several months to achieve the desired maintenance dose

Possible adverse effects
- Dizziness (common with the vasodilating beta-blockers such as carvedilol, often decreases if persist with treatment)
- Hypotension – usually a sign of intolerance (decrease dose or stop)
- Worsening heart failure – mainly increasing congestion. Manage by increasing diuretics and continuing beta-blocker if possible
- Heart block

Target doses
- Aim for metoprolol 150–200 mg daily (exact dose depends on preparation of metoprolol used), carvedilol 25 mg bid, bisoprolol 10 mg daily

Spironolactone

Check
- For contraindications such as hyperkalaemia, renal failure (creatinine >0.25 mmol/l)
- Renal function at baseline and after 3–4 days and 1 week

Initiation/titration
- Use in patients with moderate to severe symptoms (NYHA class III/IV)
- Start at 12.5 or 25 mg daily
- Dose above 50 mg per day may result in serious hyperkalaemia

Possible adverse effects
- Hyperkalaemia
- Worsening renal function
- Gynaecomastia or breast pain in men

* enalapril given as an example only

patients are only mildly symptomatic or need little diuretic therapy.[6–8] In patients with mild to moderate heart failure approximately 26 patients need to be treated for approximately 3 years to prevent one death,[7] while this number is even lower in patients with severe heart failure.[6]

Recommended angiotensin-converting enzyme inhibitors and dosages

Several ACE inhibitors, including captopril,[9] enalapril,[6–8] lisinopril,[10] ramipril[11] and trandolapril,[12] have been studied in clinical outcome studies in patients with heart failure or asymptomatic LV dysfunction. While the different ACE inhibitors may have slightly different pharmacological properties, it is generally accepted that the clinical effects of ACE inhibitors are a class effect and thus no specific ACE inhibitor is recommended. However, the dose of ACE inhibitor does appear important. Most of the large-scale clinical trials have used reasonably high target doses, for example, captopril 50 mg bid[9] or enalapril 10–20 mg twice daily.[6–8] The ATLAS Trial[10] compared low-dose (2.5–5.0 mg per day) and high-dose (32.5–35 mg daily) lisinopril for patients with symptomatic heart failure. There was a lower rate of death and hospitalization in the high-dose arm compared with the low-dose arm. Based on these data, the general recommendations are that higher doses of ACE inhibitors should be aimed for whenever possible.

Adverse effects of angiotension-converting enzyme inhibitors

Cough occurs in up to 10% of patients with heart failure treated with ACE inhibitors. Cough may also be a sign of heart failure and thus it is important to differentiate drug-induced cough from early worsening heart failure. Re-challenge after stopping the agent is often required. ACE inhibitors should only be stopped if the cough is intolerable. In general there is little value in changing between ACE inhibitors. Instead an angiotensin II receptor antagonist should be considered for ACE-intolerant patients (see below, Spironolactone).

Hypotension, hyperkalaemia and worsening renal dysfunction can occur with ACE inhibitors. Risk factors for first-dose hypotension include pretreatment hypotension (e.g. systolic blood pressure < 90 mmHg), over-diuresis, hyponatraemia. ACE inhibitors can cause rapid worsening of renal function in patients with bilateral renal artery stenosis, although fortunately this is not common in

patients with heart failure. Renal function should be checked about 1 week after starting ACE inhibitor therapy and thereafter at least every 3 months.

Beta-blockers

The renin–angiotensin–aldosterone (RAA) neurohormonal system is the target of therapy with ACE inhibitors. However, the sympathetic nervous system is activated earlier and often to a greater degree in chronic heart failure than the RAA system.[13] The degree of activation of the sympathetic nervous system is maladaptive and is an independent predictor of survival.[14] The rationale for interrupting this system with beta-blockers in patients with chronic heart failure is now well established.[15] Recently, large-scale clinical trials have demonstrated conclusive evidence of the beneficial effects of beta-blocker therapy on survival in chronic heart failure.[16–18] As a result of these data, beta-blocker therapy has become part of standard therapy for patients with chronic heart failure (in addition to ACE inhibitors and diuretics). The treatment is, in general, well tolerated, although patients require careful clinical follow-up (see Table 8.1 and below).

Expected benefits of beta-blockers

Unlike the ACE inhibitors, short-term improvements in symptoms should not be expected with beta-blocker therapy. The aim of therapy is directed more towards improvement in the longer-term (months to years) natural history of the disease. Thus, although patients may ultimately gain symptomatic benefits, these will not necessarily occur early during treatment. Indeed, patients may experience symptoms such as fatigue and should be prepared to continue therapy longer term.

In patients with mild-to-moderate heart failure beta-blockers have been shown to decrease mortality from about 13% in placebo-treated patients to about 8.6% per year with beta-blockers, an absolute risk reduction of approximately 4.4% (relative risk reduction 34%).[16,17,19] The number of patients needed to be treated for 1 year to prevent one death is about 23. In severe heart failure carvedilol reduced mortality by a similar proportion (relative risk reduction 35%), although the absolute risk is greater in such patients with risk of death in 1 year reduced from about 18.5% to about 11.4% with carvedilol.[18] In addition, beta-blockers improve LV size and function[20] and reduce hospital admissions.[16,17]

Recommended type of beta-blockers

The survival benefit with beta-blockers has been demonstrated with bisoprolol,[16] metoprolol[17] and carvedilol.[18,21] The recent COMET trial has demonstrated that carvedilol has a greater survival benefit than metoprolol tartrate.[22] All cause mortality was 34% with carvedilol compared with 40% for metoprolol (*P* = 0.0017).

Bucindolol is a 'third generation' non-selective beta-blocker with vasodilatory properties (probably due to alpha$_1$ blockade).[23] Bucindolol has been shown to improve LV function in patients with heart failure, although no effect was seen on exercise tolerance or quality of life.[24] The BEST Trial (Beta-Blocker Evaluation of Surival Trial) enrolled patients with New York Heart Association (NYHA) Class III/IV heart failure.[25] This trial, unlike CIBIS-II,[16] MERIT-HF[17] and COPERNICUS,[18] did not show a significant reduction in mortality. Subgroup analyses suggest that there was a differential effect of bucindolol on outcome according to race, and that this, in part, may have accounted for the overall neutral effect in this study.[26]

Recommended regime for initiation of beta-blocker therapy

Once patients have been selected for beta-blocker therapy according to the above criteria, beta-blockers can usually be initiated in an outpatient setting. The beta-blocker should be started at low dose, e.g. metoprolol CR 11 mg, bisoprolol 1.25 mg or carvedilol 3.125 mg or 6.25 mg. The first dose can be administered in the clinic setting and the patient observed for about 2 hours. If blood pressure and heart rate are satisfactory then the same dose can be dispensed for the patient to continue.

Following initiation of treatment, further titration can continue with the dosage increments at fortnightly intervals according to tolerability. The main message is to start at low dose and increase slowly with regular clinical review, looking for any signs of intolerance. Generally, patients should be reviewed at 3-monthly intervals, or more often as required. As is evident, for clinicians to use beta-blockers in patients with heart failure safely and effectively, careful monitoring and regular review is required to ensure that the safety and tolerability that have been demonstrated in the trials under conditions of close supervision are reproduced.

Adverse effects of beta-blockers

Possible adverse effects include bradycardia, hypotension, worsening heart failure and atrioventricular block. Signs of increasing congestion may be controlled with adjustment of diuretic dose and do not necessarily imply long-term intolerance of the drug. However, symptomatic hypotension is more difficult and often suggests intolerance. With this graduated approach, 70–80% of patients should be satisfactorily established on maintenance treatment with the dosages employed in the clinical trials (e.g. carvedilol 25 mg bd, metoprolol 150–200 mg per day)

Once on established beta-blocker therapy, subsequent deterioration, for example with worsening heart failure, does not necessarily imply intolerance and should be controlled with an increase in standard antifailure treatment.

Spironolactone

Until recently it has been assumed that the suppression of the RAA system by an ACE inhibitor alone would suppress the formation of aldosterone. In addition, there has been concern that the concurrent use of an aldosterone-receptor blocker and an ACE inhibitor could lead to dangerous hyperkaleamia. However, there are data showing that aldosterone levels are increased in chronic heart failure despite the use of ACE inhibitors.[27] Spironolactone is a competitive inhibitor of aldosterone. The RALES trial,[4] a single yet large and well-designed trial, found that the use of spironolactone in people with severe heart failure was not only safe but conferred substantial survival benefits (Table 8.1).

Expected benefits of spironolactone

The patients in the RALES trial[4] had symptoms of severe heart failure (NYHA classification III or IV) and LV ejection fraction < 35% (severe LV impairment). Spironolactone 25 mg daily was added to the usual therapy, which included ACE inhibitors and loop diuretics, although few patients were receiving beta-blockers. All-cause mortality at 2 years was reduced from 46% in the placebo group to 35% in the spironolactone group, an absolute risk reduction of 11%. The number of patients needed to be treated to prevent one death over 2 years is only nine. In addition, there were fewer hospital admissions, improved symptoms and no significant increase in the risk of hyperkalaemia. There was, however, a 10%

incidence of male patients experiencing gynaecomastia or breast pain, some of whom need to stop therapy because of these adverse effects.

Recommended regime for spironolactone

Contraindications to spironolactone include serum creatinine > 0.25 mmol/l and potassium > 5.0 mmol/l. Spironolactone should be added to ACE inhibitor and diuretic therapy at a dose of 12.5 or 25 mg daily. Creatinine and electrolytes should be checked after approximately 3–4 days, 1 week and 1 month after initiation and then as indicated by renal function (e.g. 6-monthly in stable patients).

Angiotensin receptor antagonists

Mortality for patients with heart failure remains high despite the survival benefits demonstrated with ACE inhibitor therapy. In clinical practice, ACE inhibitors may be stopped because of side-effects or not tolerated at the higher doses used in the clinical trials. In addition, there is increasing evidence that long-term ACE inhibitor therapy may only partially suppress angiotensin II levels, probably as a result of non-ACE enzyme pathways involved in the conversion of angiotensin-I to angiotensin-II.[28] The angiotensin receptor antagonists (or AII antagonists) block the renin–angiotensin system directly at the AII receptor and thus may provide more complete blockade of the effects of angiotensin II.

The Evaluation of Losartan in the Elderly trial[29] (ELITE I) was the first trial to compare the effects of losartan with an ACE inhibitor (captopril) in patients with heart failure. There was no difference between the two agents with respect to the primary endpoint of renal dysfunction. However, an unexpected finding was of a reduction in mortality with losartan compared with captopril: 4.8% vs 8.7% respectively, risk reduction 46% (95% confidence interval 5–69%). The ELITE II trial[30] was thus carried out to determine prospectively whether losartan conferred significant survival benefits over captopril. Overall, there was no statistically significant difference between losartan and captopril with respect to total mortality. These results suggest that ACE inhibitors should remain the cornerstone of treatment for patients with heart failure and angiotensin II antagonists be used for patients who are intolerant of ACE inhibitors, for example due to cough or angioedema.

Further questions remain regarding the use of angiotensin II antagonists in patients with heart failure, in particular whether patients with heart failure who are already treated with ACE inhibitors will benefit from the addition of an angiotensin II antagonist. Several smaller trials have demonstrated that angiotensin II antagonists can be used safely in addition to ACE inhibitors in patients with heart failure.[31,32] However, none of the trials completed to date have been large enough to determine whether this addition will further improve major clinical endpoints.

The Val-HeFT study[33] was a large randomized, placebo-controlled trial to determine whether the addition of the angiotensin II antagonist valsartan to standard therapy (including ACE inhibitors) in patients with heart failure improved morbidity and mortality. The first results were presented at the Scientific Sessions of the American Heart Association in November 2000.[34] While valsartan did reduce mortality and morbidity these effects appeared to occur mainly in those patients not receiving a beta-blocker or ACE inhibitor. Full publication of the results from this trial is awaited but it would appear to reinforce the message that AII antagonists are of benefit for those patients who are not receiving either an ACE inhibitor or a beta-blokcer.

A further large-scale study, the CHARM Study[35] (Candesartan in Heart Failure – Assessment of Reduction in Mortality and Morbidity), determined the effect of candesartan in a broad spectrum of patients with heart failure. The study included three major groups of patients: (a) patients with LV ejection fraction ≤ 40% who are already receiving an ACE inhibitor (n = 2300); (b) patients with LV ejection fraction ≤ 40% who are intolerant of ACE inhibitors (n = 1700); and (c) patients with LV ejection fraction > 40% who are not receiving ACE inhibitors (n = 2500). The overall CHARM programme demonstrated that candesartan was generally well tolerated and reduced cardiovascular deaths and hospital admissions for heart failure across this broad spectrum of patients with clinical heart failure.[36]

Digoxin

Digoxin has multiple modes of action including mild positive inotropic effects, suppression of renin secretion and increasing vagal tone. Digoxin has been used for the treatment of heart failure for 200 years, but only recently have reliable data become available on the clinical effects in heart failure. Much of the controversy around digoxin has centred on its use in those patients who remain in sinus rhythm.

Digoxin in heart failure patients with atrial fibrillation

Digoxin is frequently used to help to control the ventricular rate in patients with heart failure who are in atrial fibrillation. However, it should be noted that while digoxin alone may control the ventricular rate at rest it frequently does not provide sufficient rate control with exercise. Thus, other medications to help to control the ventricular response are often required, such as diltiazem, beta-blockers or amiodarone.

Digoxin in heart failure patients who remain in sinus rhythm

The DIG trial[37] examined the role of digoxin in patients with heart failure who were in sinus rhythm. In this randomized trial, digoxin or placebo was added to ACE inhibitor and diuretics. All-cause mortality was similar in the two treatment groups. However, the combined endpoint of death or hospital admission for worsening heart failure was reduced with digoxin. Most of this benefit appeared to occur in those patients with moderate to severe heart failure. This single trial has left uncertainty around the use of digoxin in heart failure with sinus rhythm. However, as there was no overall effect on all-cause mortality it is reasonable to reserve the use of digoxin for patients who remain symptomatic despite treatment with ACE inhibitors, diuretics, beta-blockers and spironolactone (all in appropriate dosages).

Recommended regime for digoxin

If digoxin is used then loading doses of digoxin are generally not required. In the presence of normal renal function a dose of 0.25 mg daily may suffice. In the elderly or in those with renal impairment a reduced dose such as 0.125 mg or 0.0625 mg daily is necessary. Digoxin levels should be checked after about 1 week in those with normal renal function, although steady state may take longer to be achieved in those with renal impairment.

Adverse effects of digoxin

Signs of digoxin toxicity include confusion, nausea, anorexia, visual disturbance and either tachy- or bradyarrhythmias. Digoxin toxicity should be suspected in a patient presenting with any of the above symptoms or unusual symptoms, particularly in the elderly. Some drugs may increase plasma digoxin levels, for example amiodarone, diltiazem, verapamil, antibiotics and quinidine.

Anticoagulation and antiplatelet therapy in heart failure

Patients with heart failure are potentially at high risk of thromboembolism, for example, one early report of patients with idiopathic dilated cardiomyopathy showed a cummulative incidence of 18%, or 3.5 events per 100 patient years.[38] A review of the studies of patients with heart failure in which separate data for those not receiving anticoagulation were available showed that the overall incidence of arterial thromboembolism ranged from 0.9 to 5.5 events per 100 patient-years.[39] Patients with atrial fibrillation and heart failure are at high risk of thromboembolic complications and anticoagulation with warfarin has been shown to decrease the risk of stroke.[40] Thus, warfarin should be considered for all patients with heart failure and atrial fibrillation. However, the risks and benefits of routine anticoagulation for patients with heart failure who remain in sinus rhythm are uncertain.

A recent large-scale trial comparing the effects of warfarin, aspirin and placebo in patients with heart failure in sinus rhythm was stopped early after 290 of the planned 6000 patients had been entered into the study because of problems with recruitment.[41] The primary endpoint of this study was a composite of non-fatal stroke, peripheral or pulmonary embolism, myocardial infarction, worsening heart failure and all-cause mortality. The trial had no major sponsorship, the participating centres were covering costs through their own resources and the study drug was supplied by donation.[41] Follow-up of the 290 patients is being continued and will provide pilot data but will not be powered for the main endpoint results.

A further trial, the WASH study,[42] was designed as a pilot study to test the feasibility of conducting a larger trial comparing aspirin (300 mg daily) and warfarin (target INR 2.5) and no antithrombotic therapy in patients with heart failure. Two hundred and seventy-nine patients were randomized in 17 centres in the UK and three in the US; mean follow-up was 27 months. There was no difference between the three treatment groups with regard to the combined primary endpoint of all-cause mortality, non-fatal myocardial infarction and non-fatal stroke. However, there was an excess of hospitalizations in the aspirin group. Recently there have been concerns of potential adverse interactions between aspirin and ACE inhibitors in patients with heart failure;[43] these results reinforce some of these concerns. A large-scale trial, the WATCH study, is currently underway comparing warfarin (target INR 2.5–3), aspirin (162.5 mg daily) and clopidogrel (75 mg daily) in patients with heart failure. This trial will provide further data on the role of anticoagulation and antiplatelet therapy in patients with heart failure.

Current recommendations

Until further clinical trials are completed the following recommendations can be made:

- anticoagulation with warfarin (target INR 2–3) for patients with heart failure and coexisting atrial fibrillation;
- anticoagulation with warfarin for patients with heart failure who are in sinus rhythm with risk factors for thromboembolism such as prior embolism or documented LV thrombus;
- low-dose aspirin for patients with heart failure and concomitant coronary artery, peripheral vascular or cerebrovascular disease.

Newer pharmacological strategies undergoing clinical research studies

Natriuretic peptides

The natriuretic peptides are a group of peptides which are synthesized and secreted from the heart and which are elevated in heart failure in proportion to the severity of the cardiac dysfunction. Atrial natriuretic peptide (ANP) is a 28-amino acid peptide that is synthesized and secreted mainly from the cardiac atria. Brain natriuretic peptide (BNP) is a 32-amino acid peptide synthesized and secreted primarily from the cardiac ventricles. High levels of ANP[44] and BNP[45] have been observed in patients with heart failure. However, these high levels appear to have reduced clinical effect in chronic heart failure, perhaps due to receptor downregulation or haemodynamic tolerance.

The natriuretic peptides may have a variety of different roles in the management of patients with heart failure, including potential for aiding diagnosis and assessing prognosis,[46] as well as in the treatment of heart failure. Intravenous preparations of ANP and BNP are available and are being assessed in ongoing trials. Intravenous administration of ANP in patients with heart failure has

been shown to have beneficial haemodynamic effects.[47] Clinical studies have shown that intravenous exogenous BNP, nesiritide, results in vasodilatation, duiresis and natriuresis and antagonism of the renin–angiotensin system.[48,49] A recent placebo-controlled study[50] has demonstrated that a 24-hour infusion of nesiritide in patients with advanced heart failure resulted in rapid and sustained beneficial effects on haemodynamics. While these results support the use of these agents in the treatment of heart failure, further clinical trials are required to more clearly determine the short- and longer-term effects of these agents.

The natriuretic peptides are inactivated in the circulation by the enzyme neutral endopeptidase. Omapatrilat, a novel vasopeptidase inhibitor, inhibits both neutral endopeptidase and angiotensin-converting enzyme, thus increases levels of the natriuretic peptides as well as decreasing angiotensin II levels.[51] The IMPRESS trial[52] compared the effects of omapatrilat with lisinopril in 573 patients with chronic heart failure treated for 24 weeks. The results suggest that omapatrilat was superior to lisinopril in improving symptoms and mortality/morbidity in heart failure.[52] However, the larger OVERTURE trial did not show that omapatrilat was superior to ACE inhibitor therapy alone in reducing the risk of death or hospital admission for heart failure, although some secondary endpoints were in favour of omapatrilat.[53] Currently, these results would not support the widespread use of omapatrilat in place of ACE inhibitors.

Cytokines, tumour necrosis factor alpha

Proinflammatory cytokines, including interleukin 1, interleukin 6 and tumour necrosis factor alpha (TNF-α), have been shown to be elevated in patients with chronic heart failure.[54] These cytokines have been associated with progression of the disease process in heart failure, including cachexia[55] and progressive LV remodeling.[56,57] These observations have led to the cytokine hypothesis of heart failure:[58] namely that the overexpression of the inflammatory cytokines contributes to the development and progression of heart failure.

This hypothesis has led to a new potential for treatment with agents that block the effects of the inflammatory cytokines. Etanercept is a soluble p75 TNF receptor fusion protein that binds to and functionally inactivates TNF-α.[59] Deswal et al[60] recently reported the results of a small, phase II trial of etanercept, in patients with advanced heart failure and elevated TNF-α levels. This study demonstrated that etanercept decreased biological activity of TNF-α, with no appreciable side-effects. Quality of life scores, 6-minute walk distance and ejection fraction increased in the etanercept group although the study was too small for these changes to reach conventional statistical significance compared with placebo. Two large-scale, randomized, placebo-controlled trials, RENAISSANCE and RECOVER, together known as the RENEWAL studies were terminated in March 2001 because it was clear that the studies would not demonstrate benefit on mortality and morbidity endpoints.[61] Overall, there do not appear to be data to support the routine use of etanercept in patients with heart failure.

Endothelin antagonists

Three endothelin peptides, ET-1, ET-2 and ET-3, each with diverse actions and two distinct receptor subtypes, types A and B, have been identified. Plasma levels of endothelin, a potent vasocontrictor, are elevated in heart failure and inversely correlate with ejection fraction and exercise capacity.[62,63] Because of the role of endothelin in the pathophysiology of heart failure, endothelin receptor antagonists have been proposed for the treatment of heart failure.

Bosentan is a non-peptide competitive antagonist, which blocks the effects of endothelin at both A and B receptors. The REACH-1 trial was a multicentre, placebo-controlled trial of bosentan in patients with severe (NYHA IIIb/IV) heart failure.[64] The trial involved 370 patients and the primary endpoint was a composite of symptoms and major events at 6 months. The trial was stopped early by the Data and Safety Monitoring Board because of concern regarding elevated hepatic transaminases.[64] At that time all patients had completed 3 months of treatment but only 47% had completed 6 months. Overall, for the entire study population there was no difference between the bosentan and placebo groups with regard to the clinical composite endpoint. However, for those patients who had reached 6 months of treatment, there was a higher proportion of patients in the bosentan group who had improved and fewer who had worsened compared with the placebo group. These results suggest that the endothelin antagonist bosentan may have beneficial long-term effects in patients with heart failure, although the abnormalities of liver function

are a concern and final publication of these results from REACH-1 are awaited.

Prevention of sudden death – amiodarone and implantable defibrillators

Sudden death, usually due to a sudden ventricular arrhythmia, is a frequent mode of death in patients with heart failure. Trials of antiarrhythmic agents in patients with heart failure have to date provided conflicting results and clinical trials are ongoing. Of the class I and class III antiarrhythmics only amiodarone appears to have any promise in heart failure although the results of the studies with amiodarone have been conflicting. The GESICA study[65] showed a reduction in overall mortality with amiodarone compared with placebo while the CHF-STAT trial[66] did not. However, subgroup analysis from the CHF-STAT trial[66] showed a trend to a reduction in mortality in patients with underlying non-ischaemic cardiomyopathy who received amiodarone.

The SWORD trial[67] investigated the effects of D-sotalol, a specific potassium channel blocker without significant beta-blocking activity, on mortality in patients with LV dysfunction following myocardial infarction (either recent or remote). The trial was stopped early due to an increase in mortality in the D-sotalol group compared with placebo (78 vs 48 deaths respectively, relative risk 1.65, p = 0.006).[67] This excess death rate was presumed to be secondary to arrhythmias. Thus, class I antiarrythmics (such as encainide and flecainide)[68] and D-sotalol[67] increase mortality in patients post myocardial infarction with LV impairment, while the effects of amiodarone are still uncertain. Further trials are underway to clarify the role of amiodarone in patients with heart failure.

The implantable defibrillators (ICD) have an established role in the management of patients with life-threatening ventricular arrhythmias.[69] However, the role of the ICDs in the primary prevention of ventricular arrhythmias and sudden death in patients with heart failure is uncertain. The Sudden Cardiac Death in Heart Failure Trial, SCD-HeFT, will determine the effects of amiodarone, ICD or placebo on total mortality in patients with heart failure (LV ejection fraction ≤ 35%) and no history of ventricular tachycardia or fibrillation. This study will provide definitive evidence of the role of amiodarone and ICDs in the primary prevention of sudden death in patients with heart failure.

References

1 Dougherty AH, Naccarelli GV, Gray EL. Congestive heart failure with normal systolic function. *Am J Cardiol* 1984; **54:** 778–82.

2 Ramachandran SV, Benjamin EJ, Levy D. Prevalence, clinical features and prognosis of diastolic heart failure: an epidemiologic perspective. *J Am Coll Cardiol* 1995; **26:** 1565–74.

3 Tresch DD, McGough MF. Heart failure with normal systolic function: a common disorder in older people. *J Am Geriatr Soc* 1995; **43:** 1035–42.

4 Pitt B, Zannad F, Remme WJ et al. The effects of spironolactone on morbidity and mortality in patients with severe heart failure. Randomized Aldactone Evaluation Study Investigators. *N Engl J Med* 1999; **341:** 709–17.

5 Francis GS, Benedict C, Johnstone DE et al, for the SOLVD Investigators. Comparison of neuroendocrine activation in patients with left ventricular dysfunction with and without congestive heart failure. A substudy of the Studies of Left Ventricular Dysfunction (SOLVD). *Circulation* 1990; **82:** 1724–9.

6 The CONSENSUS Trial Study Group. Effects of enalapril on mortality in severe congestive heart failure. Results of the Cooperative North Scandinavian Enalapril Survival Study (CONSENSUS). *N Eng J Med* 1987; **316:** 1429–35.

7 The SOLVD Investigators. Effect of enalapril on survival in patients with reduced left ventricular ejection fractions and congestive heart failure. *N Eng J Med* 1991; **325:** 293–302.

8 The SOLVD Investigators. Effect of enalapril on mortality and the development of heart failure in asymptomatic patients with reduced left ventricular ejection fractions. *N Eng J Med* 1992; **327:** 685–91.

9 Pfeffer MA, Braunwald E, Moye LA et al, on behalf of the SAVE Investigators. Effect of captopril on mortality and morbidity in patients with left ventricular dysfunction after myocardial infarction. Results of the Survival and Ventricular Enlargement Trial. *N Eng J Med* 1992; **327:** 669–77.

10 Packer M, Poole-Wilson PA, Armstrong PW et al. Comparative effects of low and high doses of the angiotensin-converting enzyme inhibitor, lisinopril, on morbidity and mortality in chronic heart failure. ATLAS Study Group. *Circulation* 1999; **100:** 2312–18.

11 The Acute Infarction Ramipril Efficacy (AIRE) Investigators. Effect of ramipril on mortality and morbidity of survivors of acute myocardial infarction with clinical evidence of heart failure. *Lancet* 1993; **342:** 821–28.

12 Kober L, Torp-Pedersen C, Carlsen JE et al, for the Trandolapril Cardiac Evaluation (TRACE) Study Group. A clinical trial of the angiotensin-converting enzyme inhibitor trandolapril in patients with left ventricular dysfunction after myocardial infarction. *N Engl J Med* 1995; **333:** 1670–6.

13 Francis GS, Cohn JN, Johnson G, Rector TS, Goldman S, Simon A, for the V-HeFT VA Cooperative Study Group. Plasma norepinephrine, plasma renin activity and congestive heart failure. Relationship to survival and effects of therapy in V-HeFT II. *Circulation* 1993; **87(Suppl VI):** VI40–8.

14 Cohn JN, Levine B, Olivari MT. Plasma norepinephrine as a guide to prognosis in patients with congestive heart failure. *N Eng J Med* 1984; **311:** 819–23.

15 Doughty RN, MacMahon S, Sharpe N. Beta-blockers in heart failure: promising or proved? *J Am Coll Cardiol* 1994; **23:** 814–21.

16 CIBIS-II Investigators and Committees. The Cardiac Insufficiency Bisoprolol Study II (CIBIS-II): a randomised trial. *Lancet* 1999; **353:** 9–13.

17 MERIT-HF Study Group. Effect of metoprolol CR/XL in chronic heart failure: metoprolol CR/XL randomised intervention trial in congestive heart failure (MERIT-HF). *Lancet* 1999; **353:** 2001–7.

18 Packer M, Coats AJS, Fowler MB et al, for the Carvedilol Prospective Randomised Cummulative Survival Study Group. Effect of carvedilol on survival in severe chronic heart failure. *N Engl J Med* 2001; **344:** 1651–8.

19 Doughty RN, Rodgers A, Sharpe N, MacMahon S. Effects of beta-blocker therapy on mortality in patients with heart failure. A systematic overview of randomised controlled trials. *Eur Heart J* 1997; **18:** 560–5.

20 Doughty RN, Whalley GA, Gamble G, MacMahon S, Sharpe N, on behalf of the Australia-New Zealand Heart Failure Research Collaborative Group. Left ventricular remodelling with carvedilol in patients with congestive heart failure due to ischaemic heart disease. *J Am Coll Cardiol* 1997; **29:** 1060–6.

21 Packer M, Bristow MR, Cohn JN et al, for the US Carvedilol Study Group. The effect of carvedilol on morbidity and mortality in patients with chronic heart failure. *N Eng J Med* 1996; **334:** 1349–55.

22 Poole-Wilson PA, Swedberg K, Cleland JGF et al, for the COMET investigators. Comparison of carvedilol and metoprolol on clinical outcomes in patients with chronic heart failure in the carvedilol or metoprolol European trial (COMET): randomized controlled trial. *Lancer* 2003; **362:** 7–13.

23 Hershberger RE, Wynn JR, Sundberg L, Bristow MR. Mechanism of action of bucindolol in human ventricular myocardium. *J Cardiovasc Pharmacol* 1990; **15:** 959–67.

24 Bristow MR, O'Connell JB, Gilbert EM et al, for the Bucindolol Investigators. Dose–response of chronic beta-blocker treatment in heart failure from either idiopathic dilated cardiomyopathy or ischaemic cardiomyopathy. *Circulation* 1994; **89:** 1632–42.

25 The Beta-Blocker Evaluation of Survival Trial Investigators. A trial of the beta-blocker bucindolol in patients with advanced chronic heart failure. *N Engl J Med* 2001; **344:** 1659–67.

26 Plehn JF, Krause-Steinrauf H, Anand IS, Gottlieb S, O'Connor CM. Effect of race on cause-specific cardiovacular mortality in BEST. *Circulation* 2000; **102(Suppl II):** II–779.

27 Borghi C, Boschi S, Ambrosioni E, Melandri G, Branzi A, Magnani B. Evidence of partial escape of renin–angiotensin–aldosterone blockade in patients with acute myocardial infarction treated with ACE inhibitors. *J Clin Pharmacol* 1993; **33:** 40–5.

28 Balcells E, Meng QC, Johnson WH, Oparil S, Dell'Italia LJ. Angiotensin II formation from ACE and chymase in human and animal hearts: methods and species considerations. *Am J Physiol* 1997; **273:** H1769–74.

29 Pitt B, Martinez FA, Meuers G et al, on behalf of the ELITE Study Investigators. Randomised trial of losartan versus captopril in patients over 65 with heart failure (Evaluation of Losartan in the Elderly Study, ELITE). *Lancet* 1997; **349:** 747–52.

30 Pitt B, Poole-Wilson P, Segal R, Martinez FA, Dickstein K, Camm AJ, on behalf of the ELITE II Investigators. Effect of losartan compared with captopril on mortality in patients with symptomatic heart failure: a randomised trial – the Losartan Heart Failure Survival Study ELITE II. *Lancet* 2000; **355:** 1582–97.

31 McKelvie R, Yusuf S, Perjak D, Held P. Comparison of candesartan, enalapril and their combination in congestive heart failure: randomised evaluation of strategies for left ventricular dysfunction (RESOLVD Pilot Study). (abstract) *Euro Heart J* 1998; **19:** 133.

32 Hamroff G, Katz SD, Mancini D et al. Addition of angiotensin II receptor blockade to maximal angiotensin-converting enzyme inhibition improves exercise capacity in patients with severe congestive heart failure. *Circulation* 1999; **99:** 990–2.

33 Cohn JN, Tognoni G, Glazer RD, Spormann D, Hester A. Rationale and design of the Valsartan Heart Failure Trial: a large multinational trial to assess the effects of valsartan, an angiotensin-receptor blocker, on morbidity and mortality in chronic congestive heart failure. *J Cardiac Failure* 1999; **5:** 155–60.

34 Cohn JN, Tognoni G. Effect of angiotensin receptor blocker valsartan on morbidity and mortality in heart failure: the Valsartan Heart Failure Study (Val-HeFT). *NEJM* 2001; **345:** 1667–75.

35 Swedberg K, Pfeffer M, Granger C et al, for the CHARM-Programme Investigators. Candesartan in heart failure – assessment of reduction in mortality and morbidity (CHARM): rationale and design. *J Cardiac Failure* 1999; **5:** 276–82.

36 Pfeffer MA, Swedberg K, Granger CB et al. for the CHARM Investigator and Committees. Effects of candesartan on mortality and morbidity in patients with chronic heart failure: the CHARM-overall programme. Lancet 2003; **362:** 759–66.

37 The Digitalis Investigation Group. The effect of digoxin on mortality and morbidity in patients with heart failure. *N Eng J Med* 1997; **336:** 525–33.

38 Fuster V, Gersh BT, Giuliani ER, Tajik AJ, Brandenberg RO, Frye RL. The natural history of idiopathic dilated cardiomyopathy. *Am J Cardiol* 1981; **47:** 525–31.

39 Baker DW, Wright RF. Management of heart failure. IV. Anticoagulation for patients with heart failure due to left ventricular systolic dysfunction. *J Am Med Assoc* 1994; **272:** 1614–18.

40 Stroke Prevention in Atrial Fibrillation Investigators. Stroke Prevention in Atrial Fibrillation Study: final results. *Circulation* 1991; **84:** 527–39.

41 Cokkinos DV, Toutouzas PK. Antithrombotic therapy in heart failure: a randomized comparison of warfarin vs aspirin (HELAS). *Euro J Heart Failure* 1999; **1:** 419–23.

42 The WASH Study Steering Committee Investigators. The WASH Study (Warfarin/Aspirin in Heart Failure) rational design and end-points. *Eur J Heart Fail* 1999; **1:** 95–9.

43 Cleland JGF. Anticoagulation and antiplatelet therapy in heart failure. *Curr Opin Cardiol* 1997; **12:** 276–87.

44 Burnett JC, Kao PC, Hu DC et al. Atrial natriuretic peptide elevation in congestive heart failure. *Science* 1986; **231:** 1145–7.

45 Mokoyama M, Nakao K, Hosoda K et al. Brain natriuretic peptide as a novel cardiac hormone in humans. *J Clin Investigation* 1991; **87:** 1402–12.

46 Struthers AD. How to use natriuretic peptide levels for diagnosis and prognosis. *Eur Heart J* 1999; **20:** 1374–5.

47 Nichols MG. The natriuretic peptides in heart failure. *J Intern Med* 1994; **235:** 515–26.

48 McGregor A, Richards M, Espiner E, Yandle T, Ikram H. Brain natriuretic peptide administration to man: actions and metabolism. *J Clin Endocrinol Metab* 1990; **70:** 1103–7.

49 Holmes SJ, Espiner E, Richards AM, Yandle TG, Frampton C. Renal, endocrine and haemodynamic effects of human brain natriuretic peptide in normal man. *J Clin Endocrinol Metab* 1993; **76:** 91–6.

50 Mills RM, LeJemtel TH, Horton DP et al, on behalf of the Natrecor Study Group. Sustained haemodynamic effects of an infusion of nesiritide (human B-type natriuretic peptide) in heart failure. *J Am Coll Cardiol* 1999; **34:** 155–62.

51 Burnett JC. Vasopeptidase inhibition: a new concept in blood pressure management. *J Hypertension* 1999; **17(Suppl):** S37–43.

52 Rouleau JL, Pfeffer MA, Stewart DJ et al. Vasopeptidase inhibitor or angiotensin converting enzyme inhibitor in heart failure? Results of the IMPRESS Trial. (abstract) *Circulation* 1999; **100(Suppl 1):** I–782.

53 Packer M, Califf RM, Konstam MA et al. Comparison of omapatrilat and enalapril in patients with chronic heart failure: the Omapatrilat Versus Enalapril Randomized Trial of Utility in Reducing Events (OVERTURE). *Circulation.* 2002; **106:** 920–6.

54 Levine B, Kalman J, Mayer L, Fillit HM, Packer M. Elevated circulating levels of tumor necrosis factor in severe chronic heart failure. *N Engl J Med* 1990; **323:** 236–41.

55 McMurray J, Abdullah I, Dargie HJ, Shapiro D. Increased concentrations of tumour necrosis factor in 'cachectic' patients with severe chronic heart failure. *Br Heart J* 1991; **66:** 356–8.

56 Habib FM, Springall DR, Davies GJ, Oakley CM, Yacoub MH, Polak JM. Tumour necrosis factor and inducible nitric oxide synthase in dilated cardiomyopathy. *Lancet* 1996; **347:** 1151–5.

57 Torre-Amione G, Kapadia S, Lee J et al. Tumor necrosis factor-α and tumor necrosis factor receptors in the failing human heart. *Circulation* 1996; **93:** 704–11.

58 Seta Y, Shan K, Bozkurt B, Oral H, Mann DL. Basic mechanisms in heart failure: the cytokine hypothesis. *J Cardiac Failure* 1996; **2:** 243–9.

59 Mohler KM, Torrance DS, Smith CA et al. Soluble tumor necrosis factor (TNF) receptors are effective therapeutic agents in lethal endotoxemia and function simultaneously as both TNF carriers and TNF antagonists. *J Immunol* 1993; **151:** 1548–61.

60 Deswal A, Bozkurt B, Seta Y et al. Safety and efficacy of a soluble P75 tumor necrosis factor receptor (Enbrel, Etanercept) in patients with advanced heart failure. *Circulation* 1999; **99:** 3224–6.

61 Coletta AP, Clark AL, Banerjee P, Cleland JGF. Clinical trials update: RENEWAL (RENAISSANCE and RECOVER) and ATTACH. *Euro J Heart Failure* 2002; **4:** 559–61.

62 Wei CM, Lerman A, Rodeheffer RJ et al. Endothelin in human congestive heart failure. *Circulation* 1994; **89:** 1580–6.

63 Krum H, Goldsmith R, Wilshire-Clement M, Miller M, Packer M. Role of endothelin in the exercise intolerance of chronic heart failure. *Am J Cardiol* 1995; **75:** 1282–3.

64 Packer M, Caspi A, Charlon V et al. Multicentre, double-blind, placebo-controlled study of long-term endothelin blockade with bosentan in chronic heart failure – results of the REACH-1 trial. (abstract) *Circulation* 1998; **98(Suppl 1):** 1–3.

65 Doval HC, Nul DR, Grancelli HO, Perrone SV, Bortman GR, Curiel R. Randomised trial of low dose amiodarone in severe congestive heart failure. *Lancet* 1994; **344:** 493–8.

66 Singh SN, Fletcher RD, Fisher SG et al. Amiodarone in patients with congestive heart failure and asymptomatic ventricular arrhythmia. Survival Trial of Antiarrhythmic Therapy in Congestive Heart Failure. *N Engl J Med* 1995; **333:** 77–82.

67 Waldo AL, Camm AJ, deRuyter H et al, for the SWORD Investigators. Effect of D-sotalol on mortality in patients with left ventricular dysfunction after recent and remote myocardial infarction. *Lancet* 1996; **348:** 7–12.

68 The Cardiac Arrhythmia Suppression Trial. Preliminary report: effect of encainide and flecainide on mortality in a randomised trial of arrhythmia suppression after myocardial infarction. *N Eng J Med* 1989; **321:** 406–12.

69 Antiarrhythmics Versus Implantable Investigators. A comparison of antiarrhythmic drug therapy with implantable defibrillators in patients resuscitated from near-fatal ventricular arrhythmias. *N Engl J Med* 1997; **337:** 1576–83.

9 Non-pharmacologic management of heart failure

Debra K Moser, Terry A Lennie and Lynn V Doering

Optimal management of heart failure patients is challenging because the course of heart failure often is marked by the reoccurrence of debilitating symptoms, progression of ventricular dysfunction, impaired quality of life, and the probability of early death from decompensated heart failure or a sudden cardiac death event. Thus, it is clear that the goals of treatment must be comprehensive and aimed at more than a single target such as symptom control. Poole-Wilson[1] described the following set of comprehensive treatment goals: (1) prevention; (2) relief of signs and symptoms; and (3) prognosis improvement. The goal of prevention includes both the deterrence of progression of already existing ventricular dysfunction, avoidance of additional new myocardial damage, and prevention of exacerbations of clinical failure. Treatment goals aimed at relieving the signs and symptoms of heart failure should target improving edema and fluid retention, exercise capacity, fatigue and breathlessness, and overall quality of life. Finally, the chosen treatment should improve the patient's prognosis.

Achieving this set of extensive goals was not always possible. It is only relatively recently that researchers identified drug classes that could improve survival in heart failure.[2–7] However, even with improvements in pharmacologic treatment, overall improvement in long-term survival is modest, rehospitalizations are frequent and quality of life remains poor. Coordination and optimization of *both* non-pharmacologic and pharmacologic therapy are necessary to reach these goals. Non-pharmacologic therapy includes a wide range of strategies from diet management (e.g. dietary sodium restriction, alcohol and fluid restriction, advice about correcting nutritional deficiencies), to exercise and activity recommendations, risk factor modification, and use of appropriate models for the packaging and delivery of care. The purpose of this chapter is to discuss the use of diet management and risk factor modification in the management of patients with chronic heart failure. Other important non-pharmacologic therapies, exercise and activity recommendations, education and counseling and use of appropriate models for the

packaging and delivery of care, are covered in other chapters in this book.

Diet management

Sodium restriction

Excessive dietary sodium intake contributes to the volume overload and subsequent systemic edema and pulmonary congestion seen in heart failure. Patients have reduced ability to excrete sodium, and even in patients with mild heart failure and no signs of congestion, a high salt diet results in increased ventricular end-diastolic and end-systolic volumes without a corresponding increase in ejection fraction or stroke volume.[8] Reduction in dietary sodium intake alone can produce significant hemodynamic and clinical improvement in patients with heart failure.[9] Diuretic therapy is more effective when a patient follows a reduced sodium diet and many cases of apparent refractoriness to diuretics are caused by concomitant excessive dietary sodium intake.[9–11]

Despite evidence of the effectiveness of a low sodium diet as part of the treatment regimen for patients with heart failure, recent evidence suggests that sodium overload is the most common reason for decompensation of heart failure,[12] and that failure of patients to adhere to the low sodium diet recommendation is the major reason for recurrent rehospitalizations.[13–17] Nonetheless, the role of dietary sodium restriction in the treatment of heart failure often receives little specific attention and instructions to patients are frequently given in a cursory fashion or are not given at all.[18,19] Even patients who have been hospitalized for heart failure have surprisingly poor knowledge of how to follow a low sodium diet.[19–21]

Prescribing the low sodium diet and increasing patient adherence

Although dietary sodium restriction is one of the oldest treatments for congestive heart failure, the efficacy of restricting sodium to any specific level has not been

Table 9.1. *Steps to prescribing a low sodium diet*

1. Assess patient's current sodium intake
2. Assess patient and family/caregiver knowledge of sodium content of foods
3. Educate and counsel, including getting patient and family motivated, and behavioral strategies in increasing adherence
4. Assess degree of adherence and intervene if necessary
5. Reassess patient and family/caregiver knowledge of low sodium diet

studied. Despite lack of research evidence about the optimal sodium restriction,[22] there is evidence that restricting sodium to about 2–3 grams per day produces improvement in clinical presentation and increases sensitivity to diuretics.[9] Whether to prescribe a 2- or 3-gram sodium restriction depends upon the severity of heart failure. For patients who have mild heart failure a 3-gram sodium restriction is suggested and is usually sufficient to control volume status. For most symptomatic patients with heart failure, especially those who require large doses of diuretics, 2 grams of sodium per day is usually prescribed.[22–24]

The prescription of a low sodium diet requires careful assessment, education and counseling (Table 9.1). Two preliminary assessments are of major importance when prescribing and introducing the low sodium diet to the patient: (1) a thorough assessment of the patient's current sodium intake and eating habits; and (2) an assessment of the patient's knowledge of the sodium content of foods. Too often, busy clinicians simply ask their patients if they know how to follow a low sodium diet or if they are following one and do no further assessment when the patient invariably says, 'Oh yes, I never add salt to my food'. With just a few more questions, such as, 'What did you eat for each meal and snack for the past few days' the clinician can get a much more thorough picture of the patient's sodium intake and knowledge. Many patients know not to add salt, but have no idea of the sodium content of the foods they regularly eat, what level of daily sodium they should aim for or how to keep track of their daily intake.[18–20] At a minimum, every patient should be asked to describe a full day's typical eating and they should be asked to sort several low, medium, and high sodium foods into their respective categories. This foundation will provide the clinician with the basic information to begin

education and counseling. Adherence and knowledge should be assessed after each education session so that misconceptions and problems can be identified and corrected early.

Education and counseling should be directed at both patients and their family/caregiver, particularly when the family or other caregiver buys the food and cooks meals. Patients and their families benefit from receiving thorough and specific instructions about how to achieve the prescribed sodium restriction. Instructions that patients and families/caregivers should receive are outlined in Table 9.2. Inadequate patient education is one reason patients fail to follow the prescribed diet and is a major factor contributing to rehospitalizations.[25] Although patients may be knowledgeable about very obvious sources of sodium, many are unaware of the significant sodium content of many other high sodium sources such as canned foods and convenience foods. Supplementing verbal instructions with written take-home materials is essential. Patients also can benefit from written materials such as those available from the Heart Failure Society of America and American Heart Association that present information on sodium substitutes, appetizing low sodium recipes, and following a sodium restricted diet while enjoying eating out in restaurants. The Heart Failure Society of America has a thorough and informative patient education series that includes a module on following the low sodium diet and this module is available free to clinicians for their patients' use (@ www.hfsa.org/pdf/module 2.pdf).

Clinicians can consider referral to a dietician or advanced practice nurse with expertise in diet counseling to enhance patient and family understanding of the sodium-restricted diet and of the options for making this diet palatable.[24] Referral for dietary counseling may be particularly important for patients from diverse cultural backgrounds or for those having difficulty adapting their preferences to a low salt diet.

Adhering to a low sodium diet prescription is difficult.[26] Advising patients to follow one and providing them with the basic knowledge about how to do so are requisites that despite their simplicity are often ignored. However, these strategies alone are not sufficient to promote adherence. Knowledge alone rarely translates into behavior change without provision by the clinician of counseling and support strategies that increase adherence. General education and counseling strategies to optimize adherence are described in Chapter 17. There have been few studies of interventions designed specifically to increase adherence to a low sodium diet in patients with heart failure, but

Table 9.2. Patient instructions for reducing sodium intake

1. Follow these three basic steps to reducing sodium in your diet
   - Stop adding salt to food during cooking or at the table; remove the salt shaker from the table.
   - Adapt foods that you like to eat to low sodium versions
   - Eat foods that are naturally low in sodium such as most fresh fruits, vegetables and unprocessed meats, fish and poultry. Most frozen fruits, vegetables (without added sauces and seasonings), and unprocessed meats, poultry and fish are also low sodium. Dried beans, peas, rice and lentils are other good low sodium foods when cooked without adding salt.
2. Learn to read food labels to keep track of the amount of sodium you eat
3. Use no-salt spices, herbs, and lemon to season foods in place of salt; experiment with different preparations. Marinate meats, poultry and fish in no-salt marinades to add flavor before broiling or baking. There are several commercial no-salt seasoning preparations available at the grocery store and many cookbooks contain recipes of no-salt seasonings and marinades. Avoid those seasonings and marinades with the words 'salt' or 'sodium' on the label.
4. Get a cookbook that has low sodium recipes and experiment.
5. Avoid the use of canned and processed (boxed, prepared, convenience) foods, which are the major source of sodium in the typical American diet.
6. Some canned foods are available in low sodium versions. Look for canned foods labeled sodium-free, no-salt, low sodium, light in sodium, very low sodium, reduced-sodium, less-sodium or unsalted (but always check the food label).
7. Make changes to your diet slowly, instead of trying to change your entire diet at once.
8. Know the sodium content of all foods that you eat because many foods are not obvious sources of sodium.
9. Before using salt substitutes that contain potassium, check with your physician.
10. Check the labels of over-the-counter medications such as anti-acids or some cold and headache preparations because many are composed largely of sodium-containing compounds.

studies of comprehensive heart failure disease management programs indicate that such approaches increase adherence.[27–29] Although it is difficult to pinpoint the specific component(s) of the programs that result in increased adherence, it is likely that some or all of the following are effective in that regard: (1) enhancing the patient's ability to undertake a greater personal role (self-care) in managing his or her heart failure; (2) thorough, repetitive education directed at both patient and family/caregiver; (3) counseling that includes attention to behavioral strategies to enhance compliance; (4) vigilant follow-up; (5) support from professional staff; and (6) individualized approach. This last strategy seems to be particularly important. Adherence to the low sodium diet prescription is enhanced when education and counseling are individualized to each patient's situation (Table 9.3).[30,31] In particular, it is vital to determine and address each patient's potential barriers to adherence (Table 9.3).

Alcohol recommendations

Consumption of alcoholic beverages is common in the general population and among patients with heart failure and thus it is important to address the issue of whether patients with heart failure should continue to drink.[32] Conflicting evidence regarding alcohol and the heart has contributed to confusion about whether heart failure patients should consume alcohol. On the one hand, there is evidence that moderate consumption of alcohol may play a protective role in the heart, while on the other hand heavy consumption of alcohol can cause cardiomyopathy and impairment of ventricular function and investigators have demonstrated that alcohol can depress myocardial contractility in patients with cardiac disease.[33–35] For this reason, many heart failure specialists recommend that all patients with heart failure should abstain from alcohol use.[22]

However, not all experts agree on this recommendation. Some health care providers feel that the benefits some patients obtain in terms of increased quality of life when they can continue moderate alcohol intake outweigh any potential, but as yet unproven, detrimental effect of alcohol. In an observational substudy of both the treatment and prevention arms of the Studies of Left Ventricular Dysfunction (SOLVD) trial, light-to-moderate alcohol consumption in patients with left ventricular dysfunction did not increase morbidity or mortality.[35]

Table 9.3. *Facilitating adoption of low sodium diet by individualizing patient instruction*

1. Identify the patient's and family's perceived barriers to adopting a low sodium diet and assist them in overcoming them
   - financial concerns?
   - usually eat packaged or convenience foods?
   - low literacy?
   - lack of cooking skills?
   - unable to understand or read food labels or calculate amount of sodium consumed?
   - eat out often?
   - lack of motivation or willpower?
   - eat lots of fast food?
   - palatability of low sodium diet a problem?
   - rest of family unwilling to eat low sodium diet?
   - depression, social isolation or cognitive impairment?
2. Find out who does the shopping and cooking and include them in education
3. Assist patient and family in adapting preferred foods to low sodium versions
4. Determine cultural eating patterns and assist in adaptation of those foods to low sodium versions

Light-to-moderate consumption compared with no alcohol consumption was associated with a modest reduction in risk of death and reduced risk of fatal myocardial infarction.[35]

Given the lack of strong research evidence, a common recommendation is that if patients choose to continue to drink alcohol, the best advice is that they limit intake to one drink per day. One drink is equivalent to 12 ounces of beer or 4 ounces of wine or a mixed drink with $1\frac{1}{2}$ ounces of 80-proof distilled spirits.

The data are clearer for patients with alcoholic cardiomyopathy. Patients with alcoholic cardiomyopathy must refrain from alcohol use since alcohol was instrumental in the development of their heart failure and can cause progression of failure.[36] Furthermore, patients with alcoholic cardiomyopathy who continue to drink have higher mortality than those who abstain from alcohol even when they are taking standard heart failure medications.[37,38] Cardiac function has been demonstrated to improve in patients with alcoholic cardiomyopathy who abstain from alcohol.[38] Thus, those patients who have alcoholic cardiomyopathy should be counseled strongly to abstain completely from alcohol. Patients with a history of alcohol abuse may need counseling and referral to stop drinking and remain alcohol free.

Fluid restriction

Fluid restriction is a common prescription for patients with acute heart failure and continued restriction is thought by many clinicians to be an important part of outpatient therapy. However, there is no evidence that stringent chronic fluid restriction is beneficial and patients with chronic heart failure generally do not need to rigidly control their fluid intake. Adequate symptom control with sodium restriction and current drug therapy usually negates the need for rigorous fluid restriction. However, many heart failure patients believe that they should increase their fluid intake to compensate for the excessive urination that occurs when they take diuretics, because one should increase fluids when they are ill or to 'cleanse the body'.[19,39] Patients should be educated to correct this misconception and they should be counseled to avoid excessive (more than 2–2.5 liters per day) fluid intake. Stringent fluid restriction is not indicated except in selected patients with severe heart failure and difficult to control hyponatremia may benefit from fluid restriction.[24]

Correction of nutritional deficiencies
Malnutrition and cardiac cachexia
Despite recent interest in malnutrition in heart failure, the study of nutrition and the impact of nutritional deficiencies on progression of heart failure still is in its relative infancy. As a consequence, many clinicians underestimate both the importance of nutrition in patients with heart failure and the potentially negative effects of nutritional deficiencies. Chronic malnutrition is associated with poor outcomes in patients with heart failure[40,41] and is now recognized as an independent risk factor for mortality in

these patients.[42] As many as 50–70% of hospitalized heart failure patients may suffer from malnutrition.[43–45]

Malnutrition has traditionally been divided into two types: maramus and kwashiorkor. Marasmus is defined as malnutrition due to decreased intake of all macronutrients, but one in which visceral proteins remain normal. Kwashiorkor is characterized by a loss of visceral proteins due to inadequate protein intake often in the face of adequate calories from carbohydrate and fat sources. The latter form is most often seen in countries with limited access to dietary protein. In countries with sufficient food supplies, people with inadequate food intake are more likely to experience marasmus, but many individuals, especially those who are ill, display a combined form of malnutrition.[46] Therefore, the more descriptive term of protein-energy malnutrition (PEM) is now widely accepted.

PEM is defined as insufficient intake or utilization of protein and energy to maintain normal body tissue stores. It is the most common form of malnutrition observed in persons with acute and chronic illness including patients with heart failure. In its most advanced stages, PEM associated with heart failure results in the syndrome known as cardiac cachexia. It is estimated that at least 35% and possibly as many as 50% of patients with advanced heart failure have cardiac cachexia.[44] Cardiac cachexia is defined as a clinically significant loss of metabolically active lean tissue and body fat. Evidence from a limited number of animal and human studies suggests that the consequences of PEM and cardiac cachexia may be serious. Malnutrition with muscle wasting appears to contribute to decreased functional capacity, anemia, decreased bone mass, impaired cognitive function, immune dysfunction, and may cause cardiac muscle atrophy.[47] Loss of cardiac muscle contributes to progression of heart failure, and is associated with a markedly increased risk of mortality that is additive to the already high mortality seen in patients with heart failure.[42,43,47,48]

Causes of protein energy malnutrition and cardiac cachexia

There are two general reasons why people with heart failure become malnourished. The first is that the onset of an acute illness or exacerbation of heart failure can cause physiological changes that enhance tissue catabolism. The second reason is inadequate nutrient intake due to appetite loss or disability. A number of mechanisms related to these reasons have been proposed to be responsible for development of PEM and muscle wasting in heart failure (Table 9.4).[43,47,49] Although poor dietary intake is an important

Table 9.4. Potential mechanisms for the development of malnutrition and cardiac cachexia in patients with heart failure

1. Poor dietary intake
   - anorexia from hepatic and gut edema
   - anorexia from drug toxicities
   - anorexia from proinflammatory cytokines
2. Increased energy requirements
3. Accelerated muscle protein breakdown due to catecholamine
4. Malabsorption
   - delayed emptying
   - intestinal hypomotility
   - intestinal edema
   - intestinal tissue hypoperfusion
5. Protein-losing enteropathy
6. Decreased skeletal muscle protein synthesis secondary to disuse atrophy and deconditioning
7. Effects of increased proinflammatory cytokine (TNFα, IL-1, IL-6) activity
8. Sympathetic nervous system activation
9. Effects of aging on appetite and muscle metabolism
   - decreased sense of taste and smell
   - early satiety due to increased CCK release
   - prolonged satiation due to delayed gastric emptying
   - psychosocial factors: social isolation, depression, and poverty
   - decreased mobility
   - sarcopenia

contributor to PEM, multiple factors related to the development and progression of heart failure itself operate together to produce cardiac cachexia and are probably the predominant cause.[47,50] Poor dietary intake is common in patients with advanced heart failure and is related to anorexia that is secondary to intestinal edema, inflammation, drug toxicities, and factors related to aging. Malabsorption of ingested nutrients occurs as a result of edema and hypoperfusion of the gut, and intestinal hypomotility. Muscle protein abnormalities are present and include accelerated muscle breakdown due to the effects of high levels of circulating catecholamines. For patients who are inactive, muscle wasting may be related to decreased skeletal muscle protein synthesis. Sympathethic nervous system activation can contribute to malnutrition and cachexia and is higher in cachexic heart failure patients than in heart failure patients without cachexia.[51]

Cachexia has been called cytokine-induced malnutrition because levels of inflammatory cytokines, tumor necrosis factor alpha (TNFα), interleukin-1 (IL-1) and interleukin-6 (IL-6) are elevated in patients with heart failure.[52–54] These inflammatory cytokines play a role in cachexia associated with other disorders and are thought to also play an important role in cardiac cachexia. Of these cytokines, TNFα has received the most attention in the cachexia associated with heart failure. TNFα has been shown to lead to a decline in nutritional status by decreasing appetite and food intake over an extended period. TNFα also accelerates protein catabolism of skeletal muscle as well as decreases free fatty acid synthesis and increases lipolysis resulting in diminished storage of body energy in the form of fat.

In addition to factors related to heart failure, a number of changes that occur with aging can contribute to decreased spontaneous food intake and altered body composition. Appetite is affected by age-related decreases in the sense of taste and smell resulting in diminished desire to eat.[55] Aging is also associated with release of higher amounts of cholecystokinin (CCK), a hormone excreted by endocrine cells of the small intestine when food is present.[56] The increased release of CCK produces the sensation of satiety that diminishes the desire to continue eating resulting in smaller meals.[57] Satiation, the length of time after a meal before hunger sensations return, can be prolonged by delayed gastric emptying that occurs as a normal part of growing older and can result in fewer meals eaten per day. Other factors that occur in older adults which can further decrease food intake include social isolation, depression, poverty, as well as limited ability to shop for and prepare foods.[50] Sarcopenia, or age-related loss of muscle mass due to changes in physical activity and circulating anabolic hormones,[58] can compound the loss of protein-based tissues due to heart failure.

Nutrition assessment

Proper assessment of nutritional status is vital to treatment of PEM. Early detection and treatment may reduce the incidence of severe malnutrition. Unfortunately, there is no single marker that is diagnostic or indicative of the severity of PEM. Clinicians must rely on multiple parameters to determine whether a patient is malnourished. In cases of severe PEM, only a few simple markers, such as history of weight loss and visual assessment will be required. In cases of suspected PEM, the clinician should use as many markers as can reasonably be obtained. It is important to note that the type of malnutrition may vary,

and therefore, not all markers examined may be abnormal even though the patient is malnourished. In these cases, the clinician should determine whether a majority of the evidence indicates PEM as well as rule out other causes of any abnormal parameter.

The simplest means of screening for risk of malnutrition is to follow changes in dry body weight. The level of involuntary weight loss indicating a clinically significant health risk is defined as greater than 5% loss in 30 days, greater than 7.5% loss in 90 days, or a 10% loss in 6 months.[58] Regardless of time period, a 10% involuntary weight loss typically indicates a mild level of PEM, a 15–25% weight loss is considered to be a sign of moderate PEM, while weight loss exceeding 25% is considered to indicate severe PEM.

Routine clinical assessment of nutritional status based on body weight alone, however, can underestimate the incidence of serious malnutrition.[44,45] Other indicators of body cell mass include body mass index (BMI) and anthropometric measures of body composition (Table 9.5).[59] Body mass index provides an indication of total body mass that is highly correlated with body fat and therefore, is a marker of body energy stores. Increased risk of mortality is associated with a BMI of < 23.5 kg/m^2 in men and < 22 kg/m^2 in women. A BMI < 21 kg/m^2 for either sex indicates the need for immediate nutritional intervention.[60] Anthropometric measures provide additional information about body composition. Triceps skin fold (TSF), which is a measure of subcutaneous fat, also indicates body energy stores. The average TSF for males age 54–74 years old is 1.5 cm (range, 0.9–2.5 cm) while in females it is 2.7 cm (range, 1.8–3.5 cm). Males with TSF < 0.6 cm and females with TSF of < 1.4 cm should be considered to have depleted body fat stores.[61] Midarm muscle circumference is used in conjunction with TSF to obtain midarm muscle area, which is an estimate of muscle mass.[62] The formula for estimating midarm muscle area as an indicator of body muscle mass is provided in Table 9.5. Table 9.6 provides guidelines for interpreting these measures.

Biological markers, such as the serum proteins albumin, transferrin, and prealbumin, as well as total lymphocyte count, provide additional data about nutritional status. The body places a high priority on serum proteins; therefore, in the absence of other causes, a drop in serum proteins provides an indication that the body does not have sufficient nutrients available to make these essential proteins. The clinical significance of altered levels of these markers is outlined in Table 9.7. Albumin has a half-life of

Table 9.5. *Indicators of body cell mass of patients with heart failure*

Body mass index (BMI).

Weight in kilograms/(height in meters)^2 or 704.5 × (weight in pounds/height in inches^2). A program to calculate BMI for varying heights and weights is available from the following website address: www.nhlbi.nih.gov/health/public/heart/obesity/lose_wt/index.htm (National Heart, Lung, and Blood Institute [NHLBI], 1999); a chart for determining BMI can be found in the *Clinical Guidelines on the Identification, Evaluation, and Treatment of Overweight and Obesity in Adults* (NHLBI, 1998).

Anthropometric measures

Triceps skin fold (TSF). The measurement is taken while the arm is freely hanging. The thumb and forefinger are used to grasp a fold of skin and subcutaneous fat slightly above the midpoint. A caliper is applied to the area and after 2–3 seconds a measurement is taken to the nearest 1.0 mm. The procedure is repeated two more times and the measurements averaged.[62]

Midarm circumference (MAC). The measurement is taken on the non-dominant arm at the midpoint between the olecranon process and acromion process (where the scapula joins the shoulder). Using a non-stretchable tape, the circumference is measured to the nearest mm while the forearm is flexed 90 degrees.[62]

Midarm muscle circumference formula (MAMC). The following formula is used to remove the contribution of subcutaneous fat and bone from the circumference of the arm. This provides an indication of the muscle mass of the arm.[61]

$$\text{MAMC (cm}^2) = \left(\frac{[\text{MAC cm} - (3.13 \times \text{TSF cm})]^2}{12.52} \right) - 10 \text{ (males) or } -6.5 \text{ (females)}$$

Table 9.6. *Midarm muscle area (cm^2) in adults 55–74 years old (adapted from Beers and Berkow[61] and National Kidney Foundation[130])*

Men	Women	Muscle mass
43–64	27–44	Adequate
≤ 40	≤ 25	Marginal
< 35	< 21	Depleted
< 30	< 18	Wasted

20 days and large amounts of this protein are stored in the body. Therefore, albumin is a good marker of longstanding PEM. Transferrin, which has a much shorter half-life of 10 days and a much smaller body store, is a more sensitive marker of short-term PEM. It is important to note that both of these proteins are affected by factors other than nutrition such as blood transfusions, trauma, sepsis, and other inflammatory disorders. Prealbumin has a half-life of 2–3 days and is the most sensitive marker of acute or early PEM and subsequently is also an early marker of adequate nutritional intervention.[63] In addition to the general categories outlined in Table 9.7, low serum prealbumin levels have been further divided into subcategories

to guide clinical practice. Patients with levels below 15 mg/dl should be referred for a dietary consultation. Those with levels below 11 mg/dl are at significant nutritional risk and require aggressive nutritional intervention. Those with prealbumin levels below 5 mg/dl are at high risk and require immediate nutritional intervention.[64] Total lymphocyte count has been advocated as another measure of nutritional status because PEM can have a significant impact on immune cell number. Lymphocyte values fluctuate widely and are influenced by multiple factors; therefore, total lymphocyte count should only be interpreted in relation to other markers of PEM.[62] That is, if total lymphocyte count is low in conjunction with other biological markers of nutritional status, then it is

Table 9.7. *Biological markers of protein energy malnutrition (PEM) severity[58]*

	Mild	Moderate	Severe
Albumin (g/dl)	2.8–3.5	2.1–2.7	< 2.1
Transferrin (mg/dl)	151–200	100–150	< 100
Prealbumin (mg/dl)	15–30	10–15	0–10
Total lymphocyte count (mm^3)	1200–1500	800–1199	< 800

likely that PEM has progressed to the point where immune function is also impaired.

Interventions

Treatment of PEM and cardiac cachexia is complicated by a lack of definitive research findings about successful strategies, and by the multiple nutritional and pathophysiologic causes of these disorders. Improving anorexia and nutritional intake alone is insufficient to correct severe malnutrition and cachexia, but it is an important component. Table 9.8 outlines a number of interventions aimed at improving anorexia associated with chronic illness. Most of these strategies are self-explanatory, but several are highlighted below. One important principle to keep in mind when planning treatment for weight loss is that it takes at least three times as long to replace tissue lost during illness than it took to lose it.[60] This is because the

rate at which protein and fat are utilized during illness is 5–10-fold faster than the rate at which these tissues are restored during recovery. Patients who develop another illness or subsequent exacerbation of their disease before fully recovering will undergo additional loss of body tissue that will require even longer to restore. Those with unstable disease may develop a progressive downward spiral of weight loss because they are unable to adequately recover before the next exacerbation. A second important principle to remember is that even healthy elderly persons need 20% more calories and 50% more protein than the current recommended daily allowance (i.e. more than the amounts listed in nutrition labels on food containers).

Although there have been few studies of its effectiveness, the most widely accepted intervention for improving nutritional intake is to recommend patients eat small, frequent meals.[43] This strategy addresses the early satiety that

Table 9.8. Interventions for treatment of anorexia associated with chronic illness[131]

Intervention	Rationale	Evidence
Minimize additional stressors	Decrease release of catabolic counterregulatory hormones	CD
Eat small frequent meals	Inflammatory mediators produce early satiety	CD, SC
Increase caloric/nutrient density of food	Volume of food has greater effect on satiety than caloric density	CD, SC, SH
Use non-narcotic pain medications	Prevent gastric stasis	CD
Provide foods that vary in color, texture, taste	Appeal to appetitive factors prevents sensory-specific satiety	SH
Eat meals when hunger sensations are present	Hunger sensations are cyclic and may diminish if meal is delayed	CD
Promote socialization during meals	People eat less when alone	CD
Add flavor enhancers	Enhance enjoyment of food if taste is diminished	SC
Diet counseling and goal setting	Increase incentives to eat even if not hungry	SC
Eat diets high in carbohydrate when ill	Appeals to food preferences during illness	CD, SC
Eat diets high in omega-3 fatty acids	Decrease inflammatory response and other components of heart failure	CT
Block cytokine actions with drugs or antagonists	Decrease anorexic activity	CD, SC
Optimize medical therapy for heart failure	Reduction in gastrointestinal edema, suppression of catabolic cytokines, reduction in protein-losing enteropathy	CD, SC
Identify and treat drug toxicities	Detection and treatment of drug toxicities reduces associated anorexia	CD
Give orexigenic drugs	Increase appetite, antagonize anorexic activity of cytokines	CT

CD, clinical deduction based on causes of anorexia; CT, clinical trials; SC, small clinical studies or case reports; SH, studies using healthy subjects.

occurs with both illness and aging. Because amount of food, rather than caloric density of food, has the greatest effect on satiety in older adults, these meals should be caloric and nutrient-dense.[65] Nutrient-dense, low sodium liquid nutrition supplements can provide a good source of additional calories, protein, and other important nutrients for cachexic patients.[43] Encouraging the intake of these supplements or other nutrient-dense snacks between meals may be a particularly effective strategy for increasing total nutrient intake in older adults. Unlike younger adults, high calorie between-meal supplements given to older adults do not appear to decrease appetite or lower the amount of food eaten at the meal following supplementation.[66] Caloric intake can also be improved by recommending the patient take medications with a liquid nutrition supplement that provides 2.0 kilocalories/cc.

Severely malnourished patients who are unable to ingest enough calories orally may benefit from supplemental nasogastric feeding or parenteral nutrition. Supplements that provide 1.5–2.0 kilocalories/cc are helpful in increasing adequate nutrient intake. In particular, malnourished heart failure patients who will be undergoing major surgery (e.g. cardiac valve replacement, coronary artery bypass grafting, or cardiac transplantation) need nutrition supplementation to improve prognosis after surgery.[67] As noted above, short-term supplementation will be ineffective in reversing malnutrition.[47] At least 3 weeks of intensive supplementation is needed to produce positive effects and even then results with heart failure patients are variable.[47,67,68] One advantage to nutritional supplementation even if it does not totally correct cachexia is that it may break the vicious cycle of cachexia leading to progression of heart failure and then contributing to more cachexia. The loss of lean body mass that is seen with these conditions is far more than can be attributed to anorexia alone.[43] Even long-term nutritional supplementation is not enough to correct muscle wasting and metabolic abnormalities because malnutrition alone is not the root cause of cardiac cachexia.[47,68]

One potential nutritional treatment that can decrease inflammation, an important component of the root cause of cardiac cachexia, is to increase the amount of omega-3 fatty acids in the diet. Current diets contain a much greater proportion of omega-6 fatty acids than is thought to be beneficial. This is because omega-6 fatty acids comprise a large component of the oils (corn, safflower, cottonseed, peanut, and soybean) used for cooking and in prepared foods. In contrast, the source of omega-3 fatty acids is primarily limited to oily fish such as sardines, mackerel, herring, trout, and salmon. Omega-3 fatty acids, however, are also available in a number of fish oil supplements. When the proportion of omega-3 fatty acids in the diet increases to about one-third the amount of omega-6 fatty acids, they replace omega-6 fatty acids in cell membranes. In response to inflammatory stimuli, these cells produce a greater amount of the less inflammatory prostaglandins and thromboxanes that come from omega-3 fatty acids than the inflammatory species that come from omega-6 fatty acids.[69] Diets containing omega-3 fatty acids have decreased proinflammatory cytokine production in animal models of heart failure.[70] This limits the negative effects of these cytokines on food intake and protein synthesis. Additional positive effects attributed to omega-3 fatty acids in patients with heart failure include antivasopressor, antihypertension, and antiarrhythmic activities, decreased blood viscosity, and slowed progression of atherosclerosis.[71]

Because cardiac cachexia is a result of multiple factors, no single treatment is effective for treating malnutrition and cachexia in heart failure. In addition to treating anorexia and giving nutritional supplements, exercise training has been recommended to combat the muscle wasting and peripheral metabolic abnormalities seen.[43,47] Exercise training is discussed in detail in Chapter 10. Correcting and controlling congestion and hemodynamic abnormalities by optimizing medical therapy is an extremely important component of malnutrition treatment and may be more effective than nutrition supplementation.[44,72]

Thiamine deficiency

Thiamine is a water-soluble B-complex vitamin that is important to carbohydrate metabolism and tissue oxygenation. Clinical thiamine deficiency can cause beriberi, a cardiovascular syndrome manifested by peripheral vasodilation, sodium and water retention, and heart failure. In the United States, beriberi as a cause of heart failure is relatively rare and occurs most often in alcoholics.

Thiamine deficiency also may occur as a result of chronic treatment with loop diuretics and can exacerbate pre-existing heart failure. Recent evidence that patients with heart failure who are receiving chronic high-dose diuretic therapy have thiamine deficiencies has provoked interest in the use of thiamine replacement to improve cardiac function.[73,74] Seligmann et al compared thiamine levels in 23 elderly heart failure patients receiving high-dose, long-term furosemide therapy to levels in 16 age-matched controls without heart failure who were not on diuretics.[74] They identified thiamine deficiency in 21 of 23 heart failure patients but in only two of the controls. In six heart failure patients they treated the deficiency with intravenous thiamine to increase levels to normal. Mean ejection fraction increased by $13 \pm 2.7\%$, from $24 \pm 4.3\%$ to $37 \pm 2.4\%$. A subsequent investigation, by the same researchers, of thiamine supplementation vs placebo in 30 heart failure patients demonstrated an improvement in ejection fraction of 22% over the 6-week treatment period.[75]

Other researchers have failed to find evidence that thiamine deficiency is common in heart failure patients receiving diuretics[76,77] and there are no other investigations of the role of thiamine supplementation in heart failure. Inconsistent findings and lack of large-scale clinical trials testing thiamine supplementation preclude clinical recommendation of thiamine supplementation to improve ventricular function at this time.[73] However, supplementation with thiamine and other water-soluble vitamins is recommended in patients on diuretics to avoid vitamin deficiencies.[22] Thiamine supplementation to enhance ventricular performance is a fruitful area for research since it has potential benefits yet is inexpensive, safe, and free of side-effects.[73]

Behavioral risk factor modification

The major causes of heart failure are ischemic heart disease and hypertension.[78–81] Once a patient develops heart failure, both of these factors can contribute to ischemic events that further damage myocardium, progression of ventricular dysfunction and marked worsening of the heart failure patient's condition. Escalating left ventricular dysfunction is associated with increased mortality and functional impairment from increased symptoms. Thus, the importance of risk factor modification to address risk factors for ischemic heart disease and hypertension must be communicated to patients and they need to be given assistance with behavior modification. Yet clinicians frequently do not address this vital component of heart failure management in their patients. This section focuses on lifestyle modification to address hypertension, hyperlipidemia, obesity, smoking, and lack of exercise in patients with heart failure. Although drug therapy is also essential for the management of hypertension, hyperlipidemia and diabetes in heart failure, the focus of this chapter is non-pharmacologic management; drug therapy is discussed in other chapters.

Hypertension

Hypertension increases both left ventricular end-systolic wall stress (afterload) and left ventricular diastolic pressure. As a result, myocardial oxygen demand increases, adversely affecting the myocardial oxygen supply/demand ratio. In this way, hypertension can contribute to heart failure exacerbation in patients with existing heart failure or to precipitation of symptomatic heart failure in patients with clinically latent left ventricular dysfunction.

The goals of therapy in patients with heart failure are to prevent further myocardial damage, limit other cardiovascular morbidity and optimize cardiac function. The Joint National Committee on Prevention, Detection, Evaluation, and Treatment of High Blood Pressure recommends maintaining blood pressure below 130/80 mmHg in patients with heart failure.[82] In heart failure, myocardial performance may be best at even lower pressures.

In patients with heart failure the management of hypertension is accomplished with both drug therapy and lifestyle modification.[82,83] Lifestyle modification complements drug therapy, reduces the dosage and number of medications needed to control blood pressure, and contributes to reductions in all-cause mortality.[82] Recommendations for lifestyle modification as an adjunct therapy for hypertension are presented in Table 9.9. Management of sodium retention, as discussed above in the section on dietary sodium restriction, is an important element of hypertension management for patients with heart failure.

Hyperlipidemia

Ischemic heart disease is the etiology of heart failure in approximately two-thirds of cases and hyperlipidemia is one of the major contributors to ischemic heart disease.[84] In patients with heart failure from ischemic heart disease it is important to prevent further myocardial damage from occurring by controlling hyperlipidemia. In patients with heart failure from non-ischemic causes, it is important to prevent development of ischemic heart disease to preserve the myocardium. Again, the management of hyperlipidemia is essential. Multiple studies have demonstrated the benefits of reducing low density lipoprotein serum cholesterol levels in terms of reducing cardiovascular mortality and risk of developing heart failure.[85–89]

In patients with known ischemic heart disease, the National Cholesterol Education Panel Adult Treatment Panel II recommends lipid targets of total cholesterol < 160 mg/dl, low density lipoprotein < 100 mg/dl, and high density lipoprotein > 45 mg/dl.[90] Many heart failure centers follow these guidelines for the management of

Table 9.9. Lifestyle modifications for hypertension management

Modification	Rationale related to hypertension management
Lose weight if overweight	1. Weight reduction of as little as 10 lbs reduces BP in a large proportion of overweight persons with hypertension[132] 2. Weight reduction enhances BP-lowering effect of concurrent antihypertensive agents[133]
Limit alcohol intake to < 1 oz ethanol per day or 0.5 oz in women and lighter individuals	1. Excessive alcohol intake can cause resistance to antihypertensive therapies[134]
Increase physical activity to 30–45 minutes most days of the week	1. Regular physical activity can enhance weight loss and functional health status and reduce the risk for all-cause mortality[135]
Reduce sodium intake to < 100 mmol/day	1. Sodium intake is positively correlated with BP[136] 2. A reduction of 75–100 mmol in sodium intake lowers BP over periods of weeks to a few years[137]
Maintain adequate intake of dietary potassium (approximately 90 mmol/day)	1. High dietary potassium intake may improve BP control in patients with hypertension[138]
Stop smoking	1. A significant rise in BP accompanies the smoking of each cigarette[139]

BP, blood pressure

hyperlipidemia in their patients with heart failure. For many patients, achieving these goals will require the use of lipid-lowering medications. Non-pharmacologic management includes encouraging well-nourished heart failure patients to follow a low fat diet in which less than 30% of the total calories should come from fat. Basic information for following a low fat diet includes educating patients to consume lean meats, low fat dairy products, and to avoid fried foods and added fat such as margarine, butter, oils, and salad dressings with a high fat content. Using fats such as omega-3 rich foods (flax seed, salmon, cod) and monounsaturated fats (olive oil, canola oil) may help decrease serum cholesterol and triglycerides.[91] The goal for triglyceride levels is < 200 mg/dl. Patients can avoid table sugar and desserts high in sugar to help maintain normal triglyceride levels.

Obesity

Obesity, defined as a BMI $\geq$ 30 kg/m^2,[40] is an independent risk factor for the development of ischemic heart disease. Obesity also is associated with multiple other cardiovascular risk factors including hypertension, diabetes and hyperlipidemia.[92] Obesity increases oxygen demand, resulting in an initial increase in the cardiac output. This adaptive response is achieved by myocardial dilation and thickening. Left ventricular hypertrophy, an important risk factor for heart failure, is evident in about 50% of patients who are more than 50% overweight.[93,94] Weight reduction can produce several beneficial effects for heart failure patients: reduced mean arterial pressure and left ventricular mass,[95] along with decreased plasma norepinephrine level, plasma renin activity and aldosterone levels.[96]

Recent evidence from observational studies showed that patients with heart failure who are obese have better one and two-year survival rates than patients who are normal or underweight. Although this calls into question the beneficial role of weight loss in heart failure, recommendations that patients remain obese rather than lose weight awaits the results of randomized, controlled trials. The current goal for heart failure patients who are overweight (BMI > 25 kg/m^2) is a weight loss of 5–10%.[97] Although this level of weight loss may seem inconsequential, it has been shown to improve outcomes and is achievable for many patients who might otherwise be overwhelmed by the prospect of losing larger quantities of weight. A weight loss program to achieve a 5–10% weight loss may help relieve heart failure symptoms while maintaining lean body mass. Options for achieving weight loss include diet, exercise, behavior modification and drug therapy. These management strategies must be used in combination

125

because any one alone is likely to be extremely ineffective. For example, dietary restriction alone although effective in the short term is associated with an extremely high recidivism rate.[96] Similarly, long-term results from behavioral modification alone are discouraging with less than 5% of subjects maintaining their weight loss.[98] The combination of diet and exercise produces the most encouraging results.[99] The use of medication to treat obesity has not been well studied in patients with heart failure and medication should only be considered following a careful weighing of risk, benefits and other available treatment options.

Smoking

Smoking has multiple hemodynamic effects that produce adverse cardiovascular consequences. In general, smoking results in increases in heart rate and blood pressure with consequent increases in myocardial oxygen consumption.[100] In patients with ischemic heart disease and angina, stroke index decreases after smoking, most likely due to the negative inotropic effects of increased carboxyhemoglobin levels.[101] Smoking also increases left ventricular end-diastolic pressure.[101] In patients with heart failure, smoking increases heart rate, blood pressure, pulmonary artery pressure, ventricular filling pressures, and systemic and pulmonary vascular resistance.[102] These hemodynamic changes result in decreased stroke volume and increased afterload.[102] Smoking also damages the cardiovascular system by producing endothelial dysfunction, coagulation defects including increased coagulation and platelet dysfunction, and vasoconstriction.[100]

As a consequence of these effects, smoking is a major risk factor for ischemic heart disease and is associated with increased risk for heart failure.[103–105] Patients who already have ischemic heart disease and who smoke are at increased risk for heart failure.[106] In one study of patients with ischemic heart disease, smokers had a 50% increased risk for heart failure compared to non-smokers.[107] Furthermore, prognosis is improved in patients who stop smoking.[107] Evidence from the SOLVD prevention and treatment trials clearly demonstrates that heart failure patients who are current smokers are at markedly increased risk, independent of other risk factors, for recurrent heart failure, myocardial infarction and death compared to non-smokers and those who have quit smoking.[108] Perhaps the most striking finding from this study was that quitting smoking reduced patients' high morbidity and mortality risk in less than 2 years and that the magnitude of risk reduction was similar to or greater than that seen with many common drug therapies in heart failure.

Thus, existing evidence strongly underscores the importance of smoking cessation in patients with heart failure. Clinicians have not emphasized smoking cessation among patients with heart failure; less than 12% of heart failure patients receive advice to stop smoking.[109,110] But, as the findings from SOLVD demonstrate, 'smoking cessation in heart failure ... is never too late' (p. 1683, ref[111]). Therefore, all patients with heart failure should be advised strongly to stop smoking and should be informed that continued smoking is associated with poorer outcomes. Although many health care providers profess frustration at patients' lack of compliance with their suggestions to stop smoking, the evidence is that adherence to this aspect of care is as good as or better than adherence to angiotensin-converting enzyme inhibitor prescription.[111]

Several approaches to smoking cessation have been tested in cardiac patients (although none specifically in patients with heart failure) including nicotine replacement using the patch, behavioral counseling, and simple advice and encouragement from a health care provider.[112–116] The nicotine patch has been shown to be safe in cardiac patients and to be effective for smoking abstinence, at least in the short term.[115–117] Behavioral counseling in cardiac patients has shown equivocal results. In two studies, nurse-delivered therapies were effective in reducing some unhealthy behaviors, such as reducing dietary fat intake and increasing exercise, but showed little effect on smoking cessation.[112,113] A third study showed that a nurse-delivered smoking cessation intervention including 3 months of telephone follow-up increased self-reported smoking cessation by 15% compared with controls.[114]

Other interventions that warrant investigation in patients with heart failure include the use of antidepressants, which have shown promise in healthy smokers.[118–120] Antidepressants along with cognitive behavioral therapy have been associated with longer abstinence rates,[118] particularly in patients with mild depression. Because depression is common among smokers and patients with heart failure, the use of antidepressants alone or in combination with nicotine replacement therapies may hold particular promise.

An acute exacerbation or new diagnosis represents a key opportunity for health care providers to initiate smoking cessation measures because patients may be more receptive to making a decision to stop smoking under these circumstances.[121] Among a group of hospitalized ischemic heart disease patients,[121] 6-month and 12-month cessation rates of more than 30% and 25%, respectively, were reported. In this group, smoking cessation was more likely if patients had no prior history of heart disease and had heart failure during hospitalization.[121]

Finally, clinicians should be particularly aware of how powerful their advice to stop smoking can be. Following personal advice and encouragement to stop smoking given by physicians during a single routine consultation, an estimated 2% of all smokers stopped smoking and did not relapse up to 1 year.[122] Advice and encouragement may be most effective for smokers at special risk.[122] In fact, physician advice and encouragement is as effective as behavior modifications techniques in achieving smoking cessation.[122] Therefore, all clinicians should take time to advise their patients who smoke to quit. The patient's plans for quitting should be discussed and additional support, including nicotine replacement, should be considered. Given the overall low success rates for long-term (1-year) smoking cessation, it is imperative that clinicians re-evaluate their patients' smoking habits periodically in these high risk patients.[122]

Lack of exercise

There is no direct evidence that sedentary life style contributes to the development of heart failure. However, it is an important risk factor for the development of ischemic heart disease and it likely contributes to the progression of heart failure and the worsening of functional status in patients with existing heart failure. A number of randomized trials have demonstrated that both in-hospital and home exercise training programs are associated with positive clinical outcomes, including increased exercise capacity, decreased resting catecholamines, and improved heart rate variability and quality of life.[123–125] Additional studies have shown various exercise regimens, including walking or stationary bicycle riding, to be safe in patients with compensated heart failure and in elderly heart failure patients.[126,127]

Whether heart failure patients are instructed to exercise and to remain physically active is unclear. Many specialists now recommend regular, progressive exercise for patients with compensated heart failure and cardiac rehabilitation for heart failure patients after an acute event is included in national guidelines.[128] However, no more than 40% of all cardiac patients are referred for training[129] and the percentage of patients with heart failure referred for cardiac rehabilitation is likely even lower. This is unfortunate because heart failure patients often face considerable difficulty increasing or maintaining their activity levels due to deconditioning and it is this type of patient who may have the most to gain from cardiac rehabilitations. Guidance for helping patients with heart failure increase their activity level and maintain increased activity can be found in Chapter 10.

Summary

In the past 15 years, heart failure has emerged as a significant public health threat with adverse consequences for individual patients and for society. As our population ages, the incidence and prevalence of heart failure will increase in the US and worldwide, and its impact will worsen dramatically. As a consequence, it is crucial that we continue to work to determine optimal pharmacologic and non-pharmacologic methods of managing heart failure. The role of non-pharmacologic intervention in the management of patients with heart failure has received considerably less attention than that of pharmacologic therapy. The many effective non-pharmacologic strategies described in this chapter should be considered by all practitioners as important adjuncts to pharmacologic therapy. Indeed, pharmacologic therapy is less effective if not supplemented with non-pharmacologic strategies. Optimal management of heart failure demands that clinicians understand and use non-pharmacologic therapy in balance with pharmacologic therapy.

References

1 Poole-Wilson PA. Relation of pathophysiologic mechanisms to outcome in heart failure. *J Am Coll Cardiol* 1993; **22(4 suppl A):** 22A–29A.

2 CONSENSUS Trial Study Group. Effects of enalapril on mortality in severe congestive heart failure, results of the Cooperative North Scandinavian Enalapril Survival Study (CONSENSUS). *N Engl J Med* 1987; **316:** 1429–35.

3 The SOLVD Investigators. Effect of enalapril on survival in patients with reduced left ventricular ejection fraction and congestive heart failure. *N Engl J Med* 1991; **325:** 293–302.

4 Garg R, Yusuf S. Overview of randomized trials of angiotensin-converting enzyme inhibitors on mortality and morbidity in patients with heart failure. Collaborative Group on ACE Inhibitor Trials. *JAMA* 1995; **273:** 1450–6.

5 Hjalmarson, A, Goldstein S, Fagerberg B et al. Effects of controlled-release metoprolol on total mortality, hospitalizations, and well-being in patients with heart

failure: the Metoprolol CR/XL Randomized Intervention Trial in congestive heart failure (MERIT-HF). *JAMA* 2000; **283:** 1295–302.

6   Packer M, Bristow M, Cohn J et al. The effect of carvedilol on morbidity and mortality in patients with chronic heart failure. *New Engl J Med* 1996; **334:** 1349–55.

7   Pitt B, Zannad F, Remme W et al. The effect of spironolactone on morbidity and mortality in patients with severe heart failure. *New Engl J Med* 1999; **341:** 709–17.

8   Volpe M, Tritto C, DeLuca N et al. Abnormalities of sodium handling and of cardiovascular adaptations during high salt diet in patients with mild heart failure. *Circulation* 1993; **88(part 1):** 1620–27.

9   Cody RJ, Pickworth KK. Approaches to diuretic therapy and electrolyte imbalance in congestive heart failure. *Cardiol Clin* 1994; **12:** 37–50.

10 Kramer BK, Schweda F, Riegger GA et al. Diuretic treatment and diuretic resistance in heart failure. *Am J Med* 1999; **106:** 90–6.

11 Tang WHW, Francis GS. Polypharmacy of heart failure. Creating a rational pharmocotherapeutic protocol. *Cardiol Clin* 2001; **19:** 583–96.

12 Bennett SJ, Huster GA, Baker SL et al. Characterization of the precipitants of hospitalization for heart failure decompensation. *Am J Crit Care* 1998; **7:** 168–74.

13 Opasich C, Rapezzi C, Lucci D, Gorini M, Pozzar F et al, on behalf of the Italian Network on Congestive Heart Failure (IN-CHF) Investigators. Precipitating factors and decision-making processes of short-term worsening heart failure despite 'optimal' treatment. *Am J Cardiol* 2001; **88:** 382–7.

14 Tsuyuki RT, McKelvie RS, Arnold JMO et al. Acute precipitation of congestive heart failure exacerbations. *Arch Int Med* 2001; **161:** 2337–43.

15 Michalsen A, Konig G, Thimme W. Preventable causative factors leading to hospital admission with decompensated heart failure. *Heart* 1998; **80:** 437–41.

16 Ghali JK, Kadakia S, Cooper R, Ferlinz J. Precipitating factors leading to decompensation of heart failure. Traits among urban blacks. *Arch Intern Med* 1988; **148:** 2013–16.

17 Vinson JM, Rich MW, Sperry JC, Shah AS, McNamara T. Early readmission of elderly patients with congestive heart failure. *J Am Geriatr Soc* 1990; **38:** 1290–5.

18 Horan M, Barrett F, Mulqueen M, Maurer B, Quigley P, McDonald KM. The basics of heart failure management: are they being ignored? *Eur Heart J* 2000; **2:** 101–5.

19 Ni H, Nauman D, Burgess D, Wise K, Crispell K, Hershberger R. Factors influencing knowledge of and adherence to self-care among patients with heart failure. *Arch Intern Med* 1999; **159:** 1613–19.

20 Neily JB, Toto KH, Gardner EB, Rame JE, Yancy CW et al. Potential contributing factors to noncompliance with dietary sodium restriction in patients with heart failure. *Am Heart J* 2002; **143:** 29–33.

21 Carlson B, Riegel B, Moser DK. Self-care abilities of patients with heart failure. *Heart Lung* 2001; **30:** 351–9.

22 Dracup K, Baker DW, Dunbar SB et al. Management of heart failure. II. Counseling, education, and lifestyle modifications. *JAMA* 1994; **272:** 1442.

23 Grady KL, Dracup K, Kennedy G et al. Team management of patients with heart failure. A statement for healthcare professionals from the Cardiovascular Nursing Council of the American Heart Association. *Circulation* 2000; **102:** 2443–56.

24 Konstam M, Dracup K, Baker D et al. Heart failure: evaluation and care of patients with left-ventricular systolic dysfunction. Clinical Practice Guideline No. 11. AHCPR Publication No. 94–0612. Rockville, MD: Agency for Health Care Policy and Research, Public Health Services, U.S. Department of Health and Human Services; 1994.

25 Marcantonio ER, McKean S, Goldfinger M et al. Factors associated with unplanned hospital readmission among patients 65 years of age and older in a Medicare-managed care program. *Am J Med* 1999; **107:** 13–17.

26 Luft FC, Morris CD, Weinberger MH. Compliance to the low-salt diet. *Am J Clin Nutr* 1997; **65(suppl):** 698S–703S.

27 Rich MW. Heart failure disease management: a critical review. *J Card Fail* 1999; **5:** 64–75.

28 Moser DK. Heart failure management: optimal health care delivery programs. *Ann Rev Nurs Res* 2000; **18:** 91–126.

29 Krumholz HM, Amatruda J, Smith GL et al. Randomized trial of an education and support intervention to prevent readmission of patients with heart failure. *J Am Coll Cardiol* 2002; **39:** 83–9.

30 Dunbar SB, Jacobson LH, Deaton C. Heart failure: strategies to enhance patient self-management. *AACN Clin Issues* 1998; **9:** 244–56.

31 Cohen SJ, Weinberger MH, Fineberg NS et al. The effect of a household partner and home urine monitoring on adherence to a sodium restricted diet. *Soc Sci Med* 1991; **32:** 1057–61.

32 Piano MR. Alcohol and heart failure. *J Card Fail* 2002; **8:** 239–46.

33 Walsh Cr, Larson MG, Evans JC et al. Alcohol consumption and risk for congestive heart failure in the Framingham heart study. *Ann Intern Med* 2002; **136:** 181–91.

34 Abramson JL, Wiliams SA, Krumholz HM, Vaccarino V. Moderate alcohol consumption and risk of heart failure among older persons. *JAMA* 2001; **285:** 1971–7.

35 Cooper HA, Exner DV, Domanski MJ. Light-to-moderate alcohol consumption and prognosis in patients with left ventricular dysfunction. *J Am Coll Cardiol* 2000; **35:** 1753–9.

36 Molgard H, Kristensen BO, Baandrup U. Importance of abstinence from alcohol in alcoholic heart disease. *Int J Cardiol* 1990; **26:** 373–5.

37 Fauchier L, Babuty D, Poret P et al. Comparison of long-term outcome of alcoholic and idiopathic cardiomyopathy. *Eur Heart J* 2000; **21:** 306–14.

38 Gavazzi A, De-Maria R, Parolini M, Porcu M. Alcohol abuse and dilated cardiomyopathy in men. *Am J Cardiol* 2000; **85:** 1114–18.

39 Riegel B, Carlson B. Facilitators and barriers to heart failure self care. *Pat Educat Counsel* 2002; **46:** 287–95.

40 Anker SD, Coats AJS. Cachexia in heart failure is bad for you. *Eur Heart J* 1998; **19:** 191–3.

41 Anker SD, Coats AJS. Cardiac cachexia: a syndrome with impaired survival and immune and neuroendocrine activation. *Chest* 1999; **115:** 836–47.

42 Anker SD, Ponikowski P, Varney S et al. Wasting as independent risk factor for mortality in chronic heart failure. *Lancet* 1997; **349:** 1050–3.

43 Freeman LM, Roubenoff R. The nutrition implications of cardiac cachexia. *Nutrition Reviews* 1994; **52:** 340–7.

44 Carr JG, Stevenson LW, Walden JA et al. Prevalence and hemodynamic correlates of malnutrition in severe congestive heart failure secondary to ischemic or idiopathic dilated cardiomyopathy. *Am J Cardiol* 1989; **63:** 709–13.

45 Schwengel RH, Gottlieb SS, Fisher ML. Protein-energy malnutrition in patients with ischemic and nonischemic dilated cardiomyopathy and congestive heart failure. *Am J Cardiol* 1994; **73:** 908–10.

46 Morley JE, Thomas DR, Kamel H. Nutritional deficiencies in long-term care. Part I. Detection and diagnosis. *Ann Long-Term Care* 2002; **6:** http://www.mmhc.com/nhm/v6n5.shtml, accessed 6-28-2002.

47 Morrison WL, Edwards RHT. Cardiac cachexia. *BMJ* 1991; **302:** 301–2.

48 Cederholm T, Jagren C, Hellstrom K. Outcome of protein-energy malnutrition in elderly medical patients. *Am J Med* 1995; **98:** 67–74.

49 Berry C, Clark AL. Catabolism in chronic heart failure. *Eur Heart J* 2000; **21:** 521–32.

50 MacIntosh C, Morley JE, Chapman IM. The anorexia of aging. *Nutrition* 2000; **16:** 983–95.

51 Anker SD, Chua TP, Ponikowski P et al. Hormonal changes and catabolic/anabolic imbalance in chronic heart failure and their importance for cardiac cachexia. *Circulation* 197; **96:** 526–34.

52 Zhao S-H, Zeng L-H. Elevated levels of tumor necrosis factor in chronic heart failure with cachexia. *Int J Cardiol* 1997; **58:** 257–61.

53 Baig MK, Mahon N, McKenna WJ et al. The pathophysiology of advanced heart failure. *Am Heart J* 1998; **I35:** S216–S230.

54 Dutka DP, Elborn JS, Delamere F et al. Tumor necrosis factor α in severe congestive cardiac failure. *Br Heart J* 1993; **70:** 141–3.

55 Marcus EL, Berry EM. Refusal to eat in the elderly. *Nutr Rev* 1998; **56:** 163–71.

56 Kutchai HC. Gastrointestinal secretions. In: Berne RM, Levy MN (eds). *Physiology* St. Louis: Mosby, 1993: 652–687.

57 Ballinger A, McLoughlin L, Medbak S, Clark M. Cholecystokinin in a satiety hormone in humans at physiological post-prandial plasma concentrations. *Clin Sci* 1995; **89:** 375–81.

58 Demling RH, DeSanti L. Effect of a catabolic state with involuntary weight loss on acute and chronic respiratory disease. Medscape, 2002; http://www.medscape.com/viewprogram/1816, accessed 6-28-2002.

59 Bennett SJ, Hackward L, Blackburn SA. Nutritional management of the patient with heart failure. In: Moser DK, Riegel B (eds). *Improving Outcomes in Heart Failure: an Interdisciplinary Approach*. Gaithersburg: Aspen Publishing, 2001.

60 Evans WJ. Aging and malnutrition: treatment guidelines. *Medscape*, 2001; http://www.medscape.com/viewprogram/715, accessed 6-28-2002.

61 Beers MH, Berkow R. Nutrition: general considerations. Nutrition in clinical medicine. In: Beers MH, Berkow R (eds). *The Merck Manual of Diagnosis and Therapy*, 17th edn. 1999. http://www.merck.com/pubs/mmanual/section1/chapter1/1b.htm.

62 Dudek SG. Assessing nutritional status. *Nutrition Handbook for Nursing Practice*, 3rd edn. Philadelphia: Lippincott, 1997: 228–61.

63 Beck FK, Rosenthal TC. Prealbumin: a marker for nutritional evaluation. *Am Fam Physician* 2002; **65:** 1575–8.

64 Prealbumin in Nutritional Care Consensus Group, Measurement of visceral protein status in assessing protein and energy malnutrition: standard of care. *Nutrition* 1995; **11:** 169–71.

65 Olin AO, Osterberg P, Hadell K et al. Energy-enriched hospital food to improve energy intake in elderly patients. *J Parenter Enteral Nutr* 1966; **20:** 93–7.

66 Beckoff K, MacIntosh CG, Chapman IM et al. Effects of glucose supplementation on gastric emptying, blood glucose homeostasis, and appetite in the elderly. *Am J Physiol Regul Integr Comp Physiol* 2001; **280:** R570–R576.

67 Paccagnella A, Calò MA, Caenaro G et al. Cardiac cachexia: preoperative and postoperative nutrition management. *J Parenteral Enteral Nutrition* 1994; **18:** 409.

68 Broqvist M, Arnqvist H, Dahlström U et al. Nutritional assessment and muscle energy metabolism in severe chronic congestive heart failure – effects of long-term dietary supplementation. *Eur Heart J* 1994; **15:** 1641–50.

69 Zeigler TR, Leader LM, Jonas CR et al. Adjunctive therapies in nutritional support. *Nutrition* 1997; **13(Suppl):** 64S–72S.

70 Freeman LM, Rush JE, Kahayias JJ et al. Nutritional alterations and the effect of fish oil supplementation in

dogs with heart failure. *J Vet Intern Med* 1998; **12:** 440–8.

71 McCarty MF. Fish oil and other nutritional adjuvants for treatment of congestive heart failure. *Med Hypotheses* 1996; **46:** 400–6.

72 Adigun AQ, Ajayi AAL. The effects of enalapril–digoxin–diuretic combination therapy on nutritional and anthropometric indices in chronic congestive heart failure: preliminary findings in cardiac cachexia. *Eur J Heart Fail* 2001; **3:** 359–63.

73 Leslie D, Gheorghiade M. Is there a role for thiamine supplementation in the management of heart failure? *Am Heart J* 1996; **131:** 1248–50.

74 Seligmann H, Halkin H, Rauchfleisch S et al. Thiamine deficiency in patients with congestive heart failure receiving long-term furosemide therapy: a pilot study. *Am J Med* 1991; **91:** 151–5.

75 Shimon I, Almog S, Vered Z et al. Improved left ventricular function after thiamine supplementation in patients with congestive heart failure receiving long-term furosemide therapy. *Am J Med* 1995; **98:** 485–90.

76 Levy WC, Soine LA, Huth MM et al. Thiamine deficiency in congestive heart failure [letter]. *Am J Med* 1992; **93:** 705–6.

77 Kwok T, Falconer-Smith JF, Potter JF et al. Thiamine status of elderly patients with cardiac failure. *Age Aging* 1992; **21:** 67.

78 Bourassa MG, Gurne O, Bandiwala SI et al. Natural history and patterns of current practice in heart failure. *J Am Coll Cardiol* 1993; **22(suppl A):** 14A–19A.

79 He J, Ogden LG, Bazzano LA et al. Risk factors for congestive heart failure in US men and women. *Arch Intern Med* 2001; **161:** 996–1002.

80 Levy D, Larson MG, Vasan RS et al. The progression from hypertension to congestive heart failure. *JAMA* 1996; **275:** 1557–62.

81 Kannel WB. Vital epidemiologic clues in heart failure. *J Clin Epid* 2000; **53:** 229–35.

82 National High Blood Pressure Education Program. The Sixth Report of the Joint National Committee on Prevention, Detection, Evaluation, and Treatment of High Blood Pressure. National Heart, Lung, and Blood Institute. Bethesda, MD: U.S. Department of Health and Human Services, 1997.

83 National High Blood Pressure Education Program Working Group. Report on hypertension in diabetes. National Heart, Lung and Blood Institute. Bethesda, MD: Department of Health and Human Services, 1995.

84 Kannel WB, Castelli WP, Gordon T. Cholesterol in the prediction of atherosclerotic disease: new perspectives based on the Framingham study. *Ann Intern Med* 1979; **90:** 85–91.

85 Scandinavian Simvastatin Survival Study Group. Randomized trial of cholesterol lowering in 4444 patients with coronary heart disease. The Scandinavian Simvastatin Survival Study (4S). *Lancet* 1994; **44:** 1383–9.

86 Sacks FM, Pfeffer MA, Moye L et al. The effect of pravastatin on coronary events after myocardial infarction in patients with average cholesterol levels. *N Engl J Med* 1996; **335:** 1001–9.

87 Tonkin AM. Management of the long-term intervention with pravastatin in ischaemic disease (LIPID) study after the Scandinavian Simvastatin Survival Study (4S). *Am J Cardiol* 1995; **76:** 107C–112C.

88 Shepard J, Cobbe SM, Ford I et al. Prevention of coronary heart disease with pravastatin in men with hypercholesterolemia. *N Engl J Med* 1995; **333:** 1301–7.

89 Kjekshus J, Pederson TR, Olsson AG, Faergeman O, Pyorala K. The effects of simvastatin on the incidence of heart failure in patients with coronary heart disease. *J Card Failure* 1997; **3:** 249–54.

90 National Institutes of Health National Cholesterol Education Program (NCEP) ATP-II Guidelines: Summary of the Second Report of the NCEDP Expert Panel on Detection, Evaluation, and Treatment of High Blood Cholesterol in Adults (Adult Treatment Panel II). *JAMA* 1993; **269:** 3015–23.

91 Ney DM. The cardiovascular system. In: Zeman FJ (edn). *Clinical nutrition and dietetics*, 2nd edn. NY: Macmillan, 1991: 373.

92 National Institutes of Health Concensus Development Panel. Health implications of obesity. *Ann Intern Med* 1985; **103:** 147–51.

93 Messerli FH, Sundgaard-Riise, Eeisin ED et al. Dimorphic cardiac adaptation to obesity and arterial hypertension. *Ann Intern Med* 1983; **99:** 757–61.

94 Reisin E, Frohlich ED, Messerli FH et al. Cardiovascular changes after weight reduction in obesity hypertension. *Ann Intern Med* 1983; **98:** 315–19.

95 MacMahon SW, Wilcken DEL, MacDonald GJ. The effect of weight reduction on left ventricular mass. *N Engl J Med* 1986; **314:** 334–8.

96 Grodstein F, Levine R, Troy L et al. Three-year follow-up of participants in a commercial weight loss program: can you keep it off? *Arch Intern Med* 1996; **156:** 1302–6.

97 National Heart, Lung, and Blood Institute. Clinical Guidelines of the identification, evaluation, and treatment of overweight and obesity in adults: the evidence reports. Bethesda, MD: US Department of Health, 1998.

98 Kramer FM, Jeffrey RW, Forster HI, Sell MK. Long-term follow-up of behavioral treatment for obesity: patterns of weight regain among men and women. *Int J Obes* 1989; **13:** 123–36.

99 Tremblay A, Despres JP, Maheux J et al. Normalization of the metabolic profile in obese women by exercise and a low fat diet. *Med Sci Sports Exer* 1991; **23:** 1326–31.

100 Rabinowitz BD, Thorp K, Huber GL et al. Acute hemodynamic effects of cigarette smoking in man assessed by systolic time intervals and echocardiography. *Circulation* 1979; **60:** 752–760.

101 Aronow WS, Cassidy J, Vangrow JS et al. Effect of cigarette smoking and breathing carbon monoxide on cardiovascular hemodynamics in anginal patients. *Circulation* 1974; **50:** 340–7.

102 Nicolozakes AW, Binkley PF, Leier CV. Hemodynamic effects of smoking in congestive heart failure. *Am J Med Sci* 1988; **296:** 377–80.

103 Doll R, Peto R. Mortality in relation to smoking: twenty years observations on male British doctors. *BMJ* 1979; **ii:** 1525–36.

104 Kannel WB, Sorlie P, McNamara PM. Prognosis after initial myocardial infarction: the Framingham study. *Am J Cardiol* 1979; **44:** 53–9.

105 Eriksson H, Svardsudd K, Larsson B et al. Risk factors for heart failure in the general population: the study of men born in 1913. *Eur Heart J* 1989; **10:** 647–56.

106 Salonen JT. Stopping smoking and long-term mortality after acute myocardial infarction. *Br Heart J* 1980; **43:** 463–9.

107 Herlitz J, Bengtson A, Hjalmarson A, Karlson BW. Smoking habits in consecutive patients with acute myocardial infarction: prognosis in relation to other risk indicators and to whether or not they quit smoking. *Cardiology* 1995; **86:** 496–502.

108 Suskin N, Sheth T, Negassa A, Yusuf S. Relationship of current and past smoking to mortality and morbidity in patients with left ventricular dysfunction. *J Am Coll Cardiol* 2001; **37:** 1677–82.

109 Nohria A, Chen YT, Morton DJ, Walsh R, Vlasses PH, Krumholz HM. Quality of care for patients hospitalized with heart failure at academic medical centers. *Amer Heart J* 1999; **137:** 1028–34.

110 Krumholz HM, Wang Y, Paent EM, Mockalis J, Petrillo M, Radford MJ. Quality of care for elderly patients hospitalized with heart failure. *Arch Int Med* 1997; **157:** 2242–7.

111 Lightwood J, Fleischmann KE, Glantz SA. Smoking cessation in heart failure: it is never too late. *J Am Coll Cardiol* 2001; **37:** 1683–4.

112 Steptoe A, Doherty S, Rink E, Kerry S, Kendrick T, Hilton S. Behavioral counseling in general practice for the promotion of healthy behavior among adults at increased risk of coronary heart disease: randomised trial. *Br Heart J* 1999; **319:** 943–7.

113 Toobert DJ, Glasgow RE, Nettekoven LA, Brown JE. Behavioral and psychosocial effects of intensive lifestyle management for women with coronary heart disease. *Patient Education Counseling* 1998; **35:** 177–88.

114 Johnson JL, Budgz B, Mackay M, Miller C. Evaluation of a nurse-delivered smoking cessation intervention for hospitalized patients with cardiac disease. *Heart Lung* 1999; **28:** 55–64.

115 Tzivoni D, Keren A, Meyler S, Khoury Z, Lerer T, Brunel P. Cardiovascular safety of transdermal nicotine patches in patients with coronary artery disease who try to quit smoking. *Cardiovasc Drugs Therapy* 1998; **12:** 239–44.

116 Joseph AM, Morman SM, Ferry LH, Prochazha AV, Westman EC et al. The safety of transdermal nicotine as an aid to smoking cessation in patients with cardiac disease. *N Engl J Med* 1996; **335:** 1792–8.

117 Zevin S, Jacob P III, Benowitz NL. Dose-related cardiovascular and endocrine effects of transdermal nicotine. *Clin Pharm Therapeutics* 1998; **64:** 87–95.

118 Hitsman B, Pingitore R, Spring B, Mahableshwarkar A, Mizes JS et al. Antidepressant pharmacotherapy helps some cigarette smokers more than others. *J Consulting Clin Psych* 1999; **67:** 547–54.

119 Jarenby DE, Leschow SJ, Nides MA, Rennard SI, Johnston JA et al. A controlled trial of sustained-release bupropion, a nicotine patch or both for smoking cessation. *N Engl J Med* 1999; **340:** 685–91.

120 Hurt RD, Sachs DP, Glover ED, Offord KP, Johnston JA et al. A comparison of sustained-release bupropion and placebo for smoking cessation. *N Engl J Med* 1997; **337:** 1195–202.

121 Rigotti NA, Singer DE, Mulley AG, Thibault GE. Smoking cessation following admission to a coronary care unit. *J Gen Intern Med* 1991; **6:** 305–11.

122 Law M, Tang JL. An analysis of the effectiveness of interventions intended to help people stop smoking. *Arch Int Med* 1995; **155:** 1933–41.

123 Sullivan MJ, Higginbotham MB, Cobb FR. Exercise training in patients with severe left ventricular dysfunction: hemodynamic and metabolic effects. *Circulation* 1988; **78:** 506–15.

124 European Heart Failure Training Group. Experience from controlled trials of physical training in chronic heart failure: protocol and patient factors in effectiveness in the improvement in exercise tolerance. *Eur Heart J* 1998; **19:** 466–75.

125 Belardinelli R, Georgiou D, Cianci G, Purcaro A. Randomized, controlled trial of long-term moderate exercise training in chronic heart failure: effects on functional capacity, quality of life, and clinical outcome. *Circulation* 1999; **99:** 1173–82.

126 Gottlieb SS, Fisher ML, Freudenberger R et al. Effects of exercise training on peak performance and quality of life in congestive heart failure patients. *J Cardiac Failure* 1999; **5:** 188–94.

127 Keteyian SJ, Levine AB, Brawner CA et al. Exercise training in patients with heart failure: a randomized, controlled trial. *Ann Intern Med* 1996; **124:** 1051–7.

128 Wenger NK, Froelicher ES, Smith LK et al. Cardiac rehabilitation as secondary prevention. Agency for Health Care Policy and Research and National Heart, Lung, and Blood Institute. Clinical Practice Guideline. Quick Reference Guide for Clinicians, 1995; **17:** 1–23.

129 Mark D, Naylor CD, Hlatky MA et al. Use of medical resources and quality of life after acute myocardial infarction in Canada and the United States. *N Engl J Med* 1994; **331:** 1130–5.

130 National Kidney Foundation. Appendix VII. Methods for performing anthropometry and calculating body measurements and references tables. 2000;

http://www.kidney.org/professionals/doqi/
guidelines/nut_appx07a.html , accessed 7–1–2002.

131 Lennie TA. Anorexia in response to acute illness. *Heart Lung* 1999; **28:** 386–401.

132 Trials of Hypertension Prevention Collaborative Research Group. Effects of wieght loss and sodium reduction intervention on blood pressure and hypertension incidence in overweight people with high-normal blood pressure: the Trials of Hypertension Prevention, phase II. *Arch Intern Med* 1997; **157:** 657–67.

133 Neaton JD, Grimm RH Jr, Prineas RJ et al, for the Treatment of Mild hypertension Study Research Group. Treatment of Mild Hypertension Study: final results. *JAMA* 1993; **270:** 713–24.

134 Puddey IB, Parker M, Beilen LJ, Vandongen R, Masarei JRL. Effects of alcohol and caloric restrictions on blood pressure and serum lipids in overweight men. *Hypertension* 1992; **20:** 533–41.

135 Paffenbarger RS Jr, Hyde RT, Wing AL, Lee IM, Jung DL, Kampert JB. The association of changes in physical activity level and other lifestyle characteristics with mortality among men. *N Engl J Med* 1993; **328:** 538–45.

136 Elliot P, Stamler J, Nichols R et al, for the Intersalt Cooperative Research Group. Intersalt revisited: further analyses of 24 hour sodium excretion and blood pressure within and across populations. *BMJ* 1996; **312:** 1249–53.

137 Cutler JA, Follmann D, Allender PS. Randomized trials of sodium reduction: an overview. *Am J Clin Nutr* 1997; **65(suppl):** 643S–651S.

138 Whelton PK, He J, Culter JA et al. Effects of oral potassium on blood pressure: meta-analysis of randomized controlled clinical trials. *JAMA* 1997; **277:** 1624–32.

139 Greenberg C, Thompson SG, Brennan PJ. The relationship between smoking and the response to antihypertensive treatment in mild hypertensives in the Medical Research Council's trial of treatment. *Int J Epidemiol* 1987; **16:** 25–30.

10 The role of exercise and activity in the management of heart failure

Cynthia D Adams

Activity intolerance is a hallmark symptom in heart failure and presents a frustrating and complicated problem not only for patients, but for the health care practitioners managing their care. Advances in pharmacologic treatment over recent years have demonstrated significant improvements in survival and quality of life for these patients. Non-pharmacologic interventions such as activity recommendations and patient education, on the other hand, often continue to reflect the beliefs of the early models of heart failure, and their potential additive effect on survival and quality of life are too often overlooked. The importance of the role of nursing in advancing knowledge and research in this area cannot be overstated. In order to appreciate the potential value of exercise as an adjunctive treatment, as well as to appreciate its avoidance until recent years, it is important to understand the historical progression of insight into the syndrome of heart failure.

Over the past few decades, there has been an evolution of theory explaining the underlying pathophysiology of heart failure. In a synopsis of the changes in the conceptual model of heart failure over the past 50 years, Packer highlights the paradigm shifts that have taken place with regard to the pathological processes and treatments associated with the syndrome.[1] In the early years, heart failure management was designed strictly to rid the body of excess water and attempt to strengthen the heartbeat. The underlying theory attributed symptoms to the underperfusion of the kidneys as a result of the failing heart. Bed rest was often prescribed to allow rest for the heart, and to promote diuresis in fluid overloaded patients by increasing venous return to the heart and subsequent enhancement of renal perfusion.[2] After the discovery of diuretics, it was clear that more explanation was needed to clarify the underlying pathology, as effective diuresis and symptom control had no effect on progression of heart failure and its staggering mortality rate.

The next accepted theory of heart failure pathology was founded upon hemodynamics. As measurement of hemodynamic profiles such as chamber pressures, cardiac output, preload, and afterload became more common,

attention shifted to reducing preload and afterload to optimize cardiac output. The use of vasodilators and inotropic agents emerged during this period. Again, it was clear that while pharmacologic management that targeted reduction of preload and afterload improved hemodynamic profiles, it had little impact on overall mortality.

In the late 1980s and early 1990s, the theory of neurohormonal activation was introduced. With identification of various hormonal pathways that are activated in heart failure and result in ventricular remodeling, vasoconstriction, and sodium and water retention, pharmacologic management has shifted to target these abnormalities. As a result of this evolutionary shift, other major advances have come to light that clarify the role of biochemical compensatory mechanisms resulting in increased norepinephrine levels, altered gene expression, downregulation of sympathetic receptor sites, impairment of oxidative capacity of skeletal muscle cells, and vascular remodeling.[2–5] Clinical trials testing the outcomes associated with interventions such as angiotensin-converting enzyme (ACE) inhibition and beta blockade have shown drastic reductions in heart failure-related mortality.[6] It is the acceptance of this theoretical model of heart failure pathology that opens the door for exploration of exercise as a valuable intervention in the management of this historically perplexing syndrome.

Review of exercise terminology

For readers other than exercise professionals, it may be useful to pause briefly to review common parameters involved with exercise testing and abnormalities therein specifically related to the heart failure population. Oxygen delivery and utilization by body tissues depends on several processes. These processes include diffusion capacity in the lung, transportation via circulation, peripheral perfusion and diffusion, and mitochondrial function in the cells.[7] Heart failure can disrupt normal oxygen delivery and utilization in a number of ways (Table 10.1). New York

Table 10.1. Mechanisms of impaired oxygen consumption in heart failure

Reduced cardiac output
- – decreased blood flow through pulmonary bed
- – decreased delivery of blood flow to tissues

Abnormal distribution of blood to exercising musculature
- – independent of decreased cardiac output

Impaired metabolism by muscle fibers
- – decreased mitochondrial density
- – decreased lipolytic oxidative enzymes
- – fiber atrophy

Chronotropic incompetence may contribute

Heart Association (NYHA) class I and II patients appear to an observer to have normal exercise capacity in terms of performance of their daily activities. However, testing reveals that they have an approximate 30% reduction in exercise capacity compared to their normal counterparts.[8] The mechanism believed to be responsible for this limitation is impaired cardiac output. NYHA class III and IV patients are limited in a much more dramatic way in their ability to perform daily activities. It is postulated that the limitation of activity tolerance in these individuals is a result of abnormal perfusion and distribution of blood flow to the exercising musculature.[9] The pathology of heart failure can affect oxygen utilization in other ways that will be discussed in more detail later in this chapter.

A widely accepted measure of cardiorespiratory endurance is the direct measure of peak oxygen uptake, or VO_2max (also known as MVO_2) during exercise of increasing intensity.[10] Studies have shown a strong correlation between VO_2max and survival in heart failure.[11] In addition to serving as a measure of functional status, VO_2max is utilized as an indicator for the appropriateness and timing of cardiac transplantation.[12,13] Peak oxygen consumption is the maximum amount of oxygen used while performing dynamic exercise involving a large portion of the total muscle mass.[10,14] For reporting purposes, VO_2max values are generally expressed relative to body weight in units of ml/kg/min. For clinically interpretive purposes, a VO_2max of less than or equal to 14 ml/kg/min is a predictor of poor survival, and the point at which cardiac transplantation, if other candidacy criteria are met, becomes an option.[15] VO_2max can be affected by

gender, age, physical condition, heredity, and cardiovascular disease. In general, women have a lower VO_2max than men, and there is an estimated decrease of 5–9% per decade of life. It is estimated that VO_2max decreases approximately 25% after 3 weeks of bed rest in healthy men.[14] It is important to note that while ejection fraction and pulmonary capillary wedge pressure are valuable measures in determining the degree of left ventricular dysfunction and prognosis, there is evidence documenting the lack of predictive value of these parameters with regard to VO_2max and heart failure symptoms.[15,16]

In exercise testing and cardiac rehabilitation arenas, oxygen uptake is also commonly expressed in terms of metabolic equivalents, or METs. One MET is representative of the oxygen uptake at rest, or about 3.5 ml/kg/min. A 2 miles per hour walk on a horizontal surface is equivalent to about 2.5 METs.[10] Activities of daily living require tolerance of exertional intensity at about 5 METs. Peak exercise maximal oxygen uptake of less than 5 METs is associated with poor prognosis. Thirteen METs at peak exercise is associated with excellent prognosis. METs of 18–20 are seen in elite and world class athletes.[14] Some examples of common activities and the corresponding MET levels are detailed in Table 10.2.

Direct measurement of peak oxygen consumption requires maximal exercise testing. This testing requires use of specific exercise equipment such as a treadmill or stationary bike, and laboratory equipment to perform expired gas

Table 10.2. ACSM's Resource Manual for Guidelines for Exercise Testing and Prescription[10]

METs associated with common activities	
Activity	METs
Sleeping	0.9
Rest – sitting quietly	1.0
Sexual activity – vigorous	1.5
Making bed	2.0
Walking 2 mph	2.5
Vacuuming	2.5
Showering/toweling dry	4.0
Mowing lawn (self-propelled push mower)	4.5
Grocery shopping with cart	3.5
Carrying groceries upstairs	8.0
Golf with cart	3.5
Jogging	7.0
Running – 9 min mile	11.0

analysis. Continuous ECG monitoring and respiratory gas analysis is used to determine oxygen consumption and overall response to exercise. This type of testing, while very valuable in clinical evaluation, requires costly equipment and specialized personnel to perform the procedure. Additionally, there is evidence in the literature suggesting that performance of activities of daily living may be better predicted by submaximal than peak exercise capacity.[17]

Alternatives to peak exercise testing that evaluate submaximal exercise capacity may yield helpful information in terms of evaluating overall functional status. Submaximal exercise testing is often utilized for patients who are considered to be at high risk for complications of maximal exercise testing. During this testing, patients are exercised to a predetermined level of exertion or heart rate which is considerably less than the targets in maximal testing. An appropriate target may be a heart rate of 120 beats per minute or 5 METs. The selected endpoints vary based upon clinical evaluation of the patient. This type of testing has been useful for recommending physical activity levels and risk stratification of patients after acute coronary events.[10]

It has been suggested that the six-minute walk test may provide accurate estimates of exercise capacity and short-term survival.[18] In comparison to peak exercise testing, it is available at a much lower cost, and places substantially less strain on the patient.[13,15,17,19,20] The six-minute walk test is a self-paced corridor walk during which patients are instructed to cover as much distance as possible during a timed six-minute interval. They walk at their pace of choice, and stop for rest periods if needed throughout the test. Duration of time and distance walked are recorded, as well as the rated perceived exertion. This test has not been shown to correlate closely with maximal testing, but appears to be a better indicator of functional capacity as defined as the ability to achieve activities of daily living.[13,15] Interestingly, it has been suggested that abnormalities limiting performance at maximal exercise intensity may differ from those affecting submaximal performance.[3]

There are also questionnaires that have been developed to estimate one's functional capacity based on self-reported ability to perform specific activities. One such instrument is the Duke Activity Status Index (DASI).[68] This questionnaire lists twelve activities ranging from self-care to participation in strenuous sports. Each item corresponds to a specific weighted score. The DASI score is the sum of the weighted values assigned to the activities that the patient is able to perform. The DASI score is then used in a formula that approximates the VO$_2$max (VO$_2$max = 0.43 × DASI

Table 10.3. *Common methods for estimating functional status*

Direct measurement of peak oxygen uptake (MVO$_2$)

Metabolic equivalents (METs) able to perform

Submaximal exercise testing

New York Heart Association classification

Six-minute walk test

Questionnaires
- Duke Activity Status Index
- Minnesota Living with Heart Failure Questionnaire
- SF 36, SF 12

+ 9.6).[10,68] Other questionnaires utilized in the evaluation of functional capacity are two measures of quality of life, the Minnesota Living with Heart Failure Questionnaire (MLHFQ)[21] and the Short Form (SF) 36.[22] The MLHFQ encompasses the domains of both physical and emotional function, and is specific to the heart failure population. The instrument has been heavily utilized in clinical trials (some of which will be discussed in this chapter). The SF 36 is a non-disease-specific instrument that is commonly used across many populations to determine functional status. It is readily available and widely used. Common methods utilized to estimate functional status are outlined in Table 10.3.

Other parameters have been utilized to estimate cardiopulmonary function and response to training. Heart rate and blood pressure responses are important components in interpretation of the exercise response. A significant drop in blood pressure (generally 10 mmHg or more) with increasing workload is abnormal and calls for termination of the test. In addition to VO$_2$max, the ventilatory or anaerobic threshold can be determined by expired gas analysis. This is the point during exercise at which lactate accumulation and anaerobic metabolism begins. This point has been associated with the onset of metabolic acidosis, hyperventilation, and reduced work capacity, and can be a useful parameter in evaluating interventions in exercise.[10] It has been clearly shown that ejection fraction alone lacks reliability as a predictor of functional capacity or survival.[7,11] A possible explanation lies in the premise that exercise capacity is the result of complex physiological interactions, making it impossible to be summated by the measurement of any single resting parameter.[3]

Contraindications to exercise

The American College of Sports Medicine (2000) specifies the following contraindications for cardiac rehabilitation: unstable angina; resting systolic blood pressure (BP) > 200 or diastolic BP > 110; symptomatic orthostatic drop in BP > 20 mmHg; critical aortic stenosis; acute illness or fever; uncontrolled arrhythmias; uncompensated heart failure; 3rd degree AV block in the absence of a pacemaker; active pericarditis or myocarditis; recent thrombophlebitis or embolism; resting ST segment displacement > 2 mm; blood glucose > 400 mg/dl; severe orthopedic conditions prohibiting exercise; or other acute metabolic conditions such as electrolyte abnormalities, volume contraction, or thyroid abnormalities.[10] It is important to keep these contraindications in mind when studying the impact of exercise on the heart failure population and in considering exercise and physical activity interventions in practice.

Studies highlighting the benefit of exercise in heart failure

While it is not within the scope of this chapter to detail all of the studies in the literature exploring the benefits of exercise in heart failure, a number of comprehensive reviews have been published.[9,23,24] The studies selected for discussion here are those that present classic, new or unique perspectives in this area.

Early studies

Work conducted by Sullivan et al at Duke University in the late 1980s broke ground in this field of study and suggested that heart failure patients (NYHA class I–III) could gain significant improvements in exercise capacity after 4–6 months of training.[25] The training program involved exercise training at 75% VO_2max for 60 minutes per session, 3–5 times weekly. The investigators found significant improvements in VO_2max, as well as an overall improvement in NYHA functional class. Cardiac output did increase at maximal exercise. Resting and submaximal heart rates were reduced. There were no significant changes found in measurable cardiac function or size after training. Also noted were increased blood flow and oxygen delivery to the leg, reduction in arterial and venous lactate production, and an increase in exercise time at the fixed submaximal work rate. Importantly, there were no reported exercise-related complications.[25] While this was important work in establishing the role of exercise in heart

failure as a sound research question, the number of subjects studied was very small (n = 12), and there was no control group studied.

Randomized, controlled studies

Several randomized, controlled trials (summarized in Table 10.4)[25–40] have been undertaken since the early studies were conducted. In the first, Coats et al studied 17 men with stable moderate to severe chronic heart failure.[26] A controlled crossover design was used to randomly assign subjects to begin in either the exercise or activity restriction phases. The researchers found significant increases in exercise tolerance and peak oxygen consumption in the exercise groups compared with controls. There was an increase in cardiac output at submaximal and peak exercise, as well as a reduction in systemic vascular resistance. Importantly, this study provided empirical evidence of enhanced vagal tone and reduction in sympathetic activity as a result of training in heart failure patients.

In similar randomized crossover trials, Meyer et al studied the benefit of interval training in 18 male patients. Interval training refers to short bouts of intense exercise alternating with frequent rest periods. Again, significant improvements in VO_2max were seen. An important observation in this work was that there was a rapid detraining effect that occurred in the restricted group after the crossover from the training phase. This study supported the value of interval training as opposed to continuous aerobic training, suggesting that desired improvements in training effects may be gained with less strain on the heart.[27–29]

Hambrecht et al randomized 73 male heart failure patients to 2 weeks of inpatient ergometer exercise for 10 minutes 4–6 times daily, followed by 6 months of home-based ergometer training for 20 minutes per day at 70% of VO_2max, vs control. They found statistically significant improvements in the training group in functional class, maximal ventilation, exercise time, and exercise capacity. Other observations included decreased resting heart rate, increased resting stroke volume, and decreased cardiomegaly.[31]

Quittan et al conducted a trial wherein 27 patients were randomized to exercise vs control. The exercise group performed aerobic training for 3 hours per week for 3 months. The control group continued their usual degree of activity through their normal daily living. The main outcome variable in this study was change in perceived quality of life. Significant improvements in quality of life (determined by the German version of the SF 36) were seen in the exercise group compared with control. While significant increases in peak oxygen uptake and exercise time were seen in the training group, there was weak correlation between the biological parameters and the perceived quality of life measures. The findings in this study suggest the importance of selecting outcome variables that measure the holistic impact of interventions from the patient perspective as opposed to a strictly biological/physiological model seen in many heart failure trials.[32]

Low intensity training

A number of studies have been designed to determine the impact of low to moderate intensity training on heart failure patients.[30,33–36] The premise here is that lower intensity training may result in benefit, while limiting the discomfort associated with higher intensity training (perhaps promoting compliance with the training program), and reducing the amount of wall stress to which the ventricle is subjected during training. Theoretical models of ventricular remodeling in heart failure suggest that increased wall stress (due to exercise or other factors) could worsen remodeling and contribute to disease progression.[9]

One of the first studies to focus on low intensity exercise was conducted by Kiilavuori et al. The randomized, controlled study randomized 27 subjects to treatment vs control. The treatment consisted of a 12-week supervised training program during which the treatment group performed cycle training at 50–60% of VO_2max, followed by 12 weeks of home-based exercise at the same intensity. While not statistically significant, there was a 12% increase in VO_2max in the training group. The authors conclude that the submaximal level of training in this study may have led to benefits that were underestimated by use of VO_2max. There was an increase in submaximal exercise endurance (88% improvement), which the authors suggest represents clinically significant data, because submaximal exercise capacity correlates better with the ability to achieve activities of daily living.[37]

Subsequent randomized trials have reinforced these findings, but with statistically significant improvements in VO_2max. Additionally, they have documented lower ventricular diastolic wall stress during lower intensity exercise when compared with conventional training programs.[33] Training programs in these studies involved exercise at 40–50% VO_2max for 30–60 minutes, 3–4 times weekly for durations of 8–12 weeks. Findings have suggested greater improvement in training parameters at 12 weeks than 6 weeks and have demonstrated reduction of norepi-

nephrine levels in the trained group as well as evidence of improved cellular oxidative capacity.[33,34]

More recently, Tokmakova et al randomized 22 male patients to exercise at 50% of VO_2max for 8 weeks vs control. They found statistically significant improvements in VO_2max, anaerobic threshold, and duration of exercise only in the trained group. Additionally, they found significant improvements in quality of life scores (by the Minnesota Living with Heart Failure Questionnaire) and perceived exertion (Borg dyspnea rating score) in the trained subjects.[35]

Sturm et al conducted a randomized, controlled trial evaluating exercise vs control. These researchers incorporated a graduated exercise program that progressed finally to 100 minutes per week of step aerobics and 50 minutes per week of cycling. Exercise intensity was limited to about 50% of VO_2max. They found significant increases in VO_2max in the trained group in comparison with control.[36]

Long term exercise

Kavanagh et al conducted a study that evaluated the impact of a training program extending over the course of a longer period (52 weeks). The study was non-randomized but included a control group for comparative purposes over the first 9-week period. Both submaximal and maximal exercise capacity improved in the subjects, as did quality of life, measured by the Chronic Heart Failure Questionnaire and the Standard Gamble measure. They also noted that the training effects achieved plateaued at 16–26 weeks into the training program. Although it was not a randomized trial, this study made a unique contribution in that it enabled some insight into the impact of longer-term training.[38]

Small muscle group training

Interestingly, studies focusing on conditioning of small muscle groups have shown promise. Various approaches have involved small peripheral muscle groups, as well as selective respiratory muscle training. The basis upon which these programs were constructed is the theoretical benefit of avoiding increased wall stress and lower work-load on the heart. These studies have shown improvement in exercise performance as well as quality of life scores, and bear further investigation.[39]

Maiorana et al published results of training effects utilizing an 8-week circuit weight training program in 13 heart failure patients. Outcome variables were cardiorespiratory fitness, muscular strength, and body composition.

Table 10.4. Clinical trials of exercise in heart failure. (Updated and modified with permission from Adams and Bennett, 2000.[24]).

Study	n	Design/subjects	Training program	Duration	Findings/comments
Sullivan et al, 1988[25]	12	Non-randomized, no control group; EF 9–33%	Cycle, walking, jogging, stair climbing 60 min. 3–5 X/week	16–24 weeks	Peak VO2 increased 23%
Coats et al, 1992[26]	17	Randomized; crossover; controlled; ischemic;	Home-based; bicycle 20 minutes 50 rpms) 5 X/week; 60–80% peak heart rate	8 weeks	Exercise time increased; peak VO_2 increased by 2.4 ml/min/kg; improved symptoms; reduced sympathetic tone
Belardinelli et al, 1995[34]	27	Matched groups by clinical and functional status; Mild CHF,	30 min. cycle at 40% peak VO_2; 3 X/week;	8 weeks	17% increase in peak VO_2; Improved anaerobic threshold; decreased norepinephrine levels; no serious adverse events
Kiilavuori et al, 1996[39]	27	Randomized; controlled; NYHA II–III EF < 40%.	30 min. 3 X/week, cycle 50–60% peak VO_2	12 weeks supervised; 12 weeks at home	NYHA 2.4–1.9 at 12 weeks 12% increase in peak VO_2 (NS); increased maximal achieved work load (p < 0.05); improvement in submaximal endurance and symptoms
Kavanagh et al, 1996[37]	21	Non-randomized; control with initial 9-week period; NYHA II–III.	Progressive aerobic walking through formal cardiac rehabilitation program; 50–60% peak VO_2	52 weeks	Improvement in peak VO_2, peak heart rate, anaerobic threshold; gains plateaued at 16–26 weeks; 10–15% improvement in six-minute walk test; improved quality of life
Meyer et al, 1996, 1997[27-29]	18	Random order crossover trial; hospitalized pa-EF 20–22%; All male subjects	Interval training program; cycle and treadmill walking at varied work/rest intervals; supervised program	3 weeks at each phase	Peak VO_2 increased 23.7%; decrease in aerobic capacity during the restricted phase occurs as quickly as training effect in the active phase
Demopoulos et al, 1997[32]	16	Non-randomized; no control group; NYHA II–IV	Low intensity cycle; < 50% peak VO_2; 1 hr/day; 4 X/week	12 weeks	22–30% increase in peak VO_2; study group includes NYHA IV; lower wall stress than more intense training regimens
Bellardinelli et al, 1999[30]	110	Randomized, controlled; stable CHF	Moderate intensity 60% peak); 3/week × 8 weeks then 2/week × 1 year	12 months	Improved peak VO_2 and thallium activity; improved quality of life and functional status
Quittan et al, 1999[32]	25	Randomized, controlled; EF 10–26%	Aerobic training 3 hours weekly	12 months	QOL (per SF 36) improved; increased MVO_2; increased exercise time

Table 10.4. *(Continued)*

Study	n	Design/subjects	Training program	Duration	Findings/comments
Tokmakova et al, 1999[35]	22	Randomized, controlled; male, ambulatory	Exercise training intensity of 50% MVO$_2$	8 weeks	Increased MVO$_2$; increased anaerobic threshold; improved QOL and Borg rating
Sturm et al, 1999[36]	26	Randomized, controlled; EF 10–26%	Step aerobics 100 min/wk; cycling 50 min/wk; 50% MVO$_2$	12 weeks	Significant improvement in MVO$_2$ with moderate exercise in severe HF
Maiorana et al, 2000[40]	13	Randomized, crossover study	Circuit weight training	8 weeks	Improved functional capacity and muscle strength
Tyni-Lenne et al, 1999[41]	24	Randomized; controlled; previously trained	Randomized to cycle vs knee extension	8 weeks	Improved MVO$_2$; decreased sympathetic activity more pronounced in minor muscle-trained group

EF, ejection fraction; CHF, chronic heart failure; NYHA, New York Heart Association, QOL, quality of life; SF 36, short form health survey; HF, heart failure; MVO$_2$, peak oxygen uptake; VO$_2$, oxygen uptake; NS, not significant

Statistically significant improvements in VO$_2$max, exercise duration, and isotonic voluntary contractile strength for the targeted muscle groups were seen. Submaximal exercise heart rate was also lower after training, which supports attenuation of neurohormonal activation. The authors concluded that functional capacity and muscle strength can be improved by applying interventions that target peripheral abnormalities in heart failure.[40]

In an interesting study by Tyni-Lenne et al, previously trained heart failure patients were randomized to either major muscle mass training (by cycle ergometer), or aerobic minor muscle mass training (by knee-extensor). Twenty-four subjects were randomized and trained for 8 weeks. There were no baseline differences between the groups among any of the measured outcome variables. VO$_2$max increased and plasma norepinephrine concentrations decreased only in the knee-extensor training group. An improvement in health-related quality of life was also demonstrated. These findings suggest that greater efficiency is shown in aerobic training involving minor muscles mass exercises than in major muscle mass exercises in previously trained heart failure patients.[41]

A summary of the cited studies is outlined in Table 10.4.

Possible mechanisms of improvement with training effect in skeletal muscle abnormalities

Historically, the excessive muscle fatigue and breathlessness leading to activity intolerance in heart failure were felt to be a result of inadequate perfusion of skeletal muscle and end organs due to impaired cardiac output. In recent years, studies have revealed intrinsic changes in skeletal muscle fibers that may result in impaired metabolism and contribute to early muscle fatigue and breathlessness. These changes include reduced mitochondrial density, reduction in lipolytic oxidative enzymes, and fiber atrophy.[42–47] Drexler et al were among the first to document a significant correlation between the density of mitochondria in the muscle cells upon biopsy, and VO$_2$max.[47]

Deconditioning is also undoubtedly a factor in the activity intolerance in chronic heart failure. However, it is not the sole determinant. There have been key differences noted at the cellular level between muscle cells of deconditioned 'healthy' subjects, and those of patients with chronic heart failure.[43] Some of these changes include cellular atrophy restricted to type II fibers in chronic heart failure, which is in contrast to the generalized changes in all fiber types in simple deconditioning and specific mitochondrial changes.[43,48]

Impaired regional blood flow

In addition to skeletal muscle cell changes, underperfusion secondary to impaired regional blood flow in heart failure is believed to be a contributing factor to activity intolerance.[9,11] A differential shunting of cardiac output results in reduction in maximal skeletal-muscle flow during exercise. The long-term benefits from ACE inhibitor and vasodilator therapy are believed to be related to the increase in peripheral perfusion and their favorable effect on skeletal muscle blood flow.[49,50]

In a study by Wilson et al, 32 patients with heart failure were enrolled in a cardiac rehabilitation program, and were subdivided for analysis based upon their hemodynamic response to exercise. Subjects with normal cardiac output response to exercise tolerated the program well, and had favorable improvements in VO_2max and anaerobic threshold. Three of eleven patients with reduced cardiac output upon exercise withdrew from rehabilitation due to exhaustion, and of the remaining participants, only one showed favorable response with regard to VO_2max and anaerobic threshold.[50] The authors concluded that the findings support the importance of circulatory impairment as a primary factor in limiting the capacity for exercise in this population independent of intrinsic skeletal muscle cell abnormalities.

Neurohormonal attenuation

In view of the importance of neurohormonal activation in explicating the pathophysiology of heart failure, its attenuation as a possible mechanism in the benefit associated with exercise must be considered. Studies evaluating the level of neurohormonal activation, specifically increased sympathetic tone, have indeed shown attenuation by exercise training.[9,26,34,37] Common markers utilized to determine neurohormonal activation that have been identified as indicators of poor prognosis are levels of circulating norepinephrine and endothelin. Both overproduction of sympathetic output and endothelial dysfunction have been identified as contributing factors in the pathology of heart failure. Specifically, impairment of endothelium-mediated vasodilation is believed to result in vasoconstriction that increases peripheral vascular resistance and diminishes blood flow to the musculature.[51] Norepiniphrine and endothelin levels, as well as the degree of endothelium-mediated vasodilation have all been shown to respond favorably to exercise training in the heart failure population.[25,26,52,53] While activation of the renin–angiotensin–aldosterone system and elevated levels of arginine vasopressin occur in chronic heart failure, the question of whether they have a direct role in limiting activity tolerance remains unanswered at this point.[3]

Chronotropic incompetence

Chronotropic incompetence, or diminished heart rate variability, is a common finding in heart failure patients. Chronotropic incompetence has been defined as the inability to achieve a peak heart rate of > 85% of the age-predicted maximum upon exercise testing.[54] In the normal heart, variation of heart rate occurs in response to changes in demand. Physical activity, emotional stress, pain, and other triggers result in an increase in heart rate. In heart failure, this normal physiologic response is blunted. As a result, there is less variation seen in the R–R intervals in any given time period than in individuals with normal cardiac function. This phenomenon has been hypothesized to be the result of autonomic dysfunction.[55] Downregulation, or desensitization of the adrenergic receptor sites to norepinephrine in response to chronically high circulating levels may play a role in diminished heart rate variability. Additionally, vagal attenuation has been raised as an explanatory mechanism. This remains an area which requires further study.[56] Ponikowski et al found increased ventilatory response to exercise as an independent predictor of depressed heart rate variability in heart failure patients.[57]

Keteyian et al randomized 40 male subjects to 24 weeks of aerobic exercise vs control. The authors reported a 16.3% increase in absolute VO_2max and observed a significant increase in peak heart rate in the treatment group. An interesting outcome of the data analysis in this study was the conclusion that 46% of the improvement in VO_2max could be attributed to the increase in peak heart rate, as a result of reversal of chronotropic incompetence.[58]

Conflicting findings

While there is growing evidence that exercise is safe and may be used as an effective adjunct to conventional heart failure therapy, there have been studies that report no improvement, or present evidence of worsening cardiac function associated with exercise training. Arvan reported no improvement in exercise tolerance with training in patients with recent myocardial infarction, left ventricular dysfunction, and symptomatic ischemia upon initial exercise testing.[59] Additionally, Jugdutt et al report worsened anterior wall motion and deterioration in ejection fraction in patients who had experienced myocardial infarction 12 weeks earlier with anterior wall akinesis greater than 18%.[60] Cohen-Solal et al outlined four case studies of subjects in whom transient diminished or plateaued VO_2max occurred during exercise testing in conjunction with observed cardiac abnormalities. These included atrial fibrillation in the presence of severe mitral stenosis; hypotension secondary to acute worsening of mitral regurgitation due to papillary muscle dysfunction; probable atrial tachycardia with widening of existing bundle branch block; and worsening of 2nd degree AV block from 2:1 to 3:1 with resultant bradycardia lasting for approximately 8 minutes, after which heart rate and VO_2max increased.[61] These observations support the importance of careful screening and evaluation of the patient prior to making recommendations involving exercise training.

In a study by Gottlieb et al, of 33 elderly patients with moderate to severe heart failure, 17 tolerated 6 months of supervised and graded exercise training. While six of the 17 showed significantly improved VO_2max, corresponding improvements in quality of life scores and outpatient energy expenditure were not seen. Additionally, of those who did show benefit, neither increase in daily expenditure nor improvement in quality of life were seen.[62] These authors concluded that while elderly patients with heart failure may safely exercise, not all will benefit.

Prescription guidelines

The Agency for Health Care Policy and Research Clinical Practice Guidelines for Cardiac Rehabilitation as Secondary Prevention grade the strength of evidence supporting the value of exercise training in heart failure as 'A', meaning that 'scientific evidence from well-designed and well-conducted controlled trials (randomized and non-randomized) provides statistically significant results that consistently support the guidelines statement.'[63] Therefore, cardiac rehabilitation exercise training is recommended to maintain functional capacity and alleviation of symptoms. While there are a number of comprehensive guidelines that have been published subsequently, to guide treatment of heart failure, there is little reference made to the potential role of exercise as a valued intervention in this population. When references are made, they are non-specific in terms of recommendations and tools for implementation, reflective of the state of the current research in this area.[6,12,63,64]

A specific program design which will best fit the heart failure patient with regard to the modality and intensity is yet unknown. Most sources recommend baseline monitored graded exercise testing to serve as a basis for prescription, and to identify underlying ischemia in heart failure patients.[10,11] If stable during the baseline testing, exercise at 60–80% of the maximum heart rate or 50–70% of VO_2max has been recommended by some sources.[11,65] In general, walking, flexibility exercises, calisthenics, cycling, and stair climbing have been found to be acceptable forms of exercise training. As suggested by Meyer et al, interval training is thought to be well suited for this population.[28,29] Increasing work is being conducted to evaluate the benefit of resistance training in heart failure as well.[40] Hanson recommends beginning exercise training at 60–65% VO_2max for 10–15 minutes' duration beginning with 2–4 minutes of exercise separated by 1-minute periods of rest. The exercise interval can be gradually increased according to patient tolerance by 1–2 minutes. The eventual goal is 30–40 minutes of training. Also recommended is a 10-minute warm-up phase to achieve optimal vasodilation. The frequency of exercise should be tailored to the needs of the patient, but should be 3–5 times weekly.[66]

At minimum, patients with heart failure should be encouraged to remain as active as possible and abandon any belief that physical activity should be restricted or avoided completely. Bed rest is no longer the treatment of choice for heart failure. Too many heart failure patients (and perhaps practitioners) continue to operate under the misconception that physical activity should be avoided. Effective progression of heart failure management into the 21st century requires that we abandon beliefs that drove interventions 40 years ago and apply evidence-based insight in our recommendations. Conservative, low intensity home walking programs are often desirable for these patients, and can be encouraged with little concern regarding adverse events. Patients should be carefully instructed to modify their activity according to any symptoms they experience, and adjust their program if they experience excessive fatigue during, or on the day following, exercise, indicating overexertion.[67]

Adherence

Once a recommendation is established with regard to physical activity, it is important to consider the many potential barriers to adherence that threaten the integrity of the intervention. The majority of patients diagnosed with chronic heart failure are elderly. These patients carry with them unique age-related challenges. Many patients experience orthostatic hypotension related to vascular dysfunction which may or may not be pharmacologically induced. This may predispose them to falling, or unstable gait, which impacts the ability to perform physical activities. Additionally, the elderly often live alone, or lack resources for transportation to suitable exercise facilities. During inclement weather, activities outside the home are of particular concern due to the recommended avoidance of temperature extremes, potential for falls on slippery surfaces, and the possible lack of transportation to an exercise facility. Prescribed physical activity must be tailored to address these potential barriers to adherence. Reasonable, achievable goals must be identified and serve as a foundation for building the exercise prescription.

Practical recommendations

Engaging heart failure patients in the quest for increased physical activity is fraught with challenges. Many patients actively limit their performance of physical activities out of fear of decompensation, avoidance of symptoms of dyspnea and fatigue, or all too often because they have been instructed by health care providers to 'take it easy'. Importantly, common comorbid conditions such as osteoarthritis, chronic pulmonary disease, peripheral vascular disease, and abnormalities of vision and balance also limit their capacity to perform physical activity. When considering recommendation of increased physical activity for heart failure patients, it is important that they be stable in terms of not only their heart failure symptoms, but also, other potentially harmful conditions such as angina, aortic stenosis, infection (such as myocarditis), and diabetes.

Referral to cardiac rehabilitation programs, particularly those providing specialized programs for heart failure patients, is a very favorable option. However, third party reimbursement for cardiac rehabilitation referral on the basis of heart failure alone is questionable at best. Additionally, there are often access issues related to the availability of such programs within a reasonable geographic proximity to the patients' homes, and transportation issues if they are unable to drive or access public transportation.

In the absence of cardiac rehabilitation as a viable option, evidence suggests that recommending home-based programs may be safe and effective. It is important to consider each patient's unique circumstances when recommending physical activity. Prior to making a recommendation, it is vital to assess the patient's current level of activity. Some may be enjoying 4-mile walks in a nearby state park, while others with the same level of disease severity may not be walking to their mailbox. Once it is determined what is 'comfortable' in terms of current level of activity, it is possible to outline a plan for advancement. For patients engaging in little physical activity at baseline, it may be necessary to start with 5-minute walking intervals, perhaps more than once daily if tolerated. Patients should be encouraged to stop for rest if they become uncomfortable with fatigue or shortness of breath. After a week, the exercise intervals may be increased by 2–5 minutes per day as tolerated, and further increased as such on a weekly basis. They should be instructed to discontinue exercise if their symptoms become severe, or if the fatigue and dyspnea experienced during exercise should fail to subside within a reasonable time after the exercise is stopped. Patients should be informed that excessive fatigue experienced the day after advancement of the exercise intensity or duration may indicate that the increase was too aggressive, and requires adjustment.

Participation in sexual activities is another question in the minds of many heart failure patients. Again, discussion of such matters may be uncomfortable, particularly for elderly patients, and they may avoid asking questions. Ask about participation in and tolerance of sexual activities, and include the spouse in the conversation when possible. Recommendations for enhancing sexual activities include avoiding heavy meals or alcohol consumption within a few hours prior to sex. Avoidance of extreme temperatures is also important. Rest periods before and/or after may be of benefit. Also, having the patient assume the side-lying or supine position during sexual activity may improve their stamina and tolerance. In the event that sexual intercourse is not tolerable for the patient, alternatives to intercourse may be explored. Non-coital mutual stimulation can be suggested, as well as encouraging open communication about sex, which can enhance the experience as well.

Conclusion

The studies evaluating the role of exercise in heart failure lend strong support to its potential benefits. However, the need for a large, randomized longitudinal trial persists. The number of subjects included in most of the studies conducted to date have been small. Individual responses to training vary substantially, making it important to obtain larger study groups to avoid skewed mean values.[48,49] Furthermore, many of the studies involved subjects who were primarily, if not exclusively, male, and more often tend to include patients with ischemic as opposed to idiopathic cardiomyopathy. Further study is required to clarify the value and mechanisms involved with submaximal vs maximal training and the impact of these interventions not only on morbidity and mortality in heart failure, but also on ability to perform activities of daily living and quality of life. More study is required in severely debilitated patients (NYHA IV), to determine potential gains as well as to formulate feasible exercise programs for patients who are unable to perform maximal

training. The studies reviewed were devoid of discussion of cultural or compliance issues related to prescription of exercise in the heart failure population.

As further findings support specific exercise regimens, practical guidelines for clinicians should be developed that delineate appropriate candidates for exercise training, levels of intensity, specific exercises (such as interval training, strength training, graded protocols, or programs which isolate small muscle groups) and goals to be achieved. As more data become available correlating exercise training with morbidity, mortality, and quality of life outcomes in chronic heart failure, cost–benefit analyses should be performed to facilitate decision-making affecting funding and reimbursement for related programs.

References

1 Packer M. How should physicians view heart failure? The philosophical and physiological evolution of three conceptual models of the disease, *Am J Cardiol* 1993; **71:** 3C–11C.

2 Sullivan MJ, Hawthorne MH. Nonpharmacologic interventions in the treatment of heart failure. *J Cardiovasc Nurs* 1996; **10:** 47–57.

3 Balady GJ, Pina IL. *Exercise and Heart Failure*. New York: Futura Publishing Company, Inc. 1997.

4 Hosenpud JD, Greenbert BH. *Congestive Heart Failure: Pathophysiology, Diagnosis, and Comprehensive Approach to Management*. New York: Springer-Verlag. 1994.

5 Patterson JH, Adams KF. Pathophysiology of heart failure: changing perceptions. *Pharmacotherapy* 1996; **16:** 27S–36S.

6 Consensus recommendations for the management of chronic heart failure, *Am J Cardiol* 1999; **83:** 2A–38A.

7 Moran JF. Exercise in Heart Failure and Exercise Prescription. (Lecture text) Oak Brook, IL: Midwest Heart Specialists Heart Failure Tutorial, 1996.

8 Liang C, Stewart DK, Le Jemtel TH et al. Characteristics of peak aerobic capacity in symptomatic and asymptomatic subjects with left ventricular dysfunction. *Am J Cardiol* 1992; **69:** 1207–11.

9 Kokkinos PF, Choucair W, Graves P et al. Chronic heart failure and exercise. *Am Heart J* 2000; **140:** 21–8.

10 American College of Sports Medicine. *ACSM's Guidelines for Exercise Testing and Prescription, 3rd edn.* Baltimore: Williams & Wilkins, 1998.

11 Braith RW, Mills RM. Exercise training in patients with congestive heart failure: how to achieve benefits safely. *Postgraduate Medicine* 1994; **96:** 119–30.

12 Committee on Evaluation and Management of Heart Failure. Guidelines for the evaluation and management of heart failure. Report of the American College of

Cardiology/American Heart Association Task Force on Practice Guidelines, *Circulation* 1995; **92:** 2764–84.

13 Cahalin LP, Mathier MA, Semigran MJ et al. The six-minute walk test predicts peak oxygen uptake and survival in patients with advanced heart failure. *Chest* 1996; **110:** 325–32.

14 Fletcher GF, Froelicher VF, Hartley LH et al. Exercise standards: a statement for health professionals from the American Heart Association. *Circulation* 1990; **82:** 2286–322.

15 Higginbotham MB, Morris KG, Conn EH et al. Determinants of variable exercise performance among patients with severe left ventricular dysfunction. *Am J Cardiol* 1983; **51:** 52–60.

16 Franciosa JA, Park M, Levine TB. Lack of correlation between exercise capacity and indexes of resting left ventricular performance in heart failure. *Am J Cardiol* 1981; **47:** 33–9.

17 Faggiano P, D'Aloia A, Gualeni A et al. Assessment of oxygen uptake during the 6-minute walk test in patients with heart failure: preliminary experience with a portable device. *Am Heart J* 1997; **134:** 203–6.

18 Guyatt GH, Sullivan MJ, Thompson PJ et al. The 6-minute walk: a new measure of exercise capacity in patients with chronic heart failure. *Can Med Assoc J* 1985; **132:** 919–23.

19 Milligan NP, Havey J, Dossa A. Using a 6-minute walk test to predict outcomes in patients with left ventricular dysfunction. *Rehab Nurs* 1997; **22:** 177–81.

20 Peeters P, Mets T. The 6-minute walk as an appropriate exercise test in elderly patients with chronic heart failure. *J Gerontol Med Sci* 1996; **51A:** M147–M151.

21 Rector TS, Kubo SH, Cohn JN. Patients' self-assessment of their congestive heart failure. Part 2. Content, reliability and validity of a new measure, the Minnesota Living with Heart Failure Questionnaire. *Heart Failure* 1987; **3:** 198–209.

22 McHorney CA, Ware JE Jr, Raczek AE. The MOS 36-item short-form health survey (SF-36). II. Psychometric and clinical tests of validity in measuring physical and mental health constructs. *Med Care* 1993; **31:** 247–63.

23 Pina IL, Fitzpatrick JT. Exercise and heart failure: a review. *Chest* 1996; **110:** 1317–27.

24 Adams CD, Bennett S. Exercise in heart failure: a synthesis of current research. *Online J Knowledge Synthesis Nursing* 2000; **7(5)**. [http://www.nursingsociety.org/library]

25 Sullivan MJ, Higginbotham MB, Cobb FR. Exercise training in patients with severe left ventricular dysfuntion: hemodynamic and metabolic effects. *Circulation* 1988; **78:** 506–15.

26 Coats AJS, Adamopoulos S, Radaelli A et al. Controlled trial of physical training in chronic heart failure: exercise performance, hemodynamics, ventilation, and autonomic function. *Circulation* 1992; **85:** 2119–31.

27 Meyer K, Gornandt L, Schwaibold M et al. Predictors of response to exercise training in severe chronic congestive heart failure. *Am J Cardiol* 1997; **80:** 56–60.

28 Meyer K, Samek L, Schwaibold M et al. Interval training in patients with severe chronic heart failure: analysis and recommendations for exercise procedures. *Med Sci Sports Exercise* 1997; **29:** 306–12.

29 Meyer K, Schwaibold M, Westbrook S et al. Effects of short-term exercise training and activity restriction on functional capacity in patients with severe chronic congestive heart failure. *Am J Cardiol* 1996; **78:** 1017–22.

30 Bellardinelli R, Georgiou D, Cianci G, Purcaro A. Randomized, controlled trial of long-term moderate exercise training in chronic heart failure: effects on functional capacity, quality of life, and clinical outcome. *Circulation* 99: 1173–82.

31 Hambrecht R, Gielen S, Linke A. Effects of exercise training on left ventricular function and peripheral resistance in patients with chronic heart failure: a randomized trial. *JAMA* 2000; **283:** 3095–101.

32 Quittan M, Sturm B, Wiesinger GF et al. Quality of life in patients with chronic heart failure: a randomized controlled trial of changes induced by a regular exercise program. *Scand J Rehab Med* 1999; **31:** 223–8.

33 Demopoulos L, Bijou R, Fergus I et al. Exercise training in patients with severe congestive heart failure: enhancing peak aerobic capacity while minimizing the increase in ventricular wall stress. *J Am Coll Cardiol* 1997; **29:** 597–603.

34 Belardinelli R, Georgiou D, Scocco V et al. Low intensity exercise training in patients with chronic heart failure. *J Am Coll Cardiol* 1995; **26:** 975–82.

35 Tokmakova M, Dobreva B, Kostianev S. Effects of short-term exercise training in patients with heart failure. *Folia Medica* 1999; **41:** 68–71.

36 Sturm B, Quittan M, Wiesinger GF et al. Moderate-intensity exercise training with elements of step aerobics in patients with severe chronic heart failure. *Arch Physical Med Rehab* 1999; **80:** 746–50.

37 Kiilavuori K, Savijarvi A, Naveri H et al. Effect of physical training on exercise capacity and gas exchange in patients with chronic heart failure. *Chest* 1996; **110:** 985–91.

38 Kavanagh T, Myers MG, Baigrie RS et al. Quality of life and cardiorespiratory function in chronic heart failure: effects of 12 months' aerobic training. *Heart* 1996; **76:** 42–9.

39 Koch M, Douard H, Broustet JP. The benefit of graded physical exercise in chronic heart failure. *Chest* 1992; **101:** 231S–235S.

40 Maiorana A, O'Driscoll G, Cheetham C et al. Combined aerobic and resistance exercise training improves functional capacity and strength in CHF. *J Appl Physiol* 2000; **88:** 1565–70.

41 Tyni-Lenne R, Gordon A, Jensen-Urstad M et al. Aerobic training involving a minor muscle mass shows greater efficiency than training involving a major muscle mass in chronic heart failure patients. *J Cardiac Fail* 1999; **5:** 300–7.

42 Mancini DM, Walter G, Reichek N et al. Contribution of skeletal muscle atrophy to exercise intolerance and altered muscle metabolism in heart failure. *Circulation* 1992; **85:** 1364–73.

43 Minotti JR, Massie BM. Exercise training in heart failure patients: does reversing the peripheral abnormalities protect the heart? *Circulation* 1992; **85:** 2323–5.

44 Wilson JR, Mancini DM, Dunkman WB. Exertional fatigue due to skeletal muscle dysfunction in patients with heart failure. *Circulation* 1993; **87:** 470–5.

45 Hambrecht R, Niebauer J, Fiehn E. Physical training in patients with stable chronic heart failure: effects on cardiorespiratory fitness and ultrastructural abnormalities of leg muscles. *J Am Coll Card* 1995; **25:** 1239–49.

46 Adamopoulos S, Coats AJS, Brunotte F et al. Physical training improves skeletal muscle metabolism in patients with chronic heart failure. *J Am Coll Cardiol* 1993; **21:** 1101–6.

47 Drexler H, Riede U, Munzel T et al. Alterations of skeletal muscle in chronic heart failure. *Circulation* 1992; **85:** 1751–9.

48 Massie BM, Camacho SA. Cahners Scientific Meeting Reports: Heart Failure Review. Belle Mead, NJ: Excerpta Medica, 1995.

49 Jette M, Heller R, Landry F et al. Randomized 4-week exercise program in patients with impaired left ventricular function. *Circulation* 1991; **84:** 1561–7.

50 Wilson JR, Groves J, Rayos G. Circulatory status and response to cardiac rehabilitation in patients with heart failure. *Circulation* 1994; **94:** 1567–72.

51 Hambrecht R, Fiehn E, Weigl C et al. Regular physical exercise corrects endothelial dysfunction and improves exercise capacity in patients with chronic heart failure. *Circulation* 1999; **98:** 2709–15.

52 Rundqvist B, Eisenhofer G, Elam M et al. Attenuated cardiac sympathetic responsiveness during dynamic

exercise in patients with heart failure. *Circulation* 1997;
95: 940–5.

53 Hornig B, Volker M, Drexler H. Physical training improves
endothelial function in patients with chronic heart
failure. *Circulation* 1996; **93:** 210–14.

54 Keteyian SJ, Brawner CA, Schairer JR et al. Effects of
exercise training on chronotropic incompetence in patients
with heart failure. *Am Heart J* 1999; **138:** 233–40.

55 Nolan J, Batin PD, Andrews R et al. Prospective study of
heart rate variability and mortality in chronic heart
failure: results of the United Kingdom heart failure
evaluation and assessment of risk trial (UK-Heart).
Circulation 1998; **98:** 1510–16.

56 Davey PP, Barlow C, Hart G. Prolongation of the QT
interval in heart failure occurs at low but not at high
heart rates. *Clin Sci* 2000; **98:** 603–10.

57 Ponikowski P, Chua TP, Piepoli M. Ventilatory response
to exercise correlates with impaired heart rate variability
in patients with chronic congestive heart failure. *Am J
Cardiol* 1998; **82:** 338–44.

58 Keteyian SJJ, Levine AB, Brawner CA et al. Exercise
training in patients with heart failure: a randomized,
controlled trial. *Ann Intern Med* 1996; **124:** 1051–7.

59 Arvan S. Exercise performance of the high risk acute
myocardial infarction patient after cardiac rehabilitation.
Am J Cardiol 1988; **62:** 197–201.

60 Jugdutt BI, Michorowski BL, Kappagoda CT. Exercise
training after Q wave myocardial infarction: importance
of regional left ventricular function and topography. *J Am
Coll Cardiol* **12:** 362–72.

61 Cohen-Solal A, Aupetit JF, Page E et al. Transient fall in
oxygen intake during exercise in congestive heart
failure. *Chest* 1996; **110:** 841–4.

62 Gottlieb SS, Fisher ML, Freudenberger R et al. Effects of
exercise training on peak performance and quality of life
in congestive heart failure patients. *J Cardiac Fail* 1999;
5: 188–94.

63 Agency for Health Care Policy and Research. *Cardiac
Rehabilitation as Secondary Prevention: Clinical Practice
Guideline*. Rockville: US Department of Health and
Human Services, 1995.

64 Adams KF, Baughman KL, Dec WG et al. HFSA
guidelines for management of patients with heart failure
caused by left ventricular systolic dysfunction:
pharmacological approaches. *J Cardiac Fail* 1999; **5:**
357–82.

65 LeJemtel TH, Demopoulos L, Jondeau G et al. Exercise
training for patients with congestive heart failure.
Contemporary Intern Med 1997; **9:** 23–8.

66 Hanson P. Exercise testing and training in patients with
chronic heart failure. *Med Sci Sports Exercise* 1996;
26: 527–37.

67 Dracup K, Baker DW, Dunbar SB et al. Management of
heart failure: counseling, education, and lifestyle
modifications. *JAMA* 1994; **272:** 1442–6.

68 Hlatky MA, Boineau RE, Higginbotham MB et al. A brief
self-administered questionnaire to determine functional
capacity (the Duke Activity Status Index). *Am J Cardiol*
1989; **64:** 651–4.

11 Caring for the hospitalized heart failure patient

Anna Gawlinski

Introduction

Heart failure affects more that 4.8 million Americans with more than 400 000 new cases diagnosed annually and a resultant 900 000 hospitalizations.[1] The management of patients with severe heart failure, (New York Heart Association [NYHA] class III–IV) who require hospitalization can be extremely challenging. These patients have little physiologic cardiac reserve capacity and require close monitoring with precise management.[2] For these reasons, hemodynamic-guided evaluation and management provides clinicians with important data upon which to base initial, as well as ongoing therapy. The goals of hemodynamic-guided management are to optimize hemodynamics and apply those therapies known to improve patient survival.

Using a case study, this chapter will present guidelines for care of the hospitalized heart failure patient. These guidelines have been used successfully at University of California, Los Angeles (UCLA) Medical Center for the last 10 years. They provide clinicians with a uniform approach to patient care that can dramatically improve heart failure patient outcomes, including survival.[3,4] Finally, the emerging role of B-type natriuretic peptide (BNP) both as a heart failure diagnostic test, and a therapeutic intervention will be discussed.

Case study

Mr L is a 37-year-old male with the diagnosis of dilated cardiomyopathy. Six weeks ago he developed flu-like symptoms and became increasingly short of breath with a progressive decrease in exercise tolerance. He reports he can walk only 100 feet, and must stop due to dyspnea and fatigue. He has 3+ orthopnea, paroxysmal nocturnal dyspnea and 2+ pedal edema. He complains of dizziness when getting out of bed. His body weight has increased 15 lbs over the last 6 weeks, despite complaints of decreased appetite, early satiety and nausea. Initial exam showed:

Heart rate: 120 beats/min
Blood pressure: 86/60 mmHg
Respiratory rate: 28 breaths/min
Breath sounds: bibasalar rales
Jugular venous pulsation: 10 cm
Heart sounds: S1, S2, S3, III/VI systolic murmur at apex
Electrocardiogram: sinus tachycardia, left bundle branch block
Jugular venous pulsations: 10 cm
Hepatomegaly
Hepatojugluar reflex +

Mr L was admitted to the Cardiac Care Unit (CCU) for management of advanced heart failure (NYHA class III–IV) and evaluation for potential heart transplantation. He demonstrated symptomatic hypotension (systolic blood pressure [SBP] < 90 mmHg) with significant volume overload, which is criteria for hospitalization. Criteria for hospitalization of heart failure patients requiring initial or follow-up management are listed on Table 11.1.[5] A thermodilution pulmonary artery catheter (PAC) was inserted to determine baseline hemodynamic and oxygenation data and guide appropriate therapy (Table 11.2).

Table 11.1. *When should patients be admitted to the hospital for acute decompensation of heart failure?*

- Onset of acute myocardial ischemia
- Pulmonary edema or increasing respiratory distress
- Oxygen saturation below 90% not caused by pulmonary disease
- Complicating medical illnesses
- Symptomatic hypotension with fluid overload
- Syncope
- Heart failure refractory to outpatient treatment
- Anasarca
- Inadequate outpatient social support system

Adapted from Francis.[5]

Table 11.2. *Baseline and post treatment data for a patient with decompensated heart failure*

Parameter	Baseline	Post NTP
HR (beats/min)	120	98
BP (mmHg)	86/60	94/64
RR (breaths/min)	28	20
PAP (mmHg)	50/34	40/18
PCWP (mmHg)	32 (with large V waves)	15
RA (mmHg)	12	7
CO (liters/min)	1.9	5.6
CI (liters/min/m²)	1.1	3.1
SVR (dynes/sec/cm⁵)	2442	1036
SaO₂ (%)	98	98
SvO₂ (%)	29	64
Hb (gm/dl)	15	16
UO (cc/hr)	30	120

NTP, sodium nitroprusside

HR, heart rate

BP, blood pressure

RR, respiratory rate

PAP, pulmonary artery pressure

PCWP, pulmonary capillary wedge pressure

RA, right atrium

CO, cardiac output

CI, cardiac index

SVR, systemic vascular resistance

SaO₂, arterial oxygen saturation

SvO₂, mixed venous oxygen saturation

Hb, hemoglobin

UO, Urinary output

Mr L's hemodynamic profile is consistent with low cardiac output due to left and right ventricular failure. The low cardiac output (1.9 l/min, cardiac index [CI] of 1.1 l/min/m²) and high pulmonary capillary wedge pressure (PCWP) of 32 mmHg are consistent with the patient's symptoms and diagnosis of decompensated heart failure. Decompensated heart failure is a clinical situation in which hemodynamic dysfunction, such as low CO and elevated filling pressure, produces symptoms severe enough to require urgent interventions.[6] These patients are often NYHA class III or IV, and have a resting left ventricular ejection fraction of < 30%.[6] Tissue oxygen is compromised by a low CO indicated by symptoms of

fatigue and/or a low mixed venous oxygen saturation (SvO₂).

Therapeutic goals

The therapeutic goals for patients with decompensated heart failure are to (1) reverse hemodynamic abnormalities, (2) relieve symptoms, and (3) provide early treatment to decrease disease progression and improve long-term survival.[7] Current consensus of heart failure management guidelines by specialty organizations reflect these goals, but do not yet address specific treatment for decompensated hospitalized heart failure patients.[8,9]

The nurse used hemodynamic and oxygenation indices to guide therapy and to determine the optimal therapeutic dose response for Mr L. Specific therapies as outlined in the protocol *Hemodynamic Management of Cardiomyopathy Patients* used in the CCU at UCLA Medical Center (Figure 11.1), helped the nurse to tailor pharmacological therapy for Mr L[3] and reverse the hemodynamic abnormalities. The rationale and clinical application of each of the initial therapies are discussed in the following sections.

Preload reduction

Diuretics
Rationale
Intravenous (IV) loop diuretics in high doses are indicated in patients with severe heart failure, such as Mr L, because oral gastrointestinal absorption is impaired by gut edema in decompensated heart failure.[10,11] Furosemide is commonly used as the initial loop diuretic. Intravenous diuretics are administered to reduce preload, or right ventricular end-diastolic volume, left ventricular end-diastolic volume (LVEDV), and myocardial wall tension. The reduction in LVEDV decreases the stretch on the mitral valve annulus and results in less mitral regurgitation. Diuretics should be continued until the hemodynamic goals have been obtained (PCWP < 15 mmHg, right atrium (RA) < 7 mmHg, and systemic vascular resistance, (SVR) < 1200 dynes/sec/cm⁵, while maintaining SBP ≥ 80 mmHg), and all systemic congestion has been resolved.[3,12] The hemodynamic parameter most predictive of patient outcome is the PCWP.[4,13] Patients who achieve a PCWP < 16 mmHg have a better prognosis than those with persistently high filling pressures (1-year survival 80% vs 56%).[4,13] When the patient approaches

1. Right heart catheter placed
   - Hemodynamics are examined
   - If PCWP > 16 mmHg and/or the CI < 2.2 l/min/m^2 on two sets of hemodynamic measurements, the catheter remains in place.
2. If SVR < 1300, PCWP > 20 mmHg, RA > 10 mmHg, and CI > 2.2 l/min/m^2 then begin diuretics alone and restart previous ACEI.
3. If the hemodynamics subsequently deteriorate (SVR > 1500), discontinue oral vasodilators (except nitrates) and begin NTP.
4. If the SVR > 1300 and PCWP > 20 mmHg or CI < 2.2 l/min/m^2, begin NTP with the following hemodynamic goals:
   - SVR < 1200, PCWP < 15 mmHg, RA < 7 mmHg, while maintaining SBP > 80 mmHg.
5. If patient has low cardiac index (CI < 1.4 l/min/m^2) consider addition of inotropic agent such as dobutamine.
6. NTP 100 mg in 250 cc D$_5$W
   - Starting dose of 20 mcg/min titrating upwards by 20 mcg/min (5% dextrose in water) every 5–10″ to a maximum dose of 300 mcg/min, or until optimum hemodynamics are achieved.
   - Diuresis with intravenous furosemide should also be initiated.
7. Obtain hemodynamic goals on NTP and intravenous furosemide.
   - Maintain these optimal hemodynamics for a minimum of 2–4 hours prior to starting oral vasodilators.
8. Start captopril as the initial vasodilator in all patients
   - Captopril 6.25 mg. Increase to 12.5 mg after 2 hours, if tolerated, after an additional 2 hours 25 mg, then increase by 25 mg every 6 hours (e.g. 50 mg, 75 mg, then 100 mg) only as necessary to taper off nitroprusside and match the hemodynamics achieved on nipride
   - *Maximum captopril dose is 100 mg PO q6 hours.*
   - *Do not continue to titrate captopril dose once off NTP, unless specific indication (e.g. SVR > 1500 or SBP > 100 mmHg).*
   - Avoid hypotension or advancing ACEI dose despite low SVR due to risk of renal insufficiency.
9. Isosorbide dinitrate to be started with initial unloading therapy in patients with coronary artery disease (10 mg or their admission dose of nitrates).
   - For patients *without* coronary artery disease, once captopril dose has reached 25 mg and still on nipride or for elevated filling pressures despite diuresis, isosorbide dinitrate to be started at 10 mg tid.
   - If tolerated, may be titrated but only if indicated by high filling pressure or SVR.
   - *Do not increase nitrates beyond 20 mg tid, unless indicated.*
   - If tolerated and indicated may increase by 10–20 mg every 8 hours, as tolerated to a maximum of 80 mg tid.
10. If optimum hemodynamics are achieved and sustained for 6–8 hours (absolute minimum 4 hours) on captopril/isosorbide dinitrate regimen, right heart catheter can be discontinued.
11. If optimum hemodynamics are not achieved on captopril/isosorbide dinitrate regimen or if captopril is not tolerated due to serious side-effects (severe symptomatic hypotension, renal insufficiency, allergic reaction) the decision regarding the addition of angiotensin receptor antagonist or hydralazine or doxazosin should be made by the attending in conjunction with the cardiomyopathy staff member.
    - Continue captopril at the greatest tolerated dose (usually 100 mg every 6 hours).
    - Hydralazine is started at 25 mg, after 2 hour 50 mg, then 50 mg every 6 hours, increase by 25 mg every 6 hours (e.g. 75 mg, 100 mg, then 150 mg) as needed to maximum 150 mg PO every 6 hours. Isosorbide dinitrate is to be continued or started.
12. Digoxin is indicated if patient remains symptomatic from heart failure.
    - Start at 0.125 mg qd or continue outpatient dose.
    - Check level when at steady state (aim for level 0.5–1.1 ng/ml)
13. Diuresis is of utmost importance in these patients; furosemide should be given 2–4 times a day with supplemental potassium.
    - I/O (input/output) should be closely followed multiple times per day.
14. Potassium and magnesium to be closely followed.
    - K+ should be kept 4–4.8 meq/dl.
    - Mg+ should be kept ≥ 1.8 meq/dl.
15. Patients should receive a 2-gram sodium diet
    - 1500–2000 liter fluid restriction.

From UCLA Heart Failure Guideline.[3]
PCWP, pulmonary capillary wedge pressure; CI cardiac index; SVR, systemic vascular resistance (dynes/sec/cm^5); RA, right atrium; ACEI, angiotensin-converting enzyme inhibitors; NTP, sodium nitroprusside; SBP, systolic blood pressure; CO, cardiac output.

Figure 11.1. *Hemodynamic management of cardiomyopathy patients.*

hemodynamic goal and dry weight, the patient may be converted to an oral loop diuretic.

Clinical application

Furosemide is a potent rapidly acting diuretic that inhibits reabsorption of sodium and chloride in the ascending loop of Henle.[14] Diuresis begins approximately 10 minutes after intravenous injection; peak effect occurs in about 30 minutes and lasts for about 6 hours.[15]

As a general guide, patients are started on an intravenous dose that is equivalent to their oral dose, with subsequent doses based on the patient's response (urine output, PCWP and RA). Patients not previously treated with a diuretic should receive a first dose of furosemide 20 mg IV.[16]

Diuretics should be given every 6 hours targeting the hemodynamic goal. Recommended timing of diuretics is three to four times a day to obtain optimal diuresis and preload reduction.[16]

For patients who fail to respond to high doses of intravenous furosemide, metolazone 5 mg PO can be added 30 minutes prior to the intravenous furosemide dose. Metolazone acts on the distal loop of Henle and potentiates the diuretic reponse. Metolazone has a 12-hour half-life and should be used only one or twice a day. Metolazone results in marked urinary potassium loss. Thus, extra potassium supplements and serum potassium monitoring are required.

Continuous diuretic

When patients do not respond to regularly administered high-dose intravenous loop diuretics with the addition of metolazone, consider continuous intravenous diuretic administration. A continuous drip may be effective when bolus administration of diuretics does not produce the expected urine output or reduction in PCWP and RA.[17–19] Continuous infusion may provide more efficient delivery of the diuretic to the nephron, eliminating compensatory sodium retention or rebound that can occur during a diuretic-free interval.[5] Diuretics that may be used for continuous therapy include furosemide, bumetanide, or torasemide.

Variability exists regarding the recommended dose for continuous infusion of diuretics. Furosemide is often given at a dose of 0.25–1.0 mg/kg/h. Bumetanide dosing as a continuous drip is 0.1–0.5 mg/h. Continuous torasemide drip is given at 5–20 mg/h.[5] Persistently high levels of preload may require a combination of therapies

along with the continuous diuretic infusion. Combination therapies include:

1) a continuous diuretic (IV furosemide or torasemide drip),
2) renal dose dopamine,
3) a combination of diuretics that affect the proximal and distal tubes (i.e. acetazolamide, furosemide, metolazone, amelioride),
4) vasodilatation of the venous capacitance vessels (intravenous nitroglycerin).[16]

Dopamine (renal perfusion)
Rationale

Dopamine is classified as an inotropic agent but in low doses (< 2–3 mcg/kg/min) produces renal vasodilation and may enhance urine output. Low-dose dopamine has primarily dopaminergic effects and produces dilation of specific vascular beds such as the renal, mesenteric, and cerebral arteries.[20,21]

Clinical application

Low-dose (or renal-dose) dopamine can be used in conjunction with diuretics to promote diuresis. Urine output may increase; heart rate and blood pressures are usually unchanged.

Afterload reduction

Nitroprusside
Rationale

Sodium nitroprusside (NTP), a potent vasodilator, was initiated intravenously to decrease the high afterload, indicated by a SVR of 2442 dynes/sec/cm[5]. By vasodilating the peripheral vessels, the decrease in afterload facilitates greater forward flow (stroke volume), increases CO/CI and tissue oxygen delivery. The increased stroke volume is usually sufficient to maintain BP at or only slightly below the pretreatment level.

Numerous studies have reported improvement in left ventricular function, tissue perfusion, cardiac output, and clinical status in low CO and high SVR states.[22,23] Nitroprusside reduces PCWP to a greater extent than dobutamine because of its more potent vasodilating effects, and its ability to enhance left ventricular diastolic relaxation.[24,25]

Clinical application

Continuous infusion of NTP is started at 20 mcg/min and is titrated upwards by 20 mcg/min every 5–10 minutes to the hemodynamic goal, (PCWP < 15 mmHg, RA < 7 mmHg, SVR < 1200 dynes/sec/cm^5, while maintaining SBP ≥ 80 mmHg). Clinical parameters used to evaluate the effect of NTP include SVR and BP. Maximum dose is 300 mcg/min.[3]

NTP is metabolized by the red blood cells to hydrocyanic acid which is converted to thiocyanate by the liver and excreted by the kidneys. Therefore, NTP should be used judiciously in patients with renal insufficiency who require prolonged infusions at high doses (300 mcg/min).[26]

NTP was titrated for Mr L, starting at 20 mcg/min to an optimum hemodynamic response dose of 196 mcg/min. Cardiac output increased in response to a decrease in preload and a reduction in afterload (SVR) with NTP. The increase in CO improved tissue oxygenation indicated by an SvO$_2$ of 64% (Table 11.2).

Nitroprusside to angiotensin-converting enzyme inhibitors
Rationale

The beneficial effects of angiotensin-converting enzyme inhibitors (ACEI) on disease progression, functional status, hospitalization and mortality, warrant placing all patients with left ventricular systolic dysfunction on ACEI, unless contraindications exist.[27]

Clinical application

Once the hemodynamic goal is achieved, and maintained for 2–6 hours (absolute minimum is 2 hours), titration of oral ACEI is done as intravenous NTP is weaned, while maintaining optimum hemodynamics. The protocol uses low doses of short-acting ACEI such as captopril initally, and titrated upwards to a dose level used in clinical trails, while matching the hemodynamic goal achieved with NTP. Specific dose titration upwards of captopril while weaning NTP is outlined in Figure 11.1. Clinical parameters such as SBP, SVR, serum creatinine and potassium are monitored as patients are switched from NTP to ACEI.

Nitroprusside vs nitroglycerin
Rationale

In patients with ischemic heart disease and myocardial ischemia, intravenous nitroglycerin (NTG) may be pre-

ferred over intravenous nitroprusside.[28,29] Early reports suggested that nitroprusside has the potential to worsen myocardial ischemia via coronary 'steal', especially in the setting of acute myocardial infarction, although this has rarely been a clinical problem in the management of patients with acutely decompensated heart failure.[30,31] For patients with acute (< 48 hours) myocardial infarction or acute myocardial ischemic syndromes and decompensated heart failure, intravenous nitroglycerin may be preferred because of its more favorable effects on coronary blood flow.[32,33]

Clinical application

For preload reduction nitrates increase venous capacitance which relieves congestion. NTG may be used to reduce afterload and SVR. Large doses of NTG are sometimes required to reduce systemic vascular resistance, and tolerance of NTG's effect can also develop.

Inotropic agents

Dobutamine
Rationale

The decision to add an inotropic agent varies among clinicians. The decision should be based on assessment of hemodynamic and physical findings. Measures to improve CO by decreasing PCWP and SVR ('unloading') should already be initiated. If patient's CO and CI remain low, and SBP is consistently less than 80 mmHg, consider adding dobutamine.[5] Dobutamine is an effective inotropic agent in patients with heart failure and can be used to support hemodynamics in patients who do not respond well to 'unloading' therapy or who require hemodynamic stabilization.

Dobutamine is a synthetic catecholamine with β1, β2 and alpha adrenoceptor stimulation. It results in increased cardiac contractility and peripheral vasodilatation. Dobutamine is associated with slight increases in heart rate (HR), decreases in PCWP, and increase in CI.[5]

Clinical application

Dobutamine is administered intravenously starting at 2.5 mcg/kg/min and increased by 2.5 mcg/kg/min until the desired clinical or hemodynamic effect is achieved or until untoward side-effects occur. A lower initial dose and slower titration should be use in patients at risk for dobutamine-induced ischemia.[16] The maximum dose is 20–30 mcg/kg/min. The half-life is short (2.5–5 minutes), with peak effect within 10 minutes. Tolerance may develop with extended use due to β-receptor downregulation. Dobutamine is the inotrope of choice in heart failure patients with oliguria and renal insufficiency.[5]

Milrinone
Rationale
Milrinone is used for inotropic support of patients who respond inadequately or develop tolerance to dobutamine. Milrinone blocks the phosphodiesterase III enzyme, thus increasing intracellular cyclic adenosine monophosphate enhances cardiac contractility and produces peripheral vaodilation. Milrinone has an advantage over dobutamine in exerting positive inotropic activity when downregulation of β-adrenergic receptors occurs due to dobutamine use.[5] Milrinone can also be used in combination with dobutamine.

Clinical application
Milrinone is started with a 50 mcg/kg bolus followed by 0.375–0.75 mcg/kg/min infusions. In some patients who are hypotensive the bolus dose may be eliminated, and continuous infusion only used.[5] Unlike the immediate effects of dobutamine, maximal hemodynamic effects of milrinone are observed at 15 minutes after initiation of infusion.[5] Because milrinone has a long biological half-life the hemodynamic effects of weaning the infusion rate downwards or off may not be seen completely for 6–12 hours.[16]

Both milrinone and dobutamine affect PCWP but generally, there is a more consistent reduction in PCWP with milrinone than with dobutamine.[34] Milrinone can precipitate hypotension when left ventricular filling pressures are low. Milrinone appears to cause less myocardial oxygen demand than dobutamine, and therefore may be preferred in patients with underlying ischemic heart disease or active angina pectoris when inotropic support is needed.[5,35] Knowledge of these hemodynamic agents will help guide clinicians in their use of these therapies (Table 11.3).[5]

In-hospital initiation of beta-blocker therapy
Rationale
Initiation of beta-blocker therapy was conventionally delayed until the heart failure patient was discharged and demonstrated to be stable as an outpatient for 2–4 weeks. The COPERNICUS trial demonstrates survival benefits with the beta-blocker carvedilol in patients with severe heart failure and that therapy can be safely initiated during hospitalization.[36] Beta-blockers have been demonstrated to improve survival (35% mortality reduction) in patients with class I–IV heart failure due to systolic dysfunction. Additional benefits include reduced hospitalization, myocardial infarction, and sudden death.[37]

Clinical applications
Beta-blockers should be initiated in all patients with mild, moderate, and severe heart failure due to systolic dysfunction in the absence of contraindications or clearly documented intolerance. Beta-blocker therapy should not be delayed until patients become resistant to other therapies. Beta-blocker therapy should be initiated in patients after adequate diuresis and following initiation of ACEI treatment. Patients requiring intravenous vasodilators or inotropic agents should have beta-blocker therapy deferred for a few days until the patient has stabilized and heart failure is compensated. Contraindications are cardiogenic shock, symptomatic bradycardia without pacemaker, 2nd or 3rd degree heart block without pacemaker, severe asthma, and severe chronic obstructive pulmonary disease (COPD). The recommended initiation dose for carvedilol for heart failure is 3.125 mg PO bid, (hold for SBP < 80 mmHg and/or HR < 45 bpm), with the first dose titration taking place on the first or second outpatient visit (2–8 week intervals).[38]

Electrolyte management
Rationale
The risk of electrolyte disturbances are increased in patients with heart failure. Neurohormonal activation, aggressive diuresis and renal dysfunction all contribute to marked fluctuations in serum electrolytes. Electrolyte disturbances can increase mortality and morbidity by causing arrhythmias, decreasing ventricular function and cardiac arrest. Hospitalized heart failure patients who undergo aggressive diuresis must have frequent determinations of serum electrolytes.

Clinical application: potassium
Serum potassium should be maintained between 4.0 and 4.6 mEq/dl. Both hypokalemia and hyperkalemia can affect left ventricular function and result in lethal arrhythmia.[39] Potassium supplements should be considered, and in most cases, prescribed for each diuretic dose. The clinician must keep in mind that serum potassium levels obtained just after an oral or intravenous potassium infusion do not reflect the potassium level a few hours later. Any new onset or increased arrhythmias warrant an imme-

Table 11.3. Adrenergic receptor activity and hemodynamic profile of commonly used positive inotropic agents

Drug	β_1	β_2	α_1	Vasodilation	Blood pressure	Filling pressure	CI	HR	MvO$_2$
Nitroprusside				++++	↓↓	↓↓↓↓	↑↑↑↑	↑	↑
Dopamine	++++	++	++++	< 3 µg/kg/min	↑↑↑	↑↑	↑↑↑	↑↓	↑↑
Dobutamine	++++	+++	+	++	↑	↓↓	↑↑↑	↑↓	↑↑
Milrinone				+++	→	↓↓↓↓	↑↑↑↑	↑↓	↑

Adapted from Francis.[5]

CI, cardiac index; HR, heart rate; MvO$_2$, myocardial oxygen consumption diate determination of electrolytes to assess for hypokalemia or hyperkalemia.

Clinical application: magnesium

Serum magnesium should be maintained > 1.8 mEq/dl.[40] Hypomagnesemia results in lethal arrhythmias such as ventricular tachycardia, ventricular fibrillation and sudden death. Heart failure patients undergoing aggressive diuresis are at risk for hypomagnesemia. The clinician must remember that serum magnesium levels do not adequately reflect tissue magnesium levels.[16]

Clinical application: sodium

Serum sodium reflects activation of the renal angiotensin system and increased level of antidiuretic hormone. If patients' serum sodium decreases, more restricted free water fluid should be initiated.[41] All intravenous medications should be maximally concentrated and mixed in normal saline. No hypertonic solutions should be administered.[16]

Digoxin
Rationale

Studies have shown digoxin to improve symptoms and functional capacity in patients with heart failure. No effect on mortality has been demonstrated.

Clinical application

Digoxin is indicated in patients with heart failure who remain symptomatic after optimal target doses of ACEI, beta-blockers, and diuretics should be started on digoxin.[42] In patients with isolated diastolic dysfunction, digoxin should not be used. Digoxin levels should be kept at between 0.5 and 1.1 ng/ml. New-onset arrhythmias should be evaluated for possible digoxin toxicity until proven otherwise. Hypokalemia can potentiate digoxin toxicity.[16]

Mechanical therapy

Consideration of mechanical support, such as the intra-aortic balloon pump (IABP), is necessary if patients are maximized on inotropic therapy and continue to demonstrate symptomatic hypotension (chest pain, increasing PCWP, dizziness, altered mental status).[16] Although there are no specific guidelines for when to insert an IABP in the patient with decompensating heart failure, when the CO is < 1.5 l/min despite maximum pharmacological support, most heart failure programs will initiate IABP therapy.[5] The physiologic benefits of IABP include increased coronary artery perfusion, decreased afterload, decreased preload, reduced wall tension, reduced myocardial oxygen demand. The use of other mechanical support devices such as ventricular assist devices are beyond the scope of this chapter.

New directions for diagnosis and treatment

B-type natriuretic peptide assay
Definition

B-type natriuretic peptide (BNP) is a cardiac neurohormone secreted from membrane granules in the cardiac ventricles as a response to ventricular volume expansion and pressure overload.[43] The natriuretic peptide system allows the heart to participate in the regulation of vascular tone and extracellular volume status. The natriuretic peptide system and the renin–angiotensin system counteract each other in arterial pressure regulation. Levels of atrial natiuretic peptide (ANP) and BNP are elevated in cardiac disease states associated with increased ventricular stretch. This assay represents the first clinically available blood test to facilitate the diagnosis of heart failure.

Clinical studies

Clinical studies have indicated that the BNP test facilitates the diagnosis of heart failure, beyond existing clinical information. In a study of 250 patients presenting with dyspnea to an emergency medical center, BNP performance was compared to a gold standard of two cardiologists (blinded to BNP levels) reviewing all clinical, radiographic, and echocardiographic data.[44] Mean BNP concentration in blood in patients with congestive heart failure (CHF) was 1076 ± 138 pg/ml vs 38 ± 4 pg/ml in those without (p < 0.001). In patients with lower extremity edema diagnosed with and without heart failure, BNP levels were 1038 ± 163 vs 63 ± 16 pg/ml.[44] In patients with dyspnea secondary to COPD or heart failure, BNP levels were 86 ± 39 with COPD compared with 1076 ± 138 with heart failure.

At a blood concentration of greater than 100 pg/ml, BNP was an accurate predictor of the presence of CHF with a sensitivity of 94%, specificity of 94%, and a 96% negative predictive value. BNP was more accurate in diagnosing CHF than history, symptoms, physical exam findings, chest X-ray, and the ECG. In multivariate analysis, BNP added significant, independent diagnostic power compared with other clinical variables and diagnostic tests. The availability of BNP measurements would have potentially corrected 29 of the 30 diagnoses missed by the physicians evaluating the patient in the emergency medical center.[44]

Congestive heart failure management

BNP levels objectively reflect severity of disease in patients with heart failure. BNP levels obtained in patients with established heart failure provide prognostic information and monitoring of levels over time may facilitate titration of heart failure medications. Investigations are currently ongoing to further evaluate the clinical utility of BNP testing for these purposes. In patients being treated for heart failure, in whom volume status and the degree of compensation are not clear based on history and physical examination, BNP is likely to provide information that has greater clinical utility than chest X-ray testing. As BNP levels correlate with PCWP, the BNP test could be considered in patients where volume status is uncertain and where right heart catheterization or serial echocardiography may otherwise be performed to assess ventricular filling pressures. Heart failure patients with persistently elevated BNP levels would be expected to benefit from increased titration of diuretics and further optimization of ACEI, beta-blocker, and spironolactone dosing. In heart failure patients with persistent or worsening symptoms out of proportion to their BNP levels, alternative causes of symptoms should be considered (i.e. other medical problems such as depression, anemia, or infection).[45]

Characteristics of assay

The triage BNP test diagnostic level to exclude heart failure is BNP < 100 pg/ml (negative). A level of ≥ 100 pg/ml is considered positive and indicative of heart failure. An elevated BNP indicates elevated ventricular filling pressure (PCWP) as occurs with systolic and diastolic dysfunction heart failure. Elevations can also be seen in acute myocardial infarction severe enough to elevate ventricular pressure. BNP levels are not influenced by hypertension, diabetes, mild renal insufficiency, or COPD. Dialysis patients will have elevated levels reflecting increased ventricular filling pressure. The assay identifies patients with heart failure and correlates with severity of symptoms/NYHA class.[45]

Nesiritide use for decompenstated heart failure

Definition

Nesiritide is human BNP produced by recombinant DNA technology. Nesiritide produces dose-dependent balanced arterial and venous vasodilatation and has been shown to result in rapid reduction in ventricular filling pressures and reversal of heart failure symptoms such as dyspnea.

Nesiritide also reduces levels of deleterious neurohormones such as aldosterone and endothelin. The use of nesiritide in addition to standard decompensated heart failure care, such as diuretic therapy, has been demonstrated to lead to meaningful clinical benefits in acutely decompensated heart failure patients. Nesiritide is an attractive therapeutic option because of its more rapid and sustained hemodynamic profile with fewer adverse effects than alternative heart failure treatments such a nitroglycerine, dobutamine, or milrinone.[46]

Indications

Nesiritide is indicated for the intravenous treatment of patients with acutely decompensated CHF who have dyspnea at rest or with minimal exertion. In these patients, the use of nesiritide is expected to reduce PCWP and improve dyspnea with fewer side-effects than other intravenous agents.[47,48]

Patient selection

Nesiritide should be considered for the volume-overloaded acutely decompensated CHF patient with adequate blood pressures. It should be used in addition to intravenous diuretics and before initiating other intravenous therapies. Patient specifics include:

- Dyspnea at rest or minimal exertion due to CHF
- SBP ≥ 90 mmHg or ≥ 80 mmHg with SVR ≥ 1500 dyne/sec/cm⁵
- Patient hospitalized for acute decompensated CHF
- Patient requires intravenous therapy
- Elevated ventricular filling pressure (≥ 20 mmHg if pulmonary artery catheter in place or by clinical estimate).[47]

Patient exclusions

- Patients in cardiogenic or other forms of shock
- Patients with SBP < 90 mmHg without PAC or < 80 mmHg with PAC
- Patients with low CI ≤ 2.0 l/min/m² with normal or low SVR ≤ 1200 dyne/sec/cm⁵
- Patients with low ventricular filling pressures (PCWP ≤ 12 mmHg).[47]

Dosage/administration

Initiation

The recommended bolus dose for nesiritide is 2 mcg/kg. The bolus dose should be administered over 60 seconds.[47]

Table 11.4. Topics for patient, family/caregiver education and counseling

General counseling

Cause or probable cause of heart failure

Explanation of symptoms

Symptoms of worsening heart failure

General explanation of treatment/care plan

Role of family members/other caregivers in the treatment/care plan

Availability and value of qualified local support group

Self-management

Importance of compliance with treatment plan

Clarification of patient responsibilities

Self-monitoring with daily weights

Monitoring of symptoms and what to do if worsened

Importance of cessation of tobacco use

Importance of obtaining vaccinations against influenza and pneumococcal disease

Prognosis

Life expectancy

Advance directives

Advice for family members in the event of sudden death

Activity recommendations

Recommendations for recreation, leisure, and work activity

Importance of regular aerobic activity

Recommendations for sexual activity, coping with sexual difficulties

Dietary recommendations

Sodium restriction

Avoidance of excessive fluid intake

Alcohol restriction

Low-fat diet for patients with cardiovascular disease

Medications

Reasons for medications, dosing and schedule

Expected effects of medication on quality of life and survival

Likely side-effects and what to do if they occur

Organizing medications and behavioral strategies (e.g. pill boxes) to
    coping with complicated regimens

Availability of lower cost medications or financial assistance

Adapted from Konstam et al[1] and Moser and Frazier.[50]

Maintenance infusion

After completion of bolus infusion begin maintenance infusion of 0.01 mcg/kg/min immediately.[47]

Clinical application

Monitoring blood pressure

Check blood pressure after initiating infusion or for change in dose:

Every 30 minutes for first hour
Every hour for the next 3 hours
Every 4 hours thereafter

Notify physician if patient develops symptomatic hypotension or SBP ≤ 80 mmHg.[47]

Monitoring urine output

Strict input and output should be documented. If urine output is < 50 cc/hr in the first 3 hours after the initiation of nesiritide, notify physician.

Monitoring weight

Daily weights should be obtained and recorded.

Monitoring symptoms

Improvement of dyspnea is expected. If respiratory rate or dyspnea either do not change or worsen during the course of nesiritide therapy, notify physician.

Monitoring BNP levels

BNP levels measured during nesiritide infusion are not clinically meaningful as exogenous BNP and endogenous BNP are indistinguishable. It is recommended that BNP levels be obtained prior to hospital discharge.[47]

Non-pharmacological therapies

Preparing for transfer and discharge

The combination of hemodynamic optimization along with non-pharmacologic therapies equals comprehensive heart failure management.[49] Educating patients and families while in the intensive care unit (ICU) or CCU setting is an important nursing intervention. Patients have experienced an acute event (hospitalization) and are open and ready for instruction on strategies to prevent rehospitalization and control disease progression. Detailed topics for patient and family education and counseling are listed in Table 11.4.[50]

During hospitalization, nutritional consultations should be made for detailed education on the 2-gram sodium diet. Education should be done with the patient and family member. Referrals for physical therapy should be initiated for instruction on in-hospital exercises and progressive home-based walking program and other exercise instructions. Cardiac rehabilitation referrals should be made as needed.

Fluid restriction of 2 liters (64 oz) should be maintained in the hospital and continued at home with education on monitoring and daily weighing. Instruction and observed behaviors using a daily weight chart can start in the ICU/CCU and be reinforced in the intermediate care unit and upon discharge. Patients require education on flexible diuretic dosing based on their daily weight. Since hospitalized patients are weighed daily, this is an excellent teaching opportunity for the nurse to test and reinforce patient's knowledge regarding their actions for scenarios of a 2-liter weight gain in 24 hrs or 4 lbs in 4 days. Patients should be able to verbalize actions to double their diuretic dose and increase potassium. Patients who are on high doses of oral furosemide should be instructed on the use of PRN metolazone. Further details of patient and family education and counseling are discussed in detail in Chapter 17.

Summary

This chapter has presented a case study with guidelines for care of the hospitalized heart failure patient. Hemodynamic indices were use to guide therapy and to determine the optimal therapeutic dose response. New diagnostics tests and treatment for decompensated heart failure were presented. These guidelines provide clinicians with a uniform approach to patient care and are pivotal to improving heart failure patient survival.

References

1 Konstam M, Dracup K, Baker D et al. Heart failure: evaluation and care of patients with left-ventricular systolic dysfunction. Clinical Practice Guideline No. 11. AHCPR Publication No. 94–0612. Rockville, MD: Agency for Health Care Policy and Research, Public Health Service, US Department of Health and Human Services, June 1994.

2 Edwards JD. Oxygen transport in cardiogenic and septic shock, to ischemic or nonischemic dilated cardiomyopathy. *Crit Care Med* 1991; **19:** 658–63.

3 UCLA Heart Failure Guideline, Ahamson UCLA Cardiomyopathy Clinic. Hemodynamic Management of Cardiomyopathy Patients. Revision 1/06/00. Los Angeles, CA, USA.

4 Stevenson LW, Tillisch JH, Hamilton MA et al. Importance of hemodynamic response to therapy in predicting survival with ejection fraction < 20% secondary to ischemic or nonischemic dilated cardiomyopathy. *Am J Cardiol* 1990; **66:** 1348–54.

5 Francis GS. Management of acute and decompensated heart failure. In: Hosenpud JD, Greenberg GH, eds. *Congestive Heart Failure*, 8th edn. Philadelphia: Lippincott Williams & Wilkins; 2000: 553–69.

6 Colucci WS, Kirkwood FA, Burnett JC, Katz SD. Treatment of Acute Decompensated CHF: Symposium Highlights. Scios, Inc.

7 Francis GS, Maisel AS, Elkayam U, Fonarow G. B-Type Natriuretic Peptide: a New Approach to an Old Problem: Program Syllabus. Fort Lee, NJ: Health Care Communications, Inc. October 2001.

8 American College of Cardiology/American Heart Association Task Force on Practice Guidelines. Guidelines for the evaluation and management of heart failure. *Circulation* 1995; **92:** 2764–84.

9 Heart Failure Society of America. Heart Failure Society of America (HFSA) practice guidelines: HFSA guidelines for management of patients with heart failure caused by left ventricular systolic dysfunction – pharmacological approaches. *J Cardiac Failure* 1999; **5:** 357–82.

10 Gerlag PGG, van Meijel JJM. High-dose furosemide in the treatment of refractory congestive heart failure. *Arch Intern Med* 1988; **148:** 286–91.

11 Vasko MR, Brown-Cartwright D, Knochel JP, Nixon JV, Brater DC. Furosemide absorption altered in decompensated congestive heart failure. *Ann Intern Med* 1985; **102:** 314–18.

12 Stevenson LW. Tailored therapy to hemodynamic goals for advanced heart failure. *Eur J Heart Failure* 1999; **1:** 251–7.

13 Campana C, Gavazzi A, Berzuini C et al. Predictors of prognosis in patients awaiting heart transplantation. *J Heart Lung Trans* 1993; **12:** 756–65.

14 Weiner IM. Diuretics and other agents employed in the mobilization of edema fluid. In: Gilman AG, Rall TW, Nies AS, Taylor P, eds. *Goodman and Gilman's The Pharmacological Basis of Therapeutics*, 8th edn. New York, NY: Macmillan Publishing Co Inc; 1993: 713–31.

15 Biddle TL, Yu PN. Effect of frusemide on hemodynamics and lung water in acute pulmonary edema secondary to myocardial infarction. *Am J Cardiol* 1979; **43:** 86–90.

16 UCLA Medical Center. UCLA Advanced Heart Failure Practice Guideline. Developed by Gregg Fonarow and Division of Cardiology, UCLA Medical Center, Revised 1998.

17 Rudy DW, Voelker JR, Greene PK, Esparza FA, Brater DC. Loop diuretics for chronic renal insufficiency: a continuous infusion is more efficacious than bolus therapy. *Ann Intern Med* 1991; **115:** 360–6.

18 Martin SJ, Danziger LH. Continuous infusion of loop diuretics in the critically ill: a review of the literature. *Crit Care Med* 1994; **22:** 1323–9.

19 Dormans TPJ, van Meyel JJM, Gerlag PGG, Tan Y, Russel FGM, Smits P. Diuretic efficacy of high dose furosemide in severe heart failure: bolus injection versus continuous infusion. *J Am Coll Cardiol* 1996; **28:** 376–82.

20 Goldberg LI. Dopamine – clinical uses of an endogenous catecholamine. *N Engl J Med* 1974; **291:** 707–10.

21 Goldberg LI. Cardiovascular and renal actions of dopamine: potential clinical applications. *Pharmacol Rev* 1972; **24:** 1–29.

22 Franciosa JA, Limas CJ, Guiha NH, Rodriguera E, Cohn JN. Improved left ventricular function during nitroprusside infusion in acute myocardial infarction. *Lancet* 1972; **1:** 650–4.

23 Chatterjee K, Parmley WW, Ganz W, Forrester J, Walinsky P et al. Hemodynamic and metabolic responses to vasodilator therapy in acute myocardial infarction. *Circulation* 1973; **48:** 1183–93.

24 Fuch RM, Rutler DL, Powell WJ. Effects of dobutamine on venous capacity. *Clin Res* 1976; **24:** 218a. Abstract.

25 Grossman W, Brodie B, Mann T, McLaurin L. Effects of sodium nitroprusside on left ventricular diastolic pressure-voume relations. *Circulation* 1975; **52(suppl 2):** II–35. Abstract.

26 Cohn JN, Burke LP. Nitroprusside. *Ann Intern Med* 1979; **91:** 752–7.

27 Fonarow GC, Chelimsky-Fallick C, Stevenson LW, Luu M, Hamilton MA et al. Effect of direct vasodilation with hydrazaline versus angiotensin-converting enzyme inhibition with captopril on mortality in advanced heart failure: the Hy-C trial. *J Am Coll Cardiol* 1992; **19:** 842–50.

28 Ludbrook PA, Byrne JD, Kurnik PB, McKnight RC. Influence of reduction of preload and afterload by nitroglycerin on left ventricular diastolic pressure–volume relations and relaxation in man. *Circulation* 1977; **56:** 937–43.

29 Flaherty JT, Magee PA, Gardner TL, Potter A, MacAllister NP. Comparison of intravenous nitroglycerin and sodium nitroprusside for treatment of acute hypertension

developing after coronary artery bypass surgery. *Circulation* 1982; **65:** 1072–77.

30 Chiariello M, Herman KG, Leinbach RC, Davis MA, Maroko PR. Comparison between the effects of nitroprusside and nitroglycerin on ischemic injury during acute myocardial infarction. *Am J Cardiol* 1976; **37:** 766–73.

31 Cohn JN, Franciosa JA, Francis GS et al. Effect of short-term infusion of sodium nitroprusside on mortality rate in acute myocardial infarction complicated by left ventricular failure. *N Engl J Med* 1982; **306:** 1129–35.

32 Guiha NH, Cohn JN, Mikulic E, Franciosa JA, Limas CJ. Treatment of refractory heart failure with infusion of nitroprusside. *N Engl J Med* 1974; **291:** 587–92.

33 Miller RR, Vismara LA, Williams DO, Amsterdam EA, Mason DT. Pharmacological mechanisms for left ventricular unloading in clinical congestive heart failure: differential effects of nitroprusside, phentolamine, and nitroglycerin on cardiac function and peripheral circulation. *Circ Res* 1976; **39:** 127–33.

34 Grose R, Strain J, Greenberg M, LeJemtel TH. Systemic and coronary effects of intravenous milrinone and dobutamine in congestive heart failure. *J Am Coll Cardiol* 1986; **7:** 1107–13.

35 Monrad ES, Bain DS, Smith HS, Lanoue AS. Milrinone, dobutamine, and nitroprusside: comparative effects of hemodynamics and myocardial energetics in patients with severe congestive heart failure. *Circulation* 1986; **73(Suppl III):** III168–III174.

36 Packer M, Bristow MR, Cohn JN, Cloucci WS, Fowler MB et al. The effect of carvediol on morbidity and mortality in patients with chronic heart failure. US Carvediol Heart Failure Study Group. *N Engl J Med* 1996; **334:** 1349–55.

37 Packer M, Coats AJ, Fowler MB et al. Effect of carvediol on survival in severe chronic heart failure. *N Engl J Med* 2001; **344:** 1651–8.

38 Fonarow G. UCLA Heart Failure Clinical Guidelines, 2001: In-Hospital Initiation of Beta Blocker Therapy for Heart Failure. 2001.

39 Dargie HJ, Cleland JGF, Leckie BJ, Inglis CG, East BW, Ford I. Relation of arrhythmias and electrolyte abnormalities to survival in patients with severe chronic heart failure. *Circulation* 1987; **75:** IV98–IV107.

40 Gottlieb SS, Fisher ML, Pressel MD, Patten RD, Weinberg M, Greenberg N. Effects of intravenous magnesium sulfate on arrhythmias in patients with congestive heart failure. *Am Heart J* 1993; **125:** 1645–50.

41 Leier CV, Dei Cas L, Metra M. Clinical relevance and management of the major electrolyte abnormalities in congestive heart failure: hyponatremia, hypokalemia, and hypomagnesemia. *Am Heart J* 1989; **128:** 564–74.

42 The effect of digoxin on mortality and morbidity in patients with heart failure. The Digitalis Investigation Group. *N Engl J Med* 1997; **336:** 525–33.

43 Bonow RO. New insights into the cardiac natriuretic peptides. *Circulation* 1996; **93:** 1946–50.

44 Dao Q, Krishnaswamy P, Kazanegra R et al. Utility of B-type natriuretic peptide in the diagnosis of congestive heart failure in an urgent-care setting. *J Am Coll Cardiol* 2001; **37:** 379–85.

45 Fonarow GC. B-type natriuretic (BNP) diagnostic module. UCLA Medical Center. 2001.

46 Troughton RW, Frampton CM, Yandle TG et al. Treatment of heart failure guided by plasma amino terminal brain natriuretic pepetide (N-BNP) concentrations. *Lancet* 2000; **355:** 1126–30.

47 Fonarow GC. Nesiritide use for decompensated heart failure, UCAL Medical Center. 2001

48 Colucci WS, Elkayam U, Horton DP, Abraham WT et al. Intravenous nesiritide, a natriuretic peptide, in the treatment of decompensated congestive heart failure. *New Engl J Med* 2000; **343:** 246–53.

49 Fonarow GC, Stevenson LW, Walden JA et al. Impact of a comprehensive heart failure management program on hospital readmission and functional status of patients with advanced heart failure. *J Am Coll Cardiol* 1997; **30:** 725–32.

50 Moser DK, Frazier SK. The congestive heart failure patient In M Chulay (ed). *AACN's Protocol for Practice: Care of the Cardiac Patient Series*. Aliso Viejo, CA: American Association of Critical Care Nurses.

12 Nurse-led management programmes in heart failure

Tiny Jaarsma and Simon Stewart

Introduction

Much has been learned in the past decade about specialist nurse-led interventions for patients with heart failure. It is generally agreed that such programmes of care can improve patient outcomes with respect to health care utilization and associated costs, quality of life and survival.[1–4] At the same time, discussion on the optimal approach and the underlying mechanisms of success of these programmes is still active. Some suggest that the key elements in the success of heart failure programmes are most probably adherence to treatment and early detection and treatment of clinical decompensation.[5] Others stress the importance of optimal medical treatment, clinical stability, access to specialist care and the role of the nurse acting as the guardian of more expensive health care facilities.[1,6,7] On balance, however, the exact mechanisms of beneficial effect and issues concerning the optimal timing, intensity and duration of an intervention or the duration of the effect of these programmes are still unknown. These issues will, therefore, continue to be the subject of debate and research for some time to come.

While there are residual practical issues concerning best practice with respect to the application of these types of programme, it is important to note that many heart failure management programmes are being copied and adapted from pre-existing programmes or newly created with an optimistic outlook and minimal homework. This, of course, may lead to an innovative and creative programme, but without a proper analysis of the inherent 'bottlenecks' in the resident health care system, the target population and a clear plan of intervention, it is unlikely that such a programme will succeed.[8]

Although it is not possible to describe 'the' best, most effective nurse-led heart failure management programme, a lot can be learned from the development and implementation of the range of pre-existing programmes that have proven to be successful. This chapter provides an overview of the key outcomes and goals, in addition to the key components of intervention, that need to be incorporated into

any service of this type within the context of the various models used to organize the programme of care. It then concludes with a short list of practical considerations in setting up a nurse-led heart failure management programme.

Improving outcomes

As discussed in greater detail in Chapter 2, the burden of heart failure involves a variety of aspects to the individual, to his/her direct environment (such as family and friends), and to society overall. Heart failure is associated with a poor prognosis, with symptoms affecting daily functioning, and a treatment regimen that can have a major impact on the daily life of patients and their families.[9–12] Progression of the disease, symptoms and treatment affect important outcomes like resource utilization and health care costs.[13]

In general, health care providers aim their treatment at improving survival and improving quality of life of patients. In comparing approaches to treatment, decreasing health care cost is often an important outcome to consider. Several nurse-led heart failure management programmes have been demonstrated to positively affect these outcomes.[2–4] In designing and discussing the content and structure of a heart failure programme, considering the mechanism(s) of beneficial effect related to these outcomes is important. For example, if one aims at improving survival, one first should ask: what influences survival of patients and which component in a nurse-led heart failure management programme is expected to contribute to survival benefit? Improved medical treatment, improved compliance of patients to their prescribed regime or early and adequate response to deterioration can be factors that underlie the more abstract outcome 'survival'.

There are many preventable and often interrelated factors contributing to poorer outcomes among heart failure patients, which can be addressed through non-pharmacological means. These potentially modifiable factors can be summarized as follows:[14–19]

- inadequate or inappropriate medical treatment or adverse effects of prescribed treatment;
- inadequate knowledge of chronic heart failure and prescribed treatment;
- lack of motivation or inability to adhere to the treatment;
- intentional non-compliance with prescribed treatment;
- problems with caregivers or extended care facilities;
- poor social support.

To influence these factors positively a multifaceted approach to heart failure management with various potential outcomes is needed.

Figure 12.1 summarizes the various outcomes a nurse-led heart failure management programme can aim at. It also illustrates how complicated and interrelated the mechanisms of beneficial effect can be.

Most studies concentrate on the number of readmissions or readmission days as a primary endpoint. However, the endpoints such as compliance, medical treatment or patient's satisfaction are also incorporated in some studies. Using each 'text box' in Figure 12.1 as a guide the following sections explore the purpose of heart failure management programmes and their intended effect (i.e. from improved knowledge to improved survival).

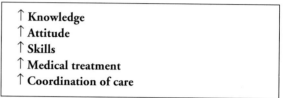

Several behaviours of patients must be changed to successfully adhere to the typically prescribed regimen. Patients need sufficient knowledge of chronic heart failure and prescribed treatment and need to be motivated for the treatment. The primary concrete target of many nurse-led

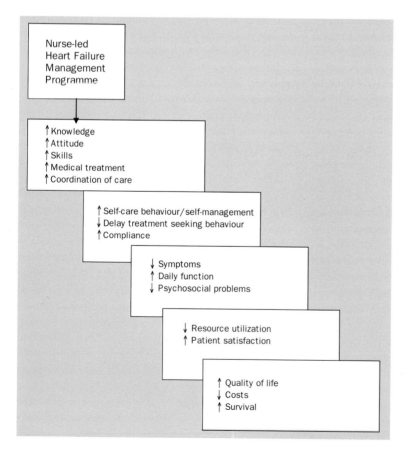

Figure 12.1. *Potential outcomes of a nurse-led heart failure management programme.*

heart failure management programmes is to improve patients' knowledge, attitude and skills and at the same time to optimize medical treatment and care. Interventions like patient education and counselling are often basic in a heart failure programme, but it is not often measured if this goal is reached. Although a lack of knowledge is often considered to be an underlying reason for negative outcomes in patients with heart failure,[20,21] only a few studies report on the effect of their intervention on the change in knowledge and attitude.[22,23]

Another important goal of a heart failure programme is optimizing medical treatment by improving physician prescribing patterns and promoting greater adherence to established treatment guidelines. Some observational data suggest that care of patients with heart failure in a specialized heart failure programme is associated with significant increase in the utilization and doses of all beneficial cardiovascular drugs, specially angiotensin-converting enzyme (ACE) inhibitors.[24–26]

A third basic factor in several nurse-led heart failure programmes is the improvement of the gap between care providers in the hospital and at home. Assessment of readiness for discharge and optimal discharge planning is often aimed for, but not often evaluated as an outcome.

Increased knowledge, skills and attitude are expected to result in improved self-care behaviour, self-management, optimal treatment-seeking behaviour and better compliance with the treatment.

> ↑Self-care behaviour/self-management
> ↓Delay treatment seeking behavior
> ↑Compliance

Patients have to learn to live with the consequences of heart failure, which means they must comply with a regimen concerning medication, diet and exercise, monitor symptoms, and seek assistance when symptoms occur. It is believed that an improvement in outcomes depends on patients' abilities to care for themselves and manage consequences of their condition. Therefore, programmes try to make patients experts in heart failure self-management and teach them to recognize deterioration and take relevant actions in case of exacerbation. As such, it has been demonstrated that a nurse-led heart failure management programme can positively affect these processes that probably affect patient outcomes.[27–29]

The amount of time between the first awareness of symptoms and the arrival at the hospital (delay-time) is often prolonged in patients with heart failure. Mean delays of 36 hours to 1 week before hospital admission are reported, with a median delay of 72 hours.[30,31] Patients who reported with the two most common symptoms of heart failure on admission (dyspnoea and oedema) had delay times approximately twice as long as those who did not have these symptoms. It is possible that these patients see these two chronic symptoms as part of their chronic condition and attempt to manage them at home before seeking health care.[31] Designing interventions that change the typical delay to treatment in heart failure is obviously important. However, delay to treatment time is not reported as an outcome in any of the studies evaluating the effect of a nurse-led heart failure management programme.

Another important objective in programmes is improved adherence to treatment. Compliance with long-term medical regimens of patients with heart failure is poor, with overall non-compliance rates ranging from 42%[18] to 64%.[32] In a study of elderly patients with heart failure, only 55% of the patients could correctly name what medication had been prescribed, 50% were unable to state the prescribed doses and 64% could not account for what medication was to be taken, i.e. at what time of day and when in relation to meals the medication was to be taken. In their overall assessment the authors found that 73% were compliant with their prescribed medicine regimen.[33] In a study on digoxin use, only 10% of the patients filled enough prescriptions to have received adequate treatment.[34]

Non-compliance extends to other aspects of the treatment regimen such as daily weighing, keeping to a salt-restricted diet, restricting fluid and alcohol intake and exercise. It seems difficult to change behaviour and to manage heart failure as expected by health care professionals. Strategies to enhance compliance include the patient but also integrate the role of physicians, nurses, other health care providers and organization into the plan to ultimately improve patient outcomes.[35,36] Only a few studies describe the effect of a nurse-led heart failure intervention programme on compliance[21,36,37] or readmissions arising from non-adherence to, or adverse effects of, prescribed treatment.[38]

It is often reasoned that as a result of better treatment and better compliance and self-care behaviour, a patient's physical state (symptoms and daily function) and psychological state will improve. Once again, there is a paucity of data to support this, although West et al showed that reported symptoms declined in intensity with statistically significant reductions in angina during exertion, cough, orthopnoea and fatigue during application of a comprehensive management programme for heart failure patients.[39]

↓ **Symptoms**
↑ **Daily function**
↓ **Psychosocial problems**

Daily function or improvement of functional capacity is also often targeted in multidisciplinary nurse-led interventions. However, in only a few studies is this outcome evaluated. In observational, non-randomized studies the increase in the ability to perform daily activities or improve exercise tolerance after participation in a heart failure programme was described.[39–41] However, one should be careful in interpreting these studies, since it is also known that patients from care-as-usual groups improve functional capacity and decrease symptoms during the post discharge period.[42,43]

In addition to decreasing physical symptoms, several programmes also aim at improving psychosocial function or adaptation of patients with heart failure.[42,44] Psychosocial factors, particularly lack of social support and depression, are associated with poorer outcomes in patients with heart failure.[45,46] It is also known that there is an association between the severity of depressive symptoms at baseline and the rate of the combined endpoint of either functional decline or death at 6 months in patients with heart failure.[47] The psychosocial aspects in heart failure are further elaborated in Chapter 15 of this book.

↓ **Resource utilization**
↑ **Patient satisfaction**

An improvement in the patient's physical and psychosocial status is expected to lead to fewer hospital admissions and better satisfaction with care. Almost all heart failure programmes are aimed at decreasing resource utilization as reflected by all-cause and heart failure-related hospital readmissions, days from hospital discharge to first event and the frequency of multiple admissions (see Tables 12.1 and 12.2).

Another outcome that is assumed to improve as a result of the above is the satisfaction of the patient with health care. Only a few studies that evaluate heart failure programmes report on patient satisfaction.[44,48] Health care providers and designers of nurse-led heart failure management programmes probably assume that by optimizing care to professional standard, patients will be more satisfied. It should be noted, however, that in a large randomized study reported by Weinberger et al, increased access to primary care was associated with both increased levels of satisfaction with the intervention and levels of health care utilization.[48]

↑ **Quality of life**
↓ **Costs**
↑ **Survival**

Increased quality of life, decreased overall costs of care and a survival advantage for patients are the ultimate goals when designing a heart failure intervention programme. Quality of life is increasingly being incorporated in the evaluation of treatment options and also in the evaluation of management programmes. Some nurse-led heart failure management programmes were explicitly reporting improved quality of life,[49–51] whereas others are satisfied with a decrease in costs while negatively affecting patient quality of life.[52]

In addition to improvement in patient outcomes, decreasing health care costs and improving survival are considered in the evaluation of almost all programmes.

It is suggested by studies of the economic burden imposed by heart failure,[53–57] that the key to cost-effectiveness of heart failure programmes is to reduce hospital stay – even at the expense of increasing levels of community-based care and pharmacotherapy.[24,26] Directly projecting the cost–benefits of the programmes of care summarized in Tables 12.1 and 12.2 to the wider health care system without adjusting for additional expenses, however, would be too simplistic and over-estimate their potential cost–benefits.[24,26] Recently the potential economic benefits from the creation of a UK-wide service based on a programme of home-based nurse management, as if it had been in operation in the year 2000, were calculated.[57] A large component of these data were derived from three key studies described in Table 12.2, which described the benefits of nurse-led, home-based interventions with a strong component of multidisciplinary involvement to optimize outcomes in older patients with heart failure in the USA,[58] Australia[59] and the UK[60] (Table 12.3). A number of assumptions were modelled on the infrastructure and impact of the city-wide Glasgow Heart Failure Liaison Service in Scotland[60] and contemporary UK data describing the burden and cost of heart failure.[53,54,61]

It was concluded that the economic consequences of applying a specialist nurse-mediated, post-discharge management service for heart failure in a country might be

Table 12.1. Randomized controlled studies examining the effects of a nurse-initiated heart failure clinic model designed to limit hospital readmission

Reference	Study cohort	Study intervention	Major endpoints	Results	Comments
Kasper EK et al[51] 2002 (USA)	200 HF pts (mean age 64 years) admitted to The John Hopkins Hospital and The John Hopkins Bayview Medical Center	Multidisciplinary management program with pre-specified schedule of contacts with a CHF nurse (mainly clinic visits) and telephone follow-up	Death from any cause plus admissions for HF, all hospital admissions and quality of life within 6 months	The primary end-point occurred less frequently in the study group compared to usual care (7 vs 13 deaths and 43 vs 59 admissions: $P = 0.09$). Overall, study pts had fewer days of readmission (4.3 vs. 6.3/pt: NS). Quality of life scores were significantly improved	This was a relatively young cohort of CHF patients: possibly because patients with renal dysfunction were excluded – event rates were low as a result
Stromberg A et al 2001[29] (Sweden)	106 HF pts (mean age 78 years) from a university hospital and two county hospitals in Linkoping	Follow-up at a hospital based nurse-led heart failure clinic	All cause mortality or all cause hospital admission, number of days in hospital, time to first readmission, quality of life, self-care behaviour within 12 months	Fewer patients with events in the intervention group compared to the control groups (29 vs 40, $P = 0.03$) and fewer deaths after 3 months (3 vs 13, $P = 0.009$) and 12 months (7 vs 20, $P = 0.005$), fewer readmissions (33 vs 56, $P = 0.0047$) and days in hospital (350 vs 593, $P = 0.045$), higher self-care	This is the first study to find significant effects on mortality in a clinic-based intervention
McDonald et al 2002 (Ireland)	98 HF patients (mean age 71 years) admitted to a university hospital in Dublin	Inpatient and outpatient education and close telephone and clinic follow-up	Hospital readmission with heart failure and/or death within 90 days and readmission within one month	No readmissions at 1 month in both care groups. After 3 months 4 endpoints were recorded in the multidisciplinary group compared with 14 endpoints in the routine care group ($P = 0.02$)	An event rate of 8.2% at 3 months is a very low reported rate for such a high-risk group
Ekman et al 1998 (Sweden)	158 HF patients (mean age 80 years) admitted to medical wards in a secondary care and regional hospital in Gothenburg	Nurse-monitored, outpatient care programme aiming at symptom management	Functional class, readmission or death and hospital days 6 months after follow-up	There was no difference in number of readmissions, mortality or survival without readmission or improvement of NYHA classification	This study also showed that 29% of the structured care patients were not able to visit the nurse, indicating that such a programme might not be appropriate for the elderly
Cline et al 1997 (Sweden)	190 CHF patients (mean age 76 years) admitted to a university-affiliated hospital in Malmo	In-hospital counselling, plus follow-up at a nurse-led, heart failure-specific outpatient clinic	Time to readmission, duration of hospital stay and health-care costs within 12 months	Mean time to first admission was prolonged in study patients ($P < 0.05$). There were no significant differences in survival, hospital stay and health care costs at 1 year	Patients were not specifically selected on the basis of risk. However, there were strong trends in favour of study patients in all outcomes studied
Weinberger et al 1996 (USA)	1396 veterans (mean age 63 years) admitted to 9 Veterans Affairs Medical Centers with diabetes, COPD or CHF (n = 504)	Clinic-based follow-up by a nurse and primary care physician for 6 months after discharge	Frequency of hospital admissions and duration of stay within 6 months	Study patients had higher rates of readmission (0.19 vs 0.14 per month $P < 0.01$) and more days of hospitalization (10.2 vs 8.8: $P < 0.05$) relative to that of usual care	This is the only reported trial of an intervention designed to reduce hospitalization in which more hospitalizations in the intervention group were documented

Table 12.2. Randomized controlled studies examining the effects of strategies with specialty care extending into home or primary care in heart failure patients

Reference	Study cohort	Study Intervention	Major endpoints	Results	Comments
Martensson et al[72] (Sweden)	**153** HF patients (mean age 79 years) registered at eight primary health care centers in south eastern Sweden	Patients and family education and monthly telephone follow-up during 12 months	Depression, Quality of life and life satisfaction	Significant differences of the nurse-led intervention between the groups were found in quality of life, life satisfaction and depression[72]	This study focused both on education of members of the HC system and education of patients and family
Harrison et al[72] 2002 (Canada)	**157 (originally 192)** HF patients admitted to two medical units in Ottawa, Ontario	Transitional care model to improve patient education and level of usual home care	Change in Quality of Life scores **within 12 weeks**	Quality of life as measured by the Minnesota, Living With Heart Failure Questionnaire was significant improved in the study group. Study patients tended to have fewer admissions (NS)	This study concentrated almost exclusively on quality of life and showed improvements with the intervention – although it also improved in the usual care group
Stewart et al[61] 2002 (Australia)	Combined analysis of **298** HF patients aged ≥ 55 years from a university hospital who were discharged to home and participated in the two reported studies	Multidisciplinary, home-based intervention with a post-discharge home visits at 7–14 days	Unplanned reacmissions plus out-of-hospital deaths during 3–6 years follow-up (median 4.2 years)	Study patients had fewer primary events (mean of 0.21 vs 0.37 events/pt/mth: $P < 0.01$). Median event-free (7 vs 3 mths: $P < 0.01$) and all-cause survival (40 vs 22 mths: $P < 0.05$) was also more prolonged)	The first study to examine the effect of this type of intervention beyond two years and provides preliminary evidence to suggest that it is possible to cost-effectively prolong survival and reduce hospital stay
Riegel et al[63] 2002 (USA)	**242 (originally 358)** HF patients (mean age 72 years) recruited from two hospitals in Southern California	Nurse-directed, telephonic case management program (average of 17 phone calls over 6 months). Additional guidelines to physicians	HF-related admissions and associatec stay within 6 months	Rate of HF-related admissions were reduced by 48% ($P < 0.05$) and associated stay by 46% ($P < 0.05$). However, all-cause stay was 28% less in the study group (NS). The cost of care also tended to be lower (NS)	In this study there was a major loss to follow-up. It does represent the first large study of telephonic-follow-up and whilst HF-related outcomes improved, it was less effective overall (all-cause events: NS)
Krumholz et al[37] 2002 (USA)	**88** HF pts (mean age 74 years) recruited from Yale-New Haven Hospital	Educational program covering 5 sequential care domains for self-care of chronic disease. 55%:45% clinic visits vs home visits plus telephone follow-up	Event-free survival, HF-related morbidity and all-cause deaths within 1 year	Event-free survival was more prolonged in the study group (HR 0.56: $P < 0.05$). Fewer study patients readmitted for HF (57% vs 82%: $P = 0.01$). Study patients tended to have fewer all-cause days of readmission/pt (10.2 vs 15.2: $P = 0.09$)	Although described as uniquely focused on education alone the study has similarities to that performed by Jaarsma et al. Whether education 'alone' was provided is debatable due to home/clinic visits and telephone 'advice'
Doughty et al[49] 2002 (New Zealand)	**197** CHF patients (mean age 73 years) from a university hospital who were discharged to home	HF management program, with vigilant follow-up, alternated between clinic and GP	Event-free survival, all-cause readmissions and stay and quality of life within 1 year	No impact on the time to first readmission but did decrease multiple readmissions	This was essentially a clinic-based intervention. Although the majority of results were disappointing, the study program did reduce hospital stay overall. The effect of decreasing multiple readmission occurred inpatients at low and high risk

Table 12.2. *Continued*

Reference	Study cohort	Study Intervention	Major endpoints	Results	Comments
Blue et al[49] 2002 (United Kingdom)	**165** CHF patients (mean age 75 years) discharged from a university-affiliated hospital to home	Nurse-led home-based program of care with multiple home visits and initiation/titration of pharmacological therapy	All-cause death and HF admission within 3–12 months. HF and all-cause stay	Patients in the study group were less likely to have a primary event (HR 0.61: $P < 0.05$). Study patients also had fewer all-cause readmissions (86 vs 114: $P < 0.05$) and associated stay ($P < 0.05$)	This is the first randomized study to examine a program of care where specialist nurses initiated and titrated pharmacotherapy. Home visits were more frequent than Stewart et al
Moser et al[64] 2000 (USA)	**136** CHF patients (mean age 70 years) discharged from a university hospital to home	Community case management with nurse-visits in hospital and at home	Readmission rate, length of stay, costs and quality of life	Lower readmission rates in the intervention group, lower health care costs, and shorter hospital lengths of stay (p < 0.01) and better quality of life	
Naylor et al[44] 1999 (USA)	**363 (60 CHF)** chronically ill patients (mean age 75 years) from a university hospital discharged to home	Comprehensive discharge planning and a home-based follow-up protocol	Hospital readmissions plus event-free survival within 24 weeks	Less study patients were readmitted (20% vs 37%: $P < 0.01$) and they had more event-free survival ($P < 0.001$)	Only 70% of intervention and 73% of usual care patients completed this study
Stewart et al[50] 1999 (Australia)	**200** HF patients aged ≥ 55 years from a university hospital who were discharged to home	Multidisciplinary, home-based intervention with at least one home visit by a cardiac nurse	Frequency of unplanned readmissions plus out-of-hospital deaths within 6 months	Usual care patients had more (129 vs 77) primary events ($P = 0.02$) and more intervention patients remained event-free (38 vs 51; $P = 0.04$) at 6 months	This is the first study to show that this type of intervention is associated with both prolonged event-free survival and fewer readmissions
Stewart et al[65,71] 1999 (Australia)	**97** HF pts admitted to a tertiary referral hospital in Adelaide, who participated in a larger study of a home intervention (n = 762)	A combination of pre-discharge education and a home visit by a nurse and pharmacist	Event free survival and hospital readmissions within 6 months and 18 months	Patients in the study group had fewer primary events (66 vs 135 events: $P < 0.05$) and fewer days of hospitalization (2.5 vs 4.5/pt: $P < 0.01$) at 6 months. At 18 month this effect was sustained	This was the first study to suggest that this type of intervention had longer-term beneficial effects on both readmission and survival
Jaarsma et al[24,43] 1999 (Netherlands)	**179** CHF patients (mean age 73 years) from a university hospital and discharged to home	A supportive education program in the hospital and home promoting self-care behaviour	Self-care behaviour and health-care utilisation within 9 months	The intervention increased self-care behaviour. There were strong associated trends towards fewer patients readmitted and fewer days of admission. No effects on quality of life	This singular strategy was beneficial overall, although none of the health-care utilisation end-points reached statistical significance
Rich et al[42] 1995 (USA)	**282** HF patients aged ≥ 70 years from the medical units of a university medical center and discharged to home	Nurse-directed, multi-disciplinary intervention involving home and clinic visits	Event-free survival, rate of readmission, quality of life, and cost of care within 3 months	Event-free survival favoured study patients ($P = 0.09$). Study patients had fewer readmissions, better quality of life and fewer health-care costs ($P < 0.05$)	This was the first, properly powered, randomised study of a nurse-led intervention in CHF

Table 12.3. Outcomes in studies examining the effects of nurse-led heart failure programmes

Knowledge	Serxner 1998; Bjork Linne 1999
Attitude	Serxner 1998
Medical treatment	
• utilization of cardiovascular drugs	West 1997; Hanumanthu 1997; Ramahi 2000; Dahl 2000
Self-care behaviour/management	West 1997; Serxner 1998 Jaarsma 2000
Compliance	Rich 1996; Sexner 1998
Symptoms	Kostis 1994; West 1997; Jaarsma 2000
Daily function	
• functional capacity	Kostis 1994; Naylor 1999; Jaarsma 2000
• exercise capacity/time	Smith 1997; West 1997; Riegel 2000
• NYHA	West 1997; Fonarow 1997; Ekman 1998; Smith 1998
• Peak oxygen consumption	Fonarow 1997 Hanumanthu 1997
Psychosocial problems	
• depression	Naylor 1999
• psychosocial adjustment to illness	Jaarsma 2000
Resource utilization	
• Number of readmissions)/days	Cintron 1983; Rich 1995; Weinberger 1996; Lasater 1996; West 1997; Smith 1997; Fonarow 1997; Stewart 1998–99; Cline 1998; Macko 1998; Ekman 1998; Shah 1998; Naylor 1999; Jaarsma 1999; Riegel 2000; Dahl 2000; Blue 2001; Doughty 2001; McDonald 2001
• Time to first admission/first event	Weinberger 1996; Cline 1998
• ER visits, clinic visits	Rich 1995; Ekman 1998; Stewart 1999; Doughty Weinberger 1996; West 1997; Jaarsma 1999
Patient satisfaction	Weinberger 1996; Naylor 1999
Quality of life	Kostis 1994; Rich 1995; Weinberger 1996; West 1997; Hanumanthu 1997; Smith 1997; Cline 1998; Jaarsma 2000; Stewart 1999; Doughty 2001
Costs	Cintron 1983; Lasater 1996; Rich 1995; Fonarow 1997; Cline 1998; Serxner 1998; Stewart 1998; Stewart 1999; Naylor 1999; Macko 1999; Riegel 2000
Survival/mortality	Cline 1998 Fonarow 1997; West 1997; Ekman 1998; Stewart 1999

huge. Reduced costs and improved efficiency of the health care system can be expected.[57]

To date there have been several studies to evaluate the effect of a nurse-led heart failure management programme designed to improve outcomes in patient with heart failure. As shown in Tables 12.1 and 12.2 these studies mostly report positive patient outcomes regarding readmissions, quality of life, cost and survival. However, some inconclusive or negative studies should not be overlooked.

As depicted in Figure 12.1, heart failure programmes have several goals, with outcomes on various levels. We know that there is a wide range in interventions that are tested in the studies presented in Tables 12.1 and 12.2. Within the intervention there are a number of components that can be considered responsible for the outcomes. These are:

- multidisciplinary approach;
- education and support (including self-management, non-compliance, continuity and early attention to signs and symptoms);
- optimization of medical therapy;
- vigilant, frequent follow-up after hospital discharge (telephone, home visit, clinic);
- increased access to health care professional;
- coordination of care;
- early attention to signs and symptoms of fluid overload;
- exercise programme.

Organizational models

The key components of these programmes, as discussed earlier, are often organized into a number of distinct models of health care delivery. Although there are a large number of within-model variations, the majority of programmes can be classified as either 'clinic-based' management or 'specialty care extending to the home'.

Clinic-based management

In the clinic model, care is delivered in an outpatient setting by practitioners with heart failure expertise to patients who attend the clinic.[62] In some cases, part of the programme starts while the patient is still in the hospital, but the primary site of care delivery is the outpatient clinic. Nurses can perform a variety of roles in these programmes. In some programmes, nurses assist cardiologists in coordinating or facilitating care. In other programmes nurses have a more independent role and manage and direct care with primary responsibility for the day-to-day care of patients. Alternatively, the nurse's major responsibility is to bridge the gap between inpatient and outpatient care.

There are several studies that examine the effect of a heart failure clinic, using a non-randomized design. They all report positive results with regard to a reduction in hospital readmission, decreased readmission rate and rehospitalization days.[26,39–41] There are a limited number of randomized controlled studies examining the effects of a clinic model in which the nurse plays an important role (Table 12.1).

The first randomized study that was published on a heart failure clinic-based model was the study of Weinberger et al.[48] They described a study in which 1396 veterans (all men) hospitalized with chronic obstructive pulmonary disease, diabetes or heart failure were randomized to either usual care or to increased access to primary care nurses and physicians. Although study patients received this extra care, they had a greater number of re-admissions to hospital, but were more satisfied with their medical care relative to usual care during 6 months' follow-up. The increased health care utilization in the study group was attributed to a combination of greater vigilance in detecting problems and the ability of those detecting such problems (the physicians) to admit patients – thereby lowering admission thresholds.

A second study, which did not show a positive effect of a heart failure clinic, was performed in Sweden by Ekman et al.[43] They studied patients who were older than 65 years of age and classified in New York Heart Association (NYHA) classes III–IV. The total in-hospital population of patients discharged with a diagnosis of heart failure during a 14-month period from a university hospital (n = 1541) was identified. Of these, 158 patients (15%) could be included in a randomized controlled study the effect of an outpatient, nurse-monitored, symptom-management programme. The study intervention consisted of a visit by a nurse before discharge and outpatient visits to a nurse for education and counselling. Nurses made follow-up telephone contacts to patients to discuss issues raised during clinic visits. The numbers of hospitalizations and hospital days did not differ between the structured-care and the usual-care groups. They also noted that no visits to the nurse occurred in 23 cases among the 79 patients randomized to the structured-care group (29%), mainly on account of death or fatigue. Ekman et al concluded that given the selection criteria and the outline of the interventions, an outpatient, nurse-monitored, symptom-management programme is often not feasible for the majority of these elderly patients with moderate-to-severe chronic heart failure, mainly because of the small proportion of eligible patients and the high drop-out rate. They suggested that management of these patients should be more adjusted to their home situation.[43]

In that same year, another Swedish study reported positive results of a heart failure clinic.[40] Cline et al reported the benefits of a clinic-based follow-up of a lower risk cohort of patients with chronic heart failure.[52] A total of 206 older patients hospitalized with heart failure were randomized to the study intervention or to usual care. The special intervention included an education programme for patients and their families, concentrating on treatment. Guidelines for adjusting treatment in response to sodium and water overload and fluid depletion were also provided. This programme was carried out over two 30-minute visits to the patient in hospital and a 1-hour group information session for the patient and family 2 weeks after discharge. Frequent and easily accessible patient-initiated follow-up was provided as a nurse-run, hospital-based clinic and telephone contact. During 12-months of follow-up, time to first readmission was one-third longer in the intervention group (106 vs 141 days; $P < 0.05$), and number of days in the hospital tended to be fewer (4.2 vs 8.2, $P = 0.07$). There was also a trend toward a mean annual reduction in health care costs per patient. No differences were found in health-related quality of life between the intervention and control group.[52]

A study from McDonald et al in Ireland also reported on the effects of a multidisciplinary heart failure clinic.[7] In this study it is proposed that in addition to the already noted effect of multidisciplinary care, a further benefit will be observed with strict application of three important components of best 'clinical practice', namely ensure maximal doses of ACE inhibitors, ensure clinical stability and involvement of the cardiology service. Consenting patients were transferred to the cardiology service and randomized into multidisciplinary care or routine care. Patients from both care groups are optimally treated according to the three components mentioned above (stability, ACE and cardiology service). Patients in the intervention group receive inpatient and outpatient education and close telephonic and clinic follow-up, while those in the routine care were returned to care of the family doctor. At 3 months, four endpoints were recorded in the multidisciplinary group (8%; one admission and three deaths) compared with 14 endpoints (29%; 12 admissions and two deaths) in the routine care group ($P = 0.02$).

A recent study from the United States[51] studied the effects of a multidisciplinary management programme with a pre-specified schedule of contacts with a heart failure nurse (mainly clinic visits) and telephone follow-up. Two hundred patients hospitalized with heart failure at increased risk of hospital readmission were included. A study cardiologist and a heart failure nurse evaluated each patient and made recommendations to the patients' primary care physician before randomization. The intervention team consisted of a cardiologist, a heart failure nurse, telephone nurse coordinator, and the patient's primary care physician. Contact with the patients was on a pre-specified schedule, mostly in a clinic, but some in the patient's home. There were 43 heart failure hospital admissions and seven deaths in the intervention group, compared with 59 heart failure

hospital admissions and 13 deaths in the non-intervention groups ($P = 0.09$). The quality of life score, percentage of patients on target vasodilator therapy and percentage of patients compliant with dietary recommendation were significantly better in the intervention groups. Cost per patient was similar in both groups.

In a study from Sweden by Strömberg et al, the effect of follow-up in a nurse-led heart failure clinic was studied in 106 patients. The first visit in the intervention group was scheduled 2–3 weeks after discharge. The intervention consisted of education aimed at assisting patients to improve their self-care regimen, non-pharmacological treatment, protocol-led changes in medication, psychosocial support and availability of nurse contact in case of problems. When those patients were stable and well informed they were referred back to their general practitioner in primary care. The study results showed that there were fewer patients with events (death or admission) after 12 months in the intervention group compared with the control group (29 vs 40, $P = 0.03$) and fewer deaths after 3 months (three vs 13, $P = 0.009$) and 12 months (seven vs 20, $P = 0.005$). The intervention group also had fewer readmissions (33 vs 56, $P = 0.0047$) and days in hospital (350 vs 593, $P = 0.045$) during the first 3 months. The intervention group had significantly higher self-care scores at 3 and 12 months compared with the control group.[29]

Specialty care extending to home

In several models, care is delivered primarily in patients' homes and sometimes include home health facilities instead of delivering the care in a clinic or outpatient setting. Instead, the health care provider comes to the home of the patient in person, calls on the telephone or both. Similar to the clinic model, the role of the nurse can be more or less independent, ranging from nurse-coordinated facilitated care – where the role of the nurse is assisting and coordinating – to nurse-directed or nurse-managed – in which the nurse has a more independent role with other responsibilities. Depending on the health care system and the available expertise, advanced practitioners, home health nurses or other health care providers are involved. During the last decade several studies have been performed to evaluate the effect of different models that provide specialist heart failure care outside the clinic setting. Several of these studies are non-randomized studies, using historical data as control.[24,63–65] All of these studies report positive findings as a result of their model. These non-experimental data are supported by experimental studies as reported in Table 12.2.

In 1995, Rich et al reported that a nurse-led, multidisciplinary intervention (which involved a component of home visits) had beneficial effects with regard to rates of hospital readmission, quality of life and cost of care within 90 days of discharge among 'high risk' chronic heart failure patients.[58] The intervention consisted of comprehensive education of the patient and family, a prescribed diet, social service consultation and planning for an early discharge, optimization of pharmacotherapy, and intensive home and clinic-based follow-up with frequent telephone contact. The intervention was successful, improved patient compliance and appeared to slow the typical cycle of recurrent hospitalization in this type of patient cohort.[36,58] At 90 days, survival without readmission was achieved in 91 of 142 (64%) intervention patients compared with 75 of 140 (54%) control patients ($P = 0.09$). There were 94 vs 53 readmissions in the control and intervention groups, respectively ($P = 0.02$). Fewer intervention group patients had more than one readmission (nine vs 23; $P = 0.01$). These results were associated with significantly better quality of life and reduced health costs among intervention patients.

After this landmark there was a hiatus of a few years before additional experimental studies were published on models delivering specialty care to heart failure patients at home. In 1999, Stewart et al reported on a large-scale randomized controlled study of chronically ill patients with a mixture of cardiac and non-cardiac disease states, commenced short before the Rich study was published.[66] They found that a nurse-led, multidisciplinary, home-based intervention was most effective in chronic heart failure patients. The next step was to prospectively examine a more heart failure-specific form of a nurse-led, home-based intervention.[50,66] Chronic heart failure patients discharged to home post-acute hospitalization were randomized to usual care (n = 100) or to a home-based intervention (n = 100). The intervention primarily consisted of a home visit at 7–14 days post discharge by a cardiac nurse to identify and address issues likely to result in unplanned hospitalization. The primary endpoint for the study was frequency of unplanned readmission plus out-of-hospital death within 6 months. During 6 months' follow-up the primary endpoint occurred more frequently in the usual care group (129 vs 77 primary events; $P = 0.02$). More intervention patients remained event-free (38 vs 51; $P = 0.04$). Overall, there were fewer unplanned readmissions (68 vs 118; $P = 0.03$) and associated days of hospitalization (460 vs 1173; $P = 0.02$) among patients assigned to the study intervention. Consequently, hospital-based costs for the intervention group tended to be lower

than usual care. They also found fewer multiple readmissions in the intervention group. In a subgroup of 68 patients, heart failure specific ($P = 0.04$) and general quality of life scores ($P = 0.01$) at 3 months were most improved among those assigned to multidisciplinary, home-based intervention. Furthermore, assignment to the study intervention was an independent predictor of survival at 6 months (adjusted relative risk 0.54; $P = 0.046$).[39]

Recently Stewart and colleagues reported a combined analysis of 297 'high risk' heart failure patients from these two studies.[50,66,67] From this pooled analysis they found that study patients had fewer primary events (mean of 0.21 vs 0.37 events per patient per month ($P < 0.01$). The median event-free (7 vs 3 months, $P < 0.01$) and all-cause survival (40 vs 22 months, $P < 0.05$) was also more prolonged.[59]

A similar intervention, in a different health care system (the Netherlands) with a patient group that seemed to be less high-risk for readmission compared to the cohort of Stewart and colleagues was evaluated by Jaarsma and colleagues.[27,42] They examined the effects of a heart failure-specific, home-based, educational programme undertaken by a specialist heart failure nurse. This study was specifically undertaken to determine whether a single-type intervention designed to increase chronic heart failure patients' self-care behaviour was sufficiently effective enough to reduce hospital readmissions by a significant margin. Despite sufficient sample size, this study demonstrated that while education alone increased self-care behaviour and had the potential to reduce hospital readmissions overall, cost-effective thresholds were not reached. For example, during a 9-month follow-up, 37% of intervention patients (n = 84) compared with 50% of usual-care patients (n = 95) were readmitted to hospital ($P = 0.06$). Patients exposed to the study intervention also tended to have fewer cardiac-related days of readmission than usual-care patients (427 vs 681 days, $P = 0.096$). Symptoms, psychosocial adjustment to illness, functional capacity and overall well-being did not change as result of the intervention.[27,42]

The research group of Krumholz tested a similar intervention, only focusing on education and support, be it somewhat more intense.[37] Patients were educated during an hour-long face-to-face in-depth session within 2 weeks of hospital discharge. Home visits were performed for 45% of intervention patients unable to travel to the hospital. Neither clinical assessment of heart failure nor modification of current medical regimen was a component of the baseline meeting. Subsequently, the nurse contacted the patient by phone on a regular basis for a total intervention period of 1 year. These calls reinforced education but did not modify current regimens or provide recommendations about treatment. However, the nurse could recommend that the patient consult his or her physician when the patient's status deteriorated abruptly or the patient experienced a significant problem with medical therapy requiring prompt attention. Among the 88 patients (44 intervention and 44 control) in the study, 25 patients (56.8%) in the intervention group and 36 patients (81.8%) in the control group had at least one readmission or died during 1-year follow-up (relative risk = 0.69, 95% confidence interval: 0.52–0.92; $P = 0.01$). The intervention was associated with a 39% decrease in the total number of readmissions (intervention group, 49 readmissions; control group, 80 readmissions; $P = 0.06$). After adjusting for clinical and demographic characteristics, the intervention group had a significantly lower risk of readmission compared with the control group (hazard ratio = 0.56, 95% confidence interval: 0.32–0.96; $P = 0.03$) and hospital readmission costs of $7515 less per patient.[37]

A more extensive home-based intervention was evaluated by a Scottish research team.[60] Blue et al have described the effects of a more intensive home-based intervention in 165 patients admitted to a tertiary referral hospital in Glasgow, Scotland. Study patients received multiple home visits and the nurses initiated and titrated pharmacotherapy according to pre-established guidelines. A home-based specialist nurse provided comprehensive education and counselling, during an early home visit and frequent visits and calls. The home-based specialist nurse was accessible in case of problems and facilitated communication among health care providers. Primary endpoints were time to death or readmission for worsening heart failure, with a median follow-up time to 9 months. Compared with usual care, those patients exposed to the study intervention had fewer readmissions for any reason (86 vs 114; $P = 0.02$), fewer admissions for chronic heart failure (19 vs 45; $P < 0.001$) and fewer days of hospitalization (mean 3.4 vs 7.5 days; $P = 0.005$).[60]

Naylor et al focused their intervention more on discharge planning.[44] They undertook a study examining the effects of a comprehensive discharge planning protocol implemented by advanced practice nurses combined with a home-based follow-up. Based upon patient, family/caregiver, and environmental assessments, an individualized plan for education and counseling, validation of learning and coordination of home services was developed. Both patients and family/caregivers were targeted for intervention. Upon discharge, all patients were visited within 48 hours and again at 7–10 days by the advanced practice

nurse. The number of home visits was not limited and visits were scheduled based on individual patient and family needs. They reported that the intervention resulted in fewer patients being readmitted (20% vs 37%, $P < 0.01$) and longer event-free survival ($P < 0.001$). After 6 months, patients in the intervention had significantly fewer readmissions, longer time to first readmission and decreased costs of care compared with the control group. There were no differences between the intervention and usual care groups in functional status, depression or patient satisfaction.[44]

A recent Canadian study focused on a transitional care model to improve patient education and the use of usual home care. The nurse-led intervention focused on the transition from hospital-to-home and supportive care for self-management 2 weeks after hospital discharge. They found better quality of life scores at 6 weeks and 12 weeks after hospital discharge, among the transitional care patients (27.2 ± 19.1 SD) compared with usual care patients ($P = 0.002$). At 12 weeks' post discharge, 31% of the usual-care patients had been readmitted compared with 23% of the transitional-care patients ($P = 0.26$).[68]

A study of a case management programme conducted in the community was presented at the American Heart Association meeting in 2000 by Moser and colleagues.[69] Importantly, this was a randomized, controlled trial (n = 136, mean age 70, 52% female) of usual care vs community-based case management for heart failure patients with both preserved and impaired left ventricular function. The intervention programme comprised a home visit and weekly calls for 1 month and then monthly calls from a specialist heart failure nurse for patient assessment, comprehensive education and counseling that included low salt diet management, daily weights, medication compliance, symptom monitoring, and social service referrals. Patients primarily received care from the community nurse case manager, but they remained under the care of their primary physicians and any specialist physicians. In the group of patients with preserved left ventricular function, intervention patients had 0.22 heart failure-related readmissions per patient compared with a rate 0.8 per patient in the control group ($P < 0.01$). In the group of patients with left ventricular dysfunction, similar results were found (0.25 vs 0.5 per patient; $P < 0.01$). Irrespective of functional status, the study intervention was also associated with lower health care costs, fewer days of readmission and better quality of life ($P < 0.01$ for both comparisons).[69]

Management of patients with heart failure may also be improved by involving general practitioners in the follow-up. Doughty et al studied the effect of an integrated heart failure management programme on hospital readmission and quality of life in the Auckland Heart Failure Management Study.[49] Although the study intervention involved a component of nurse intervention, the major emphasis was on primary care management. While failing to show any significant beneficial effects on the combined endpoint of readmission or death, the study intervention was associated with improved quality of life and fewer multiple admissions (56 intervention vs 95 control group patients; $P = 0.0015$). A yet to be published study of this type was performed by Mårtensson from Sweden, which focused intervention both at educating health care providers and educating patients. The first part of the intervention was an education programme for all primary health care nurses and primary health care physicians at the intervention centres. After that, the nurse-led intervention programme started, consisting of one intensive session at the beginning of the study including education and counselling, and telephone follow-up by a primary health care nurse for a 12-month period after the inclusion. Significant differences of the nurse-led intervention between the groups were found in quality of life, life satisfaction and depression.[70]

Although we have largely focused on experimental studies in this chapter, a recent quasi-experiment study that matched intervention and control patients on pre-admission functional status, comorbidity, and age, is certainly worth mentioning.[28] Riegel et al described that one-half (n = 5120) were given a multidisciplinary disease management intervention, whereas the other half (n = 5120) received usual care. The intervention comprised hospital education by a pharmacist and dietician, discharge assessment by a social worker, outpatient support groups, physician collaboration and home visits by a heart failure specialty team and and/or telemanagement for 6 months. Data on acute care resource use were collected 3 and 6 months after enrolment. No intervention effect was seen in the primary analysis. However, when data were analysed by pre-admission functional status (NYHA class I–IV), acute care resource use was lower in the class II–IV intervention patients. Class I intervention patients had a 288% increase in total costs and a 14-fold increase in heart failure costs.[28]

This group also reported a study of a nurse-directed telephonic case management programme (average 17 phone calls over 6 months). Guidelines were sent to physicians of patients participating in the study. In this study a total of 358 patients with heart failure were originally recruited; however, only 242 patients completed the study. Despite this important caveat, the results were positive and an important contribution to the literature. As such, a reduction in the rate of heart failure-related admission by 48% ($P < 0.005$) and associated length of stay by 46% ($P = 0.05$) were reported. Overall, total all-cause hospital stays was 28% less in the study group (not significant) and their associated cost also tended to be lower (not significant).[71]

Home telemonitoring ('telecare')

Based on promising results from pilot studies,[73] there has been increasing interest in the beneficial effects of home telemonitoring of heart failure. This intervention is quite distinct from the multidisciplinary, home-based approach detailed above. Instead, this new technology allows telephonic transmission of key data (vital signs, weight, ECG) from the patient's home to the physician. The Trans European Network – Homecare Monitoring Study (TEN-HMS),[74] randomized 427 patients to UC, UC supplemented by regular telephone contact with a specialist nurse (NT) or telemonitoring (TM). The primary endpoint was the number of days alive and out of hospital over the period of follow-up. After 400 days, the mortality rate was 26% in the UC group, 15% in the NT group and 13% in the TM group (both intervention groups $P < 0.03$ vs the UC group). The total number of admissions in the TM group was increased compared to the NT group but, because this was offset by a reduction in the duration of admission, the total number of days spent in hospital was decreased slightly in the TM group. The primary endpoint was not reduced in the TM group compared to the NT group. Clearly, a complete analysis of this study awaits publication and more trials will be needed before the place of this new technology alone, or in combination with other forms of intervention, is clarified.

From the results of randomized and non-randomized studies, it seems clear that nurse-led programmes based on a model of home care or outreach to the home situation can be effective in improving outcomes in heart failure. These programmes have the potential to prolong event-free survival, reduce the number of readmissions within 1 year of index hospitalization by approximately 50%, prolong survival, and improve quality of life. It can also be questioned if a model that only provides education in the hospital and at home, or that only provides discharge planning is enough to reduce hospital readmission and

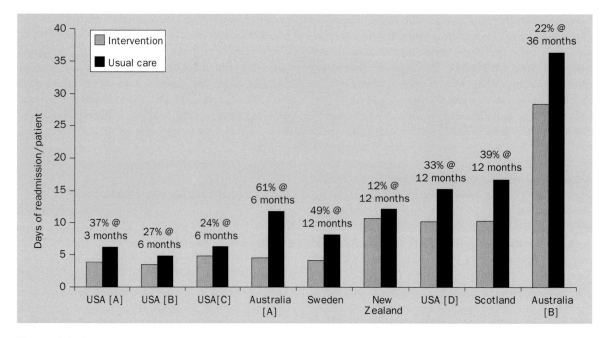

Figure 12.2. *Comparison of recurrent hospital stay (days/patient) in a range of randomized studies of post-discharge heart failure programmes.*
USA [A], Rich;[58] USA [B], Riegel;[71] USA [C], Kasper;[51] Australia [A], Stewart;[50] Sweden, Cline;[52] New Zealand, Doughty;[49] USA [D], Krumholz;[37] Scotland, Blue[60] and Australia [B], Stewart.[59] Reproduced with permission from McMurray JV, Pfeffer MA (eds). Heart Failure Updates. London: Martin Dunitz, 2003.

decrease health care costs in this predominantly vulnerable population. To date, there are no prospective studies that directly compare the relative cost-effectiveness of a clinic vs a home-based model of care. Similarly, there are no studies describing patient preferences in this regard. At the same time it is important to note that such programmes are probably most effective when both medical treatment according to official guidelines and discharge planning is applied in an optimal manner.

Nevertheless, Figure 12.2 shows that most programmes of this kind (irrespective of the exact approach implemented and the other effects summarized in Table 12.3) are effective in reducing recurrent hospital stay.

Practical considerations

After considering the desired outcomes, key components of a nurse-led heart failure management programme and the model in which these key components will be organized, it is essential to consider a number of important practicalities. For example, in considering the characteristics of successful studies presented earlier in this chapter it

is known that this approach to optimizing heart failure care should be:

- evidence-based;
- multidisciplinary with specialized staff and expert support;
- holistic;
- individualized.

In addition to the above, it is vital to consider the following questions, before actually implementing a nurse-led heart failure management programme:

- Why?
- For whom?
- By who?
- With whom?
- Where?
- How?

Why?

The objective of a nurse-led heart failure management programme should be defined, discussed and agreed on by the participants involved. In most programmes the improvement of the management of heart failure patients, improvement of the quality of life of patients and family members and reducing the hospital readmissions and costs is the primary objective. However, it can be vital for success to recognize and discuss additional hidden objectives; for example, reducing the workload of the cardiologist or shift costs from hospital to home care.

For whom?

It is important to define the type of patient that will be eligible for the intervention. Is the programme designed for patients with a high risk for readmission (for example prior admission of heart failure, elderly, lack of social support) or will every patient with heart failure be included?

Another issue to consider is whether the nurse-led heart failure management programme is suitable for women and the elderly. It is known, for example, that the elderly may be unable to come to an outpatient heart failure clinic or other outpatient service because of multiple comorbidities, impaired functional capacity, excessive fatigue and other factors.[43] Others may find it difficult to organize transportation to the clinic or to organize their household activities around the office hours of a heart failure nurse.

A patient with a language barrier or those needing another approach due to cultural problems also need the opportunity to take part in a nurse-led heart failure management programme. This means that interpreters should be available and also education materials adapted when necessary.

Depending on the payment system, it is important to consider if only patients who are discharged from a hospital and reside within the hospital's catchment area are included in the nurse-led heart failure management programme, or if patients who are treated by a general practitioner also can use the facilities of the heart failure programme, for example receive the patient education or call in case of problems.

At the same time, one should discuss if only patients with chronic heart failure due to left ventricular systolic dysfunction will be included in the programme and if patients with diastolic dysfunction should be excluded. From recent studies it is concluded that both patients with preserved left ventricular function and patients with left ventricular dysfunction have a low quality of life and can benefit form a nurse-led heart failure management programme (Tables 12.1 and 12.2).

By whom?

Various issues are at stake in deciding who will play a role in the nurse-led heart failure management programme. Depending on the objective of the programme, the target population and the resources, the composition of the team should be established. The role and responsibility of each team member should be clear, including the role of the nurse. Is the programme nurse-coordinated or nurse-managed? In other words, will the nurse have responsibility for the day-to-day care of patients and decide on the follow-up schedule, titration medication and decide on the actions to be taken if a patient deteriorates? Or does a cardiologist or other physician lead the programme and will the nurse have major responsibly in coordinating care and providing patient education?

In these discussions and preparations before starting the programme it is also necessary to decide on the degree of specialization of the nurses and physician involved in the programme. In some of the programmes specialized cardiologists and advanced nurse practitioners play the key role, while in other programmes a nurse from home-care or community nurses provide the care. Some of the nurse-led heart failure management programmes are provided by a broad multidisciplinary team including a physician (cardiologist, general practitioner, internist), nurse, physical therapist, dietitian, and social worker. In other programmes doctors and/or nurses run the programme and consult other health care providers for advice or refer the patient if needed.

All these decisions need to result in a description of the responsibilities of team members, for example who has discharge and admitting responsibilities, who has responsibilities with regard to medication titration and prescriptions and who can prescribe and execute an exercise programme.

With whom?

Formal links should be established with other specialist services and other relevant health care services. For example, in some of the hospitals or home care organizations, there is experience with similar disease management programmes, targeted on other populations (diabetes, chronic obstructive pulmonary disease). Practical advice from these colleagues, but also consultation in case of comorbidity, is vital. In addition, links with hospital staff, general practitioners and home health services are needed to secure optimal cooperation and coordination, depending on the scope of the team approach and the composition of the team that actually provides the programme to every patient with heart failure. Creating a good relationship with supporting disciplines such as dietitians, physiotherapists or social workers is essential. In addition, palliative home care teams may be involved in providing care for the patients and family in the final stages of life.

Where?

As outlined above, there are various models for the management of the patient with heart failure. Depending on the health care system, available resources and expertise and the opportunities available, it should be decided what the best approach is. The clinic approach may not be suitable for all heart failure patients, especially the elderly. However, in some situations a heart failure clinic may be the most appropriate and realistic option. Regardless of whether a hospital or home-based approach is chosen, the location of the programme needs to be clear. In several hospitals in Sweden the heart failure clinic is located on the ward where the heart failure patient was admitted. Patients feel comfortable coming to the same place, where they know familiar faces. Nurses from the cardiology unit also play a role at the heart failure clinic in the same hospital. Other potential locations for a heart failure clinic include the cardiology ward or in a separate outpatient department. As discussed in this chapter, a home-based intervention or intervention with community outreach or involvement of health care providers in the primary care can be very effective. Organizing these models also requires consideration of where the specialist nurse will be based. Will they be based in a community health care team, a general practitioner's office or perhaps in a special arrangement combining employment by the primary care organization and the acute-care hospital programme, as described by Stewart and Blue?[72]

How?

Methods to ensure key components of this type of programme (as described in Table 12.2) have to be established and guidelines for the management of the patients described. Evidence-based guidelines for diagnosis, treatment and care should be used and additional protocols for assessment and follow-up care need to be developed.

Other key issues that require extensive discussion and consideration include the extent of accessibility of health care providers to the patient, family or relevant others. For example, should there be a 24-hour coverage, or will an answer machine with relevant telephone numbers be adequate for this particular programme?

Conclusions

It seems clear that a nurse-led heart failure management programme can improve outcomes like readmission rates and costs and improve quality of life of patients with heart failure. An increasing number of descriptive, quasi-experimental and randomized studies have reported positive clinical outcomes. The number of inconclusive and negative (only one) studies are few and far between, despite the diversity of clinical settings and countries from which patients are recruited.

Looking at the available study results, we see that models that extend care to the home or base the total programme outside the hospital are most successful. A comprehensive meta-analysis of such programmes (incorporating the latest studies) is obviously overdue in this regard. There are, however, a few issues to consider when determining the clinical implication and application of models into daily practice. These issues concern the following.

The difficulty in comparing different models with different components as tested in a variety of health care systems

There is a broad range of interventions tested in the studies. All study groups designed their own new intervention, some of them explicitly stating that they were building on the models of previous studies. However, every study group needed to change the intervention to fit it into their situation.

Several important factors determine the exact composition of a nurse-led management programme and the fit of a model. These factors are related to health care systems (differences between countries, regions, etc.), differences in the level of education in health care (in nursing), differences in insurance systems or differences in availability of cardiologists and nurses in a country. As a result, there is a marked heterogeneity with respect to the specific management model, number of components, intensity and health care providers involved in those programmes of care that have been developed and applied. Even within the important component of patient follow-up, there is marked heterogeneity in the intensity of contact (ranging from weekly telephone calls to three clinic visits within 12 months).

The studies also differ considerably in the population used, with regard to the number of women or in the grade of risk for readmission of the patients. This variety in programmes and population makes it hard to decide which component or approach could have led to the effects and which management programme would be best for someone to implement in their local situation.

Lack of insight into the underlying mechanism of the intervention

Although several key components from successful heart failure management programmes are formulated, the components differ in each study. It is often not clear which mechanisms the management programme is aiming to change to reach the desired outcomes. It is known that a change of behaviours of both heart failure patients and health care providers is necessary to improve outcomes. However, special interventions to change behaviours are seldom used (or reported) in heart failure management programmes. Improvement of compliance of patients with the treatment regime and improvement of prescription compliance in health care providers is also often described as a target or a mechanism of beneficial effect in a heart failure management programme. However, few heart failure management programmes actually explain how they attain this change in behaviours or what interventions they use to achieve such change. Strategies to enhance compliance should improve patient education and include several behavioural strategies. They should include the patients, health care providers and the health care organization.

As long as it not known what underlies the positive outcomes, it is not possible to make rational and responsible decisions as to which components of a heart failure management programme should be expanded and which components may be seen as optional.

Lack of randomized, comparable and adequately powered trials

As mentioned earlier, to date, there are only a limited number of comparable randomized and adequately powered studies that study the effectiveness of nurse-led heart failure management programmes. There are several studies that compare outcomes after the implementation of the programme to those before it started. This can lead to an inflation of the magnitude of the impact. For example, readmission rates were reduced by 60–89% in several pre-post test studies. In studies in which patients are randomized to a control group, readmission rates were reduced by 43–56%. These rates of reduction from the randomized studies provide a better estimation on which to base cost–benefit analyses and inform important decisions with respect to translating research into practice.

It is, however, increasingly difficult in several countries to use a randomized controlled design, since a heart failure clinic or disease management model is widely used in some countries and has become part of the gold standard of care. However, it is important to look critically at the effectiveness of the programmes that need a controlled situation.

A limitation in the studies at this moment is that no study compares different heart failure management models and the intensity of programme needed. This represents the next logical step in research examining the optimal effectiveness of nurse-led heart failure management programmes.

Lack of insight into patient preferences and the need for tailored programmes

Only a few studies report on patient satisfaction with the heart failure management programme. It is often assumed that patients might prefer more intensive follow-up by a nurse specialist compared with a clinic visit to a cardiologist once a year, or that they prefer a home visit compared with a clinic visit. One can imagine that some patients prefer a visit from a specialized nurse in their home situation, as this requires less energy from the patient and no arrangements to travel to a clinic. However, others might be unwilling to let a nurse come into their homes, bringing the medical atmosphere and confrontation with disease into their safe homes. We do not know enough about what patient preferences are.

It is also stressed in several programmes that heart failure management needs to be tailored to the individual patient situation and that there is no 'one-size-fits-all' model. Therefore it is sometimes difficult for the health care provider in daily practice to find the most optimal evidence-based model of care delivery that suits this patient. Should they prefer a new (and maybe what they feel to be a superficial) model that is positively evaluated (maybe abroad) or should they use a model that – although it is not tested – seems to fit this patient?

Both researchers and health care providers are challenged to determine in the near future what the optimal approach for the patient with chronic heart failure is.

References

1 McMurray JJV, Stewart S. Nurse led, multidisciplinary intervention in chronic heart failure. *Heart* 1998; **80:** 430–1.

2 Rich MW. Heart failure disease management: a critical review. *J Cardiac Failure* 1999; **5:** 64–75.

3 Philbin EF. Comprehensive multidisciplinary programmes for the management of patients with congestive heart failure. *J Gen Internal Med* 1999; **14:** 130–5.

4 McAlister FA, Lawson FM, Teo KK, Armstrong PW. A systematic review of randomized trials of disease management programmes in heart failure. *Am J Med* 2001; **110:** 378–84.

5 Stewart S, Horowitz JD. Detecting early clinical deterioration in patients with chronic heart failure patients post acute hospitalisation: a critical component of multidisciplinary, home-based intervention. *Eur J Heart Fail* 2002; **4:** 345–51.

6 Balk AH. The heart failure nurse to help us close the gap between what we can and what we do achieve. *Eur Heart J* 1999; **20:** 632–3.

7 McDonald K, Ledwidge M, Cahill J, Quigley P, Maurer B. Heart failure management: multidisciplinary care has intrinsic benefit above the optimization of medical care. *J Card Fail* 2002; **8:** 142–8.

8 Riegel B, Rich MW. Multidisciplinary disease management models of heart failure care. In: Moser DK, Riegel B (eds). *Improving outcomes in heart failure*. MD: Aspen Publishers, Inc. 2001.

9 Ho KKL, Anderson KM, Karmel WB et al. Survival after the onset of congestive heart failure in the Framingham Heart Study subjects. *Circulation* 1993; **88:** 107–15.

10 Stewart S, MacIntyre K, Hole DA, Capewell S, McMurray JJV. More malignant than cancer? Five-year survival following a first admission for heart failure in Scotland. *Eur J Heart Fail* 2001; **3:** 315–22.

11 Stewart AL, Greenfield S, Hays RD et al. Functional status and well-being of patients with chronic conditions: results from the medical outcomes study. *JAMA* 1989; **262:** 907–13.

12 Jaarsma T, Halfens R, Huijer-Abu Saad H, Dracup K, Stappers J, van Ree J. Quality of life in older patients with systolic and diastolic heart failure. *Eur J Heart Fail* 1999; **1:** 151–60.

13 McMurray JJ, Petrie MC, Murdoch DR, Davie AP. Clinical epidemiology of heart failure: public and private health burden. *Eur Heart J* 1998; **19:** 9–16.

14 Wolinski FD, Smith DM, Stump TE, Everhoge JM, Lubitz RM. The sequelae of hospitalization for congestive heart failure among older adults. *J Am Geriatr Soc* 1997; **45:** 558–63.

15 Krumholz HM, Parent EM, Tu N et al. Readmission after hospitalization for congestive heart failure among Medicare beneficiaries. *Arch Intern Med* 1997; **157:** 99–104.

16 Vinson JM, Rich MW, Sperry JC. Early readmission of elderly patients with congestive heart failure. *J Am Geriatr Soc* 1990; **38:** 1290–5.

17 Happ MB, Naylor MD, Roe-Prior P. Factors contributing to rehospitalization of elderly patients with heart failure. *J Cardiovasc Nurs* 1997; **11:** 75–84.

18 Michalsen A, Konig G, Thimme W. Preventable causative factors leading to hospital admission with decompensated heart failure. *Heart* 1998; **80:** 437–41.

19 Tsuyuki RT, McKelvie RS, Arnold JM, Avezum A Jr, Barretto AC et al. Acute precipitants of congestive heart failure exacerbations. *Arch Intern Med* 2001; **161:** 2337–42.

20 Jaarsma T, Abu-Saad HH, Dracup K, Halfens R. Self-care behaviour of patients with heart failure. *Scand J Caring Sci* 2000; **14:** 112–19.

21 Riegel B, Carlson B. Facilitators and barriers to heart failure self-care. *Patient Educ Counseling* 2002; **46:** 287–95.

22 Serxner S, Miyaji M, Jeffords J. Congestive heart failure disease management: a patient education intervention. *Congest Heart Fail* 1998; **4:** 23–8B.

23 Linne AB, Liedholm H, Israelsson B. Effects of systematic education on heart failure patients' knowledge after 6 months. A randomised, controlled trial. *Eur J Heart Fail* 1999; **1:** 219–27.

24 Hanumanthu S, Butler J, Chomsky D, Davis S, Wilson JR. Effects of a heart failure programme on hospitalization frequency and exercise tolerance. *Circulation* 1997; **96:** 2842–8.

25 Ramahi TM, Longo MD, Rohlfs K, Sheynberg N. Effect of heart failure programme on cardiovascular drug utilization and dosage in patients with chronic heart failure. *Clin Cardiol* 2000; **23:** 881–2.

26 Dahl J, Penque S. The effects of an advance practice nurse directed heart failure programme. *Nurse Practitioner* 2000; **25:** 61–77.

27 Jaarsma T, Halfens R, Huijer Abu-Saad H, Dracup K, Gorgels T et al. Effects of education and support on self-care and resource utilization in patients with heart failure. *Eur Heart J* 1999; **20:** 673–82.

28 Riegel B, Carlson B, Glaser S, Hoaglund P. Which heart failure patients respond best to a multidisciplinary disease management approach? *J Cardiac Fail* 2000; **6:** 290–9.

29 Stromberg A, Martensson J, Fridlund B, Levin LA, Karlsson JE, Dahlstrom U. Nurse-led heart failure clinics improve survival and self-care behaviour in patients with heart failure. Results from a prospective randomised study. *Eur Heart J* 2003; **24:** 1014–23.

30 Friedman MM. Older adults' symptoms and their duration before hospitalization for heart failure. *Heart Lung* 1997; **26:** 169–76.

31 Evangelista LS, Dracup K, Doering L. Treatment-seeking delays in heart failure patients. *J Heart Lung Transplant* 2000; **19:** 932–8.

32 Ghali JK, Kadakia S, Cooper R, Ferlinz J. Precipitating factors leading to decompensation of heart failure. *Arch Intern Med* 1988; **148:** 2013–17.

33 Cline CM, Bjorck-Linne AK, Israelsson BY, Willenheimer RB, Erhardt LR. Non-compliance and knowledge of prescribed medication in elderly patients with heart failure. *Eur J Heart Fail* 1999; **1:** 145–9.

34 Monane M, Bohn RL, Gurwitz JH, Glynn RJ, Avorn J. Noncompliance with congestive heart failure therapy in the elderly. *Arch Int Med* 1994; **154:** 433–7.

35 Burke LE, Dunbar-Jacobs J. Adherence to medication, diet, activity recommendations: from assessment to maintenance. *J Cardiovasc Nurs* 1995; **9:** 62–79.

36 Rich MW, Gray DB, Beckham V, Wittenberg C, Luther P. Effect of a multidisciplinary intervention on medication compliance in elderly patients with congestive heart failure. *Am Med J* 1996; **101:** 270–6.

37 Krumholz HM, Amatruda J, Smith GL, Mattera JA, Roumanis SA et al. Randomized trial of an education and support intervention to prevent readmission of patients with heart failure. *J Am Coll Cardiol* 2002; **39:** 83–9.

38 Stewart S, Pearson S. Uncovering a multitude of sins: medication management in the home post acute hospitalisation among the chronically ill. *Aust NZ J Med* 1999; **29:** 220–7.

39 West JA, Miller NH, Parker KM et al. A comprehensive management system for heart failure improves clinical outcomes and reduces medical resources. *Am J Cardiol* 1997; **79:** 58–63.

40 Fonarow GG, Stevenson LW, Walden JA et al. Impact of a comprehensive heart failure management programme on hospital readmission and functional status of patients with advanced heart failure. *J Am Coll Cardiol* 1997; **30:** 725–32.

41 Smith LE, Fabbri SA, Pai R, Ferry D, Heywood JT. Symptomatic improvement and reduced hospitalization for patients attending a cardiomyopathy clinic. *Clin Cardiol* 1997; **20:** 949–54.

42 Jaarsma T, Halfens R, Tan F, Abu-Saad HH, Dracup K, Diederiks J. Self-care and quality of life in patients with advanced heart failure: the effect of a supportive educational intervention. *Heart Lung* 2000; **29:** 319–30.

43 Ekman I, Andersson B, Ehnfors M, Matejka G, Persson B, Fagerberg B. Feasibility of a nurse-monitored, outpatient programme for elderly patients with moderate-to-severe chronic heart failure. *Eur Heart J* 1998; **19:** 1254–60.

44 Naylor MD, Brooten D, Campbell R, Jacobsen BS, Mezey MD et al. Comprehensive discharge planning and home follow-up of hospitalized elders. *JAMA* 1999; **281:** 613–20.

45 Moser DK, Worster PL. Effect of psychosocial factors on physiologic outcomes in patients with heart failure. *J Cardiovasc Nurs* 2000; **14:** 106–15.

46 Moser DK. Psychosocial factors and their association with clinical outcomes in patients with heart failure: why clinicians do not seem to care. *Eur J Cardiovasc Nurs* 2002; **1:** 183–8.

47 Vaccarino V, Kasl SV, Abramson J, Krumholz HM. Depressive symptoms and risk of functional decline and death in patients with heart failure. *J Am Coll Cardiol* 2001; **38:** 199–205.

48 Weinberger M, Oddone EZ, Henderson WG. Does increased access to primary care reduce hospital readmissions? *New Engl J Med* 1996; **334:** 1441–7.

49 Doughty RN, Wright SP, Walsh HJ et al. Randomised, controlled trial of integrated heart failure management: the Auckland Heart Failure Management Study. *Eur Heart J* 2001: 2002; **23:** 139–46.

50 Stewart S, Marley JE, Horowitz JD. Effects of a multidisciplinary, home-based intervention on unplanned readmission and survival among patients with chronic congestive heart failure: a randomized controlled study. *Lancet* 1999; **354:** 1077–83.

51 Kasper EK, Gerstenblith G, Hefter G, Van Anden E, Brinker JA et al. A randomized trial of the efficacy of multidisciplinary care in heart failure outpatients at high risk of hospital readmission. *J Am Coll Cardiol* 2002; **39:** 471–80.

52 Cline CMJ, Israelsson BYA, Willenheimer RB, Broms K, Erhardt LR. Cost-effective management programme for heart failure reduces rehospitalisation. *Heart* 1998; **80:** 442–6.

53 McMurray JJV, Hart W, Rhodes G. An evaluation of the cost of heart failure to the National Health Service in the UK. *Br J Med Econ* 1993; **6:** 91–8.

54 Stewart S, Jenkins A, Buchan S et al. The current cost of heart failure in the UK – an economic analysis. *Eur J Heart Fail* 2002; **4:** 361–71.

55 Mark DB. Economics of treating heart failure. *Am J Cardiol* 1997; **80:** 33H–38H.

56 Weintraub WS, Cole J, Tooley JF. Cost and cost-effectiveness studies in heart failure research. *Am Heart J* 2002; **143:** 565–76.

57 Stewart S, Blue L, Walker A et al. An economic analysis of specialist heart failure management in the UK – can we afford not to implement it? *Eur Heart J* 2002; **17:** 1369–78.

58 Rich MW, Beckham V, Wittenberg C, Leven CL, Freedland KE, Carney RM. A multidisciplinary intervention to prevent readmission of elderly patients with congestive heart failure. *N Engl J Med* 1995; **333:** 1190–5.

59 Stewart S, Horowitz JD. Home-based intervention in congestive heart failure: long-term implications on readmission and survival. *Circulation* 2002; **105:** 2861–6.

60 Blue L, Strong E, Murdoch DR et al. Improving long-term outcome with specialist nurse intervention in heart failure: a randomized trial. *BMJ* 2002; **323:** 1112–15.

61 Stewart S, MacIntyre K, McCleod MC, Bailey AE et al. Trends in heart failure hospitalisations in Scotland, 1990–1996: an epidemic that has reached its peak? *Eur Heart J* 2000; **22:** 209–17.

62 Grady KL, Dracup K, Kennedy G, Moser DK, Piano M et al. Team management of patients with heart failure. A statement of health care professionals from the Cardiovascular Nursing council of the American Heart Association. Circulation 2000;102:2443–56.

63 Cintron G, Bigas C, Linares E, Aranda JM, Hernandez E. Nurse practitioner role in a chronic congestive heart failure clinic: in-hospital time, costs, and patient satisfaction. *Heart Lung* 1983; **12:** 237–40.

64 Lasater M. The effect of a nurse-managed congestive heart failure clinic on patient readmission and length of stay. *Home Health Nurse* 1996; **14:** 351–6.

65 Kornowski R, Zeeli D, Averbuch M et al. Intensive home-care surveillance prevents hospitalization and improves morbidity rates among elderly patients with severe congestive heart failure. *Am Heart J* 1995; **129:** 762–6.

66 Stewart S, Vandenbroek AJ, Pearson S, Horowitz JD. Prolonged beneficial effects of a home-based intervention on unplanned readmissions and mortality among patients with congestive heart failure. *Arch Intern Med* 1999; **159:** 257–61.

67 Stewart S, Pearson S, Horowitz JD. Effects of a home-based intervention among patients with congestive heart failure discharged from acute hospital care. *Arch Intern Med* 1998; **158:** 1067–72.

68 Harrison MB, Browne GB, Roberts J. Quality of life of individuals with heart failure: a randomized trial of the effectiveness of two models of hospital-to-home transition. *Med Care* 2002; **40:** 271–82.

69 Moser DK, Macko MJ, Worster P. Community case management decreases rehospitalization rates and costs, and improves quality of life in heart failure patients with preserved and non-preserved left ventricular function: a randomized controlled trial. *Circulation* 2000; **102:** II749.

70 Mårtensson J. The life situation of patients with heart failure in primary health care. Doctoral thesis. Gothenburg, 2002.

71 Riegel B, Carlson B, Kopp Z et al. Effect of a standardized nurse case-management telephone intervention on resource use in patients with chronic heart failure. *Arch Intern Med* 2002; **162:** 705–12.

72 Stewart S, Blue L (eds). *Improving Outcomes in Chronic Heart Failure with Specialist Nurse Intervention: A Practical Guide*. London: BMJ Publishers, 2000.

73 Shah NB, Der E, Ruggerio C, Heidenreich PA, Massie BM. Prevention of hospitalizations for heart failure with an interactive home monitoring programme. *Am Heart J* 1998; **135:** 373–8.

74 Coletta AP, Louis AA, Clark AL et al. Clinical trials update from the European Society of Cardiology: CARMEN, EARTH, OPTIMAAL, ACE, TEN-HMS, MAGIC, SOLVD-X and PATH-CHF II. *Eur J Heart Failure* 2002; **4:** 661–6.

75 Kostis JB, Rosen RC, Cosgrove NM, Shindler DM, Wilson AC. Nonpharmacologic therapy improves functional and emotional status in congestive heart failure. *Chest* 1994; **106:** 996–1001.

13 Caring for the older person with heart failure

Mark C Petrie

Introduction

As described in Chapter 1, remarkably, the average age of patients with chronic heart failure (CHF) in the community is currently almost 80 years old.[1] With a continually ageing population, this is likely to rise even further. The profile of most patients with CHF is dramatically different from the large-scale clinical trials. It is important, therefore, to interpret data from the reports of these trials and the management guidelines generated from them carefully when attempting to optimize the therapeutic management of the older individual.

Rather than limiting ourselves to strict age criteria, this chapter, through a series of key questions, will specifically consider how increasing age influences all aspects of heart failure.

How common is chronic heart failure in older patients?

The number of patients in the population with CHF approximately doubles with every decade.[2] Between 50 and 59 years of age approximately 1 in 100 men and women suffers from CHF.[2] This figure rises to 1 in 10 in those men and women aged between 80 and 89 years.[2] Significantly, almost one-half of newly diagnosed cases of CHF occur in patients aged greater than 80 years.[3]

Are the causes of chronic heart failure different in the older patient?

Coronary heart disease and hypertension are the most common causes of CHF in all age groups. The effect of age on these causes is minimal. Older patients with hypertension in the population,[4] and indeed in clinical trials,[5,6] do consistently develop CHF more often than their younger counterparts. Older patients following a myocardial infarction are also more likely to develop CHF.[7–10] Everyday clinical practice tells us that valvular heart disease is not an uncommon cause of CHF in elderly patients.

Is diagnosing chronic heart failure more difficult in the older patient?

As discussed in Chapter 6, making a clinical diagnosis of heart failure is problematic in all age groups as the symptoms and signs of CHF are shared with a variety of other conditions. This is particularly the case in the elderly who more commonly suffer from diseases that can mimic CHF. In the elderly the strongest predictors of the presence of CHF are a history of myocardial infarction or angina.[11] The most commonly seen physical sign is basal crackles but the most discriminatory physical sign is a raised jugular venous pressure greater than 5 cm.[11]

How should we investigate the older patient with suspected heart failure?

Elderly patients with suspected heart failure should be investigated in the same manner as their younger counterparts. If a patient has a normal electrocardiogram it is unlikely that they have CHF. Patients with abnormal electrocardiograms should have an echocardiogram. Disappointingly, older patients with CHF in the community have been found to less often undergo echocardiography.[12]

Is systolic or diastolic heart failure more prevalent in the older population?

How often systolic and diastolic abnormalities of left ventricular function are responsible for CHF is currently one of the most controversial areas in cardiology. How common diastolic heart failure (or 'heart failure with preserved left ventricular systolic function') is depends on several factors including how preserved left ventricular function is defined. The measurement commonly used is termed left ventricular 'ejection fraction'. The lower range of normal use is anywhere between 35% and 50%. Depending on the 'cut-off' used (and which technique is used to measure 'ejection fraction'), varying proportions of patients have preserved and impaired left ventricular function (or 'diastolic' or 'systolic' heart failure).

Although the elderly are often said to suffer more frequently from diastolic CHF it is uncertain whether the increased proportion of patients in this age group with chronic symptoms of shortness of breath on exertion and ankle swelling with preserved left ventricular systolic function suffer from heart failure or a variety of other conditions.[13]

How many other diseases do elderly patients with chronic heart failure suffer from?

Few elderly patients have CHF as an isolated medical problem. Fifty percent of elderly patients with CHF have an average of more than five unrelated diseases.[14] These commonly include diabetes, chronic renal failure and chronic obstructive pulmonary disease.[15–17] Diabetes is present in approximately one-third[16,17] and renal failure[15] and chronic obstructive pulmonary disease[15,16] in around one-fifth of patients. Atrial fibrillation[18] and renovascular disease[19] are also seen in around one-third of elderly patients with CHF.

How does chronic heart failure affect the elderly patient?

Hospitalizations

CHF is the most common cause of hospitalization in the elderly.[20–22] The average age of patients hospitalized for CHF is consistently above 70 years and frequently over 80.[23–28] Hospitalization due to CHF is rising in general but this rise is predominantly seen in the elderly and very elderly populations.[25,29,30]

Once hospitalized, the length of stay of elderly patients is long. In New Zealand patients over 75 years stayed an average 19 days compared to 11 days for those under 75 years.[26]

Unfortunately readmissions are also common. Indeed, age is the most powerful predictive factor for readmission in previously hospitalized patients with CHF.[31] Between 1 in 2 and 1 in 3 of all elderly patients are readmitted within 6 months.[32–36] Many CHF readmissions in the elderly can be attributed to relatively simple factors. These include failure to take prescribed medications and diet, inadequate discharge planning or follow-up, failed social support system or failure to seek medical support promptly. Medication-related factors can also lead to readmission, e.g. omission (or submaximal dosing) of angiotensin-converting enzyme (ACE) inhibitors or coprescription of drugs that have deleterious effects in CHF (e.g. non-steroidal anti-inflammatory agents). It has been estimated that 50% of hospital admissions among older individuals with CHF are preventable.[37]

Effect on quality of life and preference for resuscitation

CHF has a profound effect on quality of life in all age groups including the elderly, although few reports have looked specifically at the degree of effect in this group.[38] Older patients hospitalized with severe CHF are less likely to want to be resuscitated than their younger counterparts though, interestingly, the majority of elderly patients do express a preference for resuscitation.[39]

Depression

Depression is remarkably common in patients hospitalized with CHF. Between 50% and 58% of such patients are depressed.[18,40] Lack of emotional support in patients aged 65 years or older who are hospitalized with CHF is associated with an increased risk of fatal and non-fatal cardiovascular events at 1 year.[41]

Death

Elderly patients with CHF have greater mortality rates than their younger counterparts.[4,23,29] This increase is seen for every decade lived and is more pronounced in women than men.[4] In New Zealand two-thirds of heart failure deaths occur in patients over 75 years of age.[26] Very elderly patients with CHF have a very high mortality. Patients over the age of 80 hospitalized in the Philadelphia Geriatric Center for CHF had a 1-year mortality of 63%.[42] In the Framingham study few patients over the age of 80 years with CHF lived for more than 5 years.[43]

What is appropriate treatment in the older patient?

Non-pharmacological therapy

The basic tenets of education, a low salt diet, fluid restriction and self-weighing are the same in the elderly as every other subgroup. A few small studies in the elderly have confirmed the benefits of exercise training programmes in this group.[44-46] Administering influenza A vaccine to patients over 64 years of age with CHF during the 1991–1992 influenza epidemic resulted in a 37% reduction in the rate of hospitalizations for heart failure.[47] Vaccination against influenza A is therefore recommended.

Pharmacological therapy
Diuretics (and which type of diuretic)

Diuretics have been the mainstay of therapy to combat salt and water retention in CHF for decades. There are undoubted symptomatic benefits of these drugs. Several factors should be borne in mind when prescribing and adjusting therapy in the elderly. These factors include a susceptibility to hypokalaemia (caused by a reduced dietary intake of potassium, decreased body stores and less effective renal conservation of potassium). The elderly kidney is also less efficient at clearing diuretics. The initial choice of diuretic is conventionally a loop diuretic (e.g. frusemide or bumetanide). Doses are usually titrated to relieve fluid retention but prevent dehydration. If a patient becomes hypokalaemic, adding a potassium-sparing diuretic is preferable to giving oral potassium supplements. Potassium-sparing diuretics used in this situation include amiloride.

Spironolactone, an aldosterone antagonist, has recently received much attention in the management of CHF. This stemmed from the RALES trial that studied the effects of spironolactone in patients with severe heart failure (with symptoms at rest or on minimal exertion).[48] Low-dose spironolactone (average dose 26 mg), added to conventional therapy (including an ACE inhibitor), decreased mortality, reduced hospital admissions and improved New York Heart Association (NYHA) class. The average age was 67 years. A similar reduction in mortality was seen in patients greater than or equal to, or less than, 67 years of age. While the risks of hyperkalaemia and renal failure in RALES (where electrolytes were checked frequently) were not high, clinical practice suggests that the incidence of these adverse effects may be greater in everyday patients, i.e. not in a trial setting. It should be emphasized that the evidence for the benefit of these agents is in patients with severe heart failure and they should not be prescribed for all patients with CHF or simply left ventricular systolic dysfunction.

Diuretics can pose practical problems in the elderly. Poor mobility may prevent easy access to toilet facilities. Consideration of such points and provision of simple aids may prevent inconvenience and embarrassment. Patients should be instructed that it is not necessary to take their diuretics at the same time every day and can be taken at a time that suits the patient.

Clinical trials of other drugs for chronic heart failure

Very few elderly patients with CHF have been included in clinical trials. Some studies have actively excluded the elderly on the basis of age alone. Others have exclusion criteria that mitigate against inclusion of the elderly. An ideal trial on which to base management would include the kinds of patients encountered everyday in clinical practice. The lack of inclusion of elderly patients in these trials means that we have less evidence on which to base prescribing in this population.

Trials with angiotensin-converting enzyme inhibitors in heart failure

The large multicentre trials of ACE inhibitors in CHF that have reported mortality and morbidity benefit have contained only a small proportion of elderly subjects. The small number of elderly patients in the landmark CONSENSUS trial meant that significant reduction in mortality was not achieved for subgroup analysis over the age of 70 years (in contrast to those aged less than 70).[49] The SOLVD trials did not report analysis by age.[50]

A meta-analysis of the ACE inhibitor trials failed to demonstrate a significant survival effect in those aged over over 60 years (young by any standards) but did show a significant benefit in this older population when a combined endpoint of total mortality and hospitalizations was examined.[51]

Trials of beta-blockers

That beta-blockers are of benefit in all stages of heart failure if used cautiously is the greatest advance in heart failure therapeutics over the last 5 years. Once again, very few elderly patients have been included in these practice-changing trials. Few studies have looked at the effect of age on this beneficial effect. The US Carvedilol group found that the statistically significant reduction in deaths was similar for CHF patients younger and older than 59 years of age.[52] The reduction of cardiovascular hospitalization was also not dependent on age. The only other large trial of beta-blockers to report the effect of age on treatment was the MERIT-HF trial.[53] Although slightly less benefit was seen in the upper age tertile, this was not significant and a beneficial treatment effect was still seen.

Trials of angiotensin II receptor antagonists

ELITE II was unusual in studying a relatively elderly population. Eighty-five percent were greater than 65 years and the average age of patients enrolled was 71.5 years.[54] While this study found that losartan was better tolerated than captopril there was a trend in both those aged above and below 71 years towards a benefit for captopril over losartan. The full publication of Val-HeFT and the completion of the CHARM projects may shed light on the relative merits of ACE inhibitors and angiotensin II receptor antagonists in this population.

Trials of hydralazine plus isosorbide dinitrate and digoxin

Both the initial trials showing a mortality benefit with the vasodilating combination of isosorbide dinitrate and hydralazine[55,56] and the studies of digoxin in CHF[57–59] recruited few elderly patients and did not report the effect of age on treatment effect.

Do older patients have more adverse effects?

In the Studies of Left Ventricular Dysfunction trial, older patients taking enalapril were more likely to report adverse events than younger patients (although very few truly elderly patients were included).[60] This increased risk with age was seen for hypotension, gastrointestinal symptoms, cough, hyperkalaemia and leukopenia. A more recent report from the Studies of Left Ventricular Dysfunction study found that older age was associated with an increased risk of developing worsening renal function.[61] The slightly increased occurrence of adverse effects is often given as an excuse for underprescribing in the elderly. The elderly should not be denied these therapies but optimal monitoring should be employed to detect the development of adverse effects.

Underprescription of angiotensin-converting enzymes inhibitors in the elderly

ACE inhibitors are generally underprescribed in CHF but this is particularly the case in the elderly.[62–64] Between one-quarter and one-third of elderly patients are prescribed ACE inhibitors but only a small proportion of these are prescribed target doses.[65]

Compliance and polypharmacy

Compliance

Non-compliance with prescribed medication is suspected to be an important cause of treatment failures in CHF.[66–68] Patients prescribed digoxin were found to only collect sufficient medication for around one-third of their first year on the drug. Improved compliance can be achieved by education and follow-up in the over 70s.[69] Intensive nurse-led home-based interventions target poor compliance and have resulted in a reduction in hospital admissions.[70,71]

Polypharmacy

The increasing number of evidence-based treatments now results in patients with CHF being prescribed many different classes of drugs. Elderly patients, as previously noted, have multiple comorbidities that often mean additional treatments. Patients should be educated as to the reasons for treatment and every effort made to supply tablets in a suitable fashion (e.g. dosette boxes). Pharmacists and nurse specialists can be particularly valuable in helping to overcome problems associated with polypharmacy.

Drugs to avoid in chronic heart failure

Non-steroidal anti-inflammatory drugs are widely used in the elderly. The use of these agents in patients aged over 55 years taking diuretics is associated with a two-fold increased risk of hospitalization for CHF.[72]

What is the optimal system of care for older patients?

The benefits of nurse-led outpatient management have been considered in Chapter 12. The success of this approach has been demonstrated in the elderly with CHF.

Ideally, such a service should be allied to a heart failure or heart function clinic staffed with physicians with a specialist interest. Family involvement is also often particularly valuable in the elderly.

Is there a role for cardiac transplantation?

Cardiac transplantation is rarely an option for the elderly patient with CHF. In the limited series available it is unclear whether older patients have a better or worse outcome than their younger counterparts.

Can we prevent heart failure in the elderly?

Several trials of treating hypertension in elderly populations have found marked decreases in the incidence of heart failure. A recent meta-analysis found that treating hypertensive patients aged over 80 years reduces the development of heart failure by 39%.[73] Primary prevention of coronary heart disease and appropriate secondary prevention following myocardial infarction should also result in a reduction in the incidence of heart failure. Few of the primary or secondary prevention trials in coronary heart disease have included large numbers of elderly patients.[74]

ACE inhibitors have recently been found to reduce the risk of developing heart failure when given to patients with either vascular disease or diabetes (with other risk factors).[75] The risk of developing heart failure was reduced by 23%. The overall benefit of ramipril was at least as large in those aged greater than or equal to 65 years as it was in patients aged less than 65 years.

Conclusions

CHF is predominantly a disease of the elderly. Studies of all aspects of CHF should focus on this patient group. In particular, the design of future trials of therapies (both pharmacological and non-pharmacological) should ensure the inclusion of adequate numbers of older patients. Networks of care involving specialist nurses and heart failure clinics should be widely instituted with the expectation of improved quality of care.

References

1 Mosterd A, Hoes AW, deBruyne MC et al. Prevalence of heart failure and left ventricular dysfunction in the general population – the Rotterdam Study. *Eur Heart J* 1999; **20**: 447–55.

2 Kannel WB, Belanger AJ. Epidemiology of heart failure. *Am Heart J* 1991; **121**: 951–7.

3 Senni M, Tribouilloy CM, Rodeheffer RJ et al. Congestive heart failure in the community – a study of all incident cases in Olmsted County, Minnesota, in 1991. *Circulation* 1998; **98**: 2282–9.

4 Ho KKL, Pinsky JL, Kannel WB, Levy D. The epidemiology of heart failure – the Framingham study. *J Am Coll Cardiol* 1993; **22**: A6–A13.

5 Kostis JB, Davis BR, Cutler J et al. Prevention of heart failure by antihypertensive drug treatment in older persons with isolated systolic hypertension. *J Am Med Assoc* 1997; **278**: 212–16.

6 Staessen JA, Fagard R, Thijs L et al. Randomised double-blind comparison of placebo and active treatment for older patients with isolated systolic hypertension. *Lancet* 1997; **350**: 757–64.

7 Herlitz J, Karlson BW, Petterson P. Risk factors for death and mode of death after acute myocardial infarction in relation to age. *Coronary Artery Dis* 1992; **3**: 1055–63.

8 Rask Madsen C, Jensen G, Kober L et al. Age-related mortality, clinical heart failure, and ventricular fibrillation in 4259 Danish patients after acute myocardial infarction. *Eur Heart J* 1997; **18**: 1426–31.

9 O'Connor CM, Hathaway WR, Bates ER et al. Clinical characteristics and long-term outcome of patients in whom congestive heart failure develops after thrombolytic therapy for acute myocardial infarction: development of a predictive model. *Am Heart J* 1997; **133**: 663–73.

10 Devlin W, Cragg D, Jacks M, Friedman H, O'Neill W, Grines C. Comparison of outcome in patients with acute myocardial infarction aged >75 years with that in younger patients. *Am J Cardiol* 1995; **75**: 573–6.

11 Morgan S, Smith H, Simpson I et al. Prevalence and clinical characteristics of left ventricular dysfunction among elderly patients in general practice setting: cross sectional survey. *BMJ* 1999; **318**: 368–72.

12 Senni M, Rodeheffer RJ, Tribouilloy CM et al. Use of echocardiography in the management of congestive heart failure in the community. *J Am Coll Cardiol* 1999; **33**: 164–70.

13 Caruana L, Petrie MC, Davie AP, McMurray JJV. Do patients with suspected heart failure but preserved left ventricular systolic function suffer from diastolic

heart failure or from misdiagnosis? *BMJ* 2000; **321:** 215–18.

14 Cocchi A, Zuccala G, Menichelli P et al. Congestive-heart-failure in the elderly – an intriguing clinical reality. *Cardiol Elderly* 1994; **2:** 227–32.

15 McDermott MM, Gheorghiade M. Heart failure between 1986 and 1994: temporal trends in drug-prescribing practices, hospital readmissions, and survival at an academic medical center. *Am Heart J* 1998; **135:** 924.

16 Ni HY, Nauman DJ, Hershberger RE. Managed care and outcomes of hospitalization among elderly patients with congestive heart failure. *Arch Int Med* 1998; **158:** 1231–6.

17 Goldberger M, Peled HB, Stroh JA, Cohen MN, Frishman WH. Prognostic factors in acute pulmonary oedema. *Arch Int Med* 1986; **146:** 489–93.

18 Fraticelli A, Gesuita R, Vespa A, Paciaroni E. Congestive heart failure in the elderly requiring hospital admission. *Arch Geront Geriatr* 1996; **23:** 225–38.

19 MacDowall P, Kalra PA, O'Donoghue DJ, Waldek S, Mamtora H, Brown K. Risk of morbidity from renovascular disease in elderly patients with congestive cardiac failure. *Lancet* 1998; **352:** 13–16.

20 Graves EJ. National Hospital Discharge Survey, 1993. National Center for Health Statistics, Vital and Health Statistics. Washington DC, US Department of Health and Human Services, 1993.

21 Gillum RF. Idiopathic cardiomyopathy in the United States. *Am Heart J* 1986; **111:** 753–5.

22 Rodriguez Artalejo F, Guallar Castillon P, Banegas JRB, Calero JD. Trends in hospitalization and mortality for heart failure in Spain, 1980–1993. *Eur Heart J* 1997; **18:** 1771–9.

23 Bourassa MG, Gurne O, Bangdiwala SI et al. Natural history and patterns of current practice in heart-failure. *J Am Coll Cardiol* 1993; **22:** A14–A19.

24 McMurray J, McDonagh T, Morrison CE, Dargie HJ. Trends in hospitalization for heart failure in Scotland 1980–1990. *Eur Heart J* 1993; **14:** 1158–62.

25 Haldeman GA, Croft JB, Giles WH, Rashidee A. Hospitalization of patients with heart failure: National Hospital Discharge Survey, 1985 to 1995. *Am Heart J* 1999; **137:** 352–60.

26 Doughty R, Yee T, Sharpe N, MacMahon S. Hospital admissions and deaths due to congestive heart failure in New Zealand, 1988–91. *NZ Med J* 1995; **108:** 473–5.

27 Chin MH, Goldman L. Correlates of major complications or death in patients admitted to the hospital with congestive heart failure. *Arch Int Med* 1996; **156:** 1814–20.

28 Lowe JM, Candlish PM, Henry DA, Wlodarcyk JH, Heller RF, Fletcher PJ. Management and outcomes of congestive heart failure: a prospective study of hospitalised patients. *Med J Australia* 1998; **168:** 115–18.

29 Kannel WB, Ho KKL, Thom T. Changing epidemiological features of cardiac disease. *Br Heart J* 1994; **72:** S3–S9.

30 Reitsma JB, Mosterd A, deCraen AJM et al. Increase in hospital admission rates for heart failure in the Netherlands, 1980–1993. *Heart* 1996; **76:** 388–92.

31 Wolinsky FD, Overhage JM, Stump TE, Lubitz RM, Smith DM. The risk of hospitalization for congestive heart failure among older adults. *Med Care* 1997; **35:** 1031–43.

32 Burns RB, McCarthy EP, Moskowitz MA, Ash A, Kane RL, Finch M. Outcomes for older men and women with congestive heart failure. *J Am Geriatr Soc* 1997; **45:** 276–80.

33 Gooding J, Jette AM. Hospital readmission among the elderly. *J Am Ger Soc* 1985; **33:** 595–601.

34 McDermott MM, Feinglass J, Lee PI et al. Systolic function, readmission rates, and survival among consecutively hospitalized patients with congestive heart failure. *Am Heart J* 1997; **134:** 728–36.

35 Rich MW, Freedland KE. Effect of DRGs on three month readmission rate of geriatric patients with congestive heart failure. *Am J Public Health* 1988; **78:** 680–2.

36 Cline CMJ, Broms K, Willenheimer RB, Israelsson BA, Erhardt LR. Hospitalisation and health care costs due to congestive heart failure in the elderly. *Am J Ger Cardiol* 1996; **5:** 10–15.

37 Michalsen A, Konig G, Thimme W. Preventable causative factors leading to hospital admission with decompensated heart failure. *Heart* 1998; **80:** 437–41.

38 Cline CMJ, Willenheimer RB, Erhardt LR, Wiklund I, Israelsson BYA. Health-related quality of life in elderly patients with heart failure. *Scand Cardiovasc J* 1999; **33:** 278–85.

39 Krumholz HM, Phillips RS, Hamel MB et al. Resuscitation preferences among patients with severe congestive heart failure – results from the SUPPORT project. *Circulation* 1998; **98:** 648–55.

40 Koenig HG. Depression in hospitalized older patients with congestive heart failure. *Gen Hosp Psych* 1998; **20:** 29–43.

41 Krumholz HM, Butler J, Miller J et al. Prognostic importance of emotional support for elderly patients hospitalized with heart failure. *Circulation* 1998; **97:** 958–64.

42 Wang R, Mouliswar M, Denman S, Kleban M. Mortality of the institutionalized old-old hospitalized with congestive heart failure. *Arch Int Med* 1998; **158:** 2464–8.

43 Ho KKL, Anderson KM, Kannel WB, Grossman W, Levy D. Survival after the onset of congestive heart failure in Framingham heart study subjects. *Circulation* 1993; **88:** 107–15.

44 Vaitkevicius PV, Ebersold C, Haydar Z, Stewart KJ, Fleg JL. The utility of exercise training to improve functional capacity of elderly heart failure patients. *Circulation* 1997; **96:** 465.

45 Owen A, Croucher L. Effect of an exercise programme for elderly patients with heart failure. *Eur J Heart Fail* 2000; **2:** 65–70.

46 Wielenga RP, Huisveld IA, Bol E et al. Exercise training in elderly patients with chronic heart failure. *Coronary Artery Dis* 1998; **9:** 765–70.

47 Nichol KL, Margolis KL, Wuorenma J, von Sternberg T. The efficacy and cost-effectiveness of vaccination against influenza among elderly persons living in the community. *N Engl J Med* 1994; **331:** 778–84.

48 Pitt B, Zannad F, Remme WJ et al. The effect of spironolactone on morbidity and mortality in patients with severe heart failure. *N Engl J Med* 1999; **341:** 709–17.

49 The CONSENSUS trial group. Effects of enalapril on mortality in severe congestive heart failure. *New Engl J Med* 1987; **316:** 1429–35.

50 The SOLVD Investigators. Effect of enalapril on survival in patients with reduced left ventricular ejection fractions and congestive heart failure. *New Engl J Med* 1991; **325:** 303–10.

51 Garg R, Yusuf S. Overview of randomized trials of angiotensin-converting enzyme inhibitors on mortality and morbidity in patients with heart failure. *J Am Med Assoc* 1995; **273:** 1450–6.

52 Packer M, Bristow MR, Cohn JN et al. The effect of carvedilol on morbidity and mortality in patients with chronic heart failure. *New Engl J Med* 1996; **334:** 1349–55.

53 Hjalmarson A, Goldstein S, Fagerberg B et al. Effect of metoprolol CR/XL in chronic heart failure: Metoprolol CR/XL Randomised Intervention Trial in Congestive Heart Failure (MERIT-HF). *Lancet* 1999; **353:** 2001–7.

54 Pitt B, Poole-Wilson PA, Segal R, Martinez FA, Dickstein N. Effect of losartan compared to captopril on mortality in patients with symptomatic heart failure: randomise trial – the Losartan Heart Failure Survival Study ELITE II. *Lancet* 2000; **355:** 1582–7.

55 Cohn JN, Archibald DG, Ziesche S et al. Effect of vasodilator therapy on mortality in chronic congestive heart failure. *N Engl J Med* 1986; **314:** 1547–52.

56 Cohn JN, Johnson G, Ziesche S et al. A comparison of enalapril with hydralazine isosorbide dinitrate in the treatment of chronic congestive-heart-failure. *New Engl J Med* 1991; **325:** 303–10.

57 The Digitalis Investigation Group. The effect of dogoxin on mortality and morbidity in patients with heart failure. *N Engl J Med* 1997; **336:** 525–533.

58 Uretsky BF, Young JB, Shahidi FE et al. Randomized study assessing the effect of digoxin withdrawal in patients with mild-to-moderate chronic congestive heart failure – results of the PROVED trial. *J Am Coll Cardiol* 1993; **22:** 955–62.

59 Packer M, Gheorghiade M, Young JB. Withdrawal of digoxin from patients with chronic heart failure treated with angiotensin-converting enzyme-inhibitors. *N Engl J Med* 1993; **329:** 1820.

60 Kostis JB, Shelton B, Gosselin G et al. Adverse effects of enalapril in the Studies of Left Ventricular Dysfunction. *Am Heart J* 1996; **131:** 350–5.

61 Ljungman S, Kjekshus J, Swedberg K. Renal-function in severe congestive heart failure during treatment with enalapril. *Am J Cardiol* 1992; **70:** 479–87.

62 Clinical Quality Improvement Investigators. Mortality and patterns of practice in 4606 acute care patients with congestive heart failure. The relative importance of age, sex and medical therapy. *Arch Int Med* 1996; **156:** 1669–73.

63 Gambassi G, Forman DE, Lapane KL et al. Management of heart failure among very old persons living in long-term care: has the voice of trials spread? *Am Heart J* 2000; **139:** 85–93.

64 OKeeffe S, Harvey G, Lye M. Use of angiotensin-converting enzyme inhibitors in elderly patients with heart failure. *Age Ageing* 1998; **27:** 297–301.

65 Gattis WA, Larsen RL, Hasselblad V, Bart BA, OConnor CM. Is optimal angiotensin-converting enzyme inhibitor dosing neglected in elderly patients with heart failure? *Am Heart J* 1998; **136:** 43–8.

66 Ghali JK, Kadakia S, Cooper R et al. Precipitating factors leading to decompenstaion of heart failure. Traits among urban blacks. *Arch Int Med* 1988; **148:** 2013–16.

67 Wagdi P, Vuilliomemet A, Kaufman U et al. Inadequate treatment compliance, patient information and drug prescription as a cause of emergency hospitalisation of patients with chronic heart failure. *Schweiz Med Wochenschr* 1993; **123:** 108–12.

68 Colley C, Lucas L. Polypharmacy: the cure becomes the disease. *J Gen Int Med* 1993; **8:** 278–83.

69 Monane M, Bohn RL, Gurwitz JH, Glynn RJ, Avorn J. Noncompliance with congestive heart failure therapy in the elderly. *Arch Int Med* 1994; **154:** 433–7.

70 Naylor M, Brooten D, Jones R, Lavizzo-Mourey R, Mezey M, Pauly M. Comprehensive discharge planning for the hospitalised elderly. *Ann Int Med* 1994; **120:** 999–1006.

71 Stewart S, Marley JE, Horowitz JD. Effects of a multidisciplinary, home-based intervention on unplanned readmissions and survival among patients with chronic congestive heart failure: a randomised controlled study. *Lancet* 1999; **354:** 1077–83.

72 Heerdink ER, Leufkens HG, Herings RMC, Ottervanger JP, Stricker BHC, Bakker A. NSAIDs associated with increased risk of congestive heart failure in elderly patients taking diuretics. *Arch Int Med* 1998; **158:** 1108–12.

73 Gueyffier F, Bulpitt C, Boissel JP et al. Antihypertensive drugs in very old people: a subgroup meta-analysis of randomised controlled trials. *Lancet* 1999; **353:** 793–6.

74 Flather MD, Yusuf S, Kober L. Long-term ACE-inhibitor therapy in patients with heart failure or left-ventricular dysfunction: a systematic overview of data from individual patients. *Lancet* 2000; **355:** 1575–81.

75 Gerstein HC, Yusuf S, Mann JFE et al. Effects of ramipril on cardiovascular and microvascular outcomes in people with diabetes mellitus: results of the HOPE study and MICRO-HOPE substudy. *Lancet* 2000; **355:** 253–9.

14 Caring for the patient with endstage heart failure

Marjorie Funk and Kimberly Hudson

Once heart failure is recognized, the mortality rate is very high. In fact, heart failure is associated with a shorter life expectancy than that of many types of cancer.[1] Data from the Framingham[2] and Rochester[3] studies indicate that 1-year mortality rates for newly diagnosed cases average between 35% and 45%. In the Framingham cohort, the median survival time after the diagnosis of heart failure was 1.7 years for men and 3.2 years for women. Data from Framingham indicate that the 1-, 2-, 5-, and 10-year survival rates were better for women, but that very few people with heart failure were still alive 10 years after initial diagnosis (11% of men and 21% of women) (see Figure 14.1).[2]

In persons with heart failure, sudden cardiac death occurs at six to nine times the rate in the general population. In their review of 27 studies, Narang et al reported that sudden death accounted for 32–34% of heart failure deaths,[4] whereas in the Framingham study 40–50% of all heart failure deaths were sudden.[5] In fact, many patients die of a fatal arrhythmia at a time when they are clinically stable. The precise mechanism implicated in sudden death in patients with heart failure remains to be elucidated, but antiarrhythmic therapy (with the possible exception of amiodarone in severe heart failure) has *not* been shown to prevent such deaths.[6] Recently, implantable defibrillators and neurohormonal inhibition have shown promise in

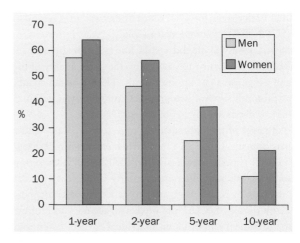

Figure 14.1. *Survival rates in patients with heart failure – the Framingham Study.*[2]

preventing sudden death in patients with advanced heart failure.

The trajectory of heart failure is less predictable than that seen in many other causes of death (see Figure 14.2). A patient dying of colon cancer, for example, has a long period of functional stability, eventually ending with a month or two of progressive disability and weight loss.

Figure 14.2. *Trajectory of dying from colon cancer or heart failure.*[7]

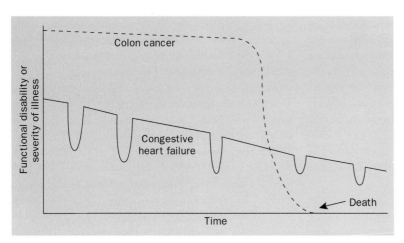

A patient with heart failure will most often exhibit a slow and lengthy decline in functional ability, with periodic bouts of severe symptoms, although death may occur suddenly from arrhythmias at any time. In general, the end of life for patients with severe heart failure may be characterized by repeated hospitalizations and a progressively declining quality of life.[7]

On the other hand, Levenson et al,[8] in their analysis of data from the Study to Understand Prognoses and Preferences for Outcomes and Risks of Treatment (SUPPORT), reported that despite increasing severity of illness, quality of life did not decline as death approached. Many patients seem to have enjoyed a good quality of life and prognosis right up until death. The estimated chance of 6-month survival was greater than 50% even within 3 days of death.

Because of the unpredictable trajectory of heart failure, it is difficult for health care providers to determine prognosis for patients with heart failure. Although a low serum sodium, declining functional capacity, and left ventricular dilatation by echocardiography have been used as prognostic indicators, they lack the predictive accuracy to indicate the imminent end of life in individual patients.[9] Without a definite prognosis, patients may underestimate the seriousness of their condition and not consider that they are nearing the end of life. Therefore, patients may benefit from more supportive care earlier in the trajectory of their illness, so they are better prepared psychologically, socially, and spiritually for death.

End-of-life care

Interest and research in the care of the dying has been increasing over the last 30 years and has resulted in better symptom control, psychological support, and choice for people dying of cancer. Although heart disease is the leading cause of death in both the United States and the United Kingdom, research into, and specialist services for, care of patients dying from heart disease has been negligible. There has been very little written about dying of heart disease. Better symptom control and psychological care should be available to patients with heart failure as they approach death. Although heart failure has traditionally been considered a chronic condition, it may also need to be seen as a terminal illness.

Terminal care has been defined as the management of patients for whom death is felt to be certain and imminent and for whom medical effort has turned away from active therapy and become concentrated on the relief of symptoms and the support of both the patient and the family.[10] Comfort measures directed at the relief of symptoms are an essential component of terminal care.

Although the concept of terminal care has traditionally been considered to be synonymous with palliative care, palliative care is now thought to be a more holistic approach to care. The World Health Organization[11] defines palliative care as

> ... the active total care of patients whose disease is not responsive to curative treatment. Control of pain, of other symptoms, and of psychological, social and spiritual problems is paramount ... Palliative care affirms life and regards dying as a normal process; neither hastens nor postpones death; provides relief from pain and other distressing symptoms; integrates the psychological and spiritual aspects of patient care; offers a support system to help patients live as actively as possible until death; offers a support system to help the family cope during the patient's illness and in their own bereavement.

The goal of palliative care is achievement of the best possible quality of life for patients and their families. Therefore, palliative care can be initiated earlier in the illness trajectory and may be more appropriate than terminal care for patients with heart failure. In addition to comfort measures, palliative care may also include therapies traditionally thought to be curative.

The backbone of palliative care is effective management of symptoms. Palliative care in cancer and heart failure may be very different. Cancer treatments, such as chemotherapy and radiation, usually cause undesirable symptoms. On the other hand, recommended treatment for heart failure (e.g. diuretics, angiotensin-converting enzyme (ACE) inhibitors, nitrates, beta-blockers, digitalis) should improve symptoms. Palliative care for patients with cancer usually involves the use of analgesics, sedatives, and antiemetics for symptom management. Palliative care for patients with heart failure may include these agents, but the focus is on maximizing therapy with medications for heart failure. Although many patients with a poor prognosis refuse medical interventions, patients with severe heart failure usually receive maximal medical therapy until death. The preferences of patients with heart failure for maximal medical therapy was supported in a recently published study by Fried et al.[12] They reported that a vast majority (> 93%) of patients with heart failure preferred interventions that had a high probability of restoring current health, even if the treatment was highly burdensome. On the other hand, most patients (> 78%) were not willing to undergo an intervention if it had a high probability of resulting in functional or cognitive impairment, even if the treatment was not burdensome.

Palliative care is often provided by a hospice – either in the home or inpatient facility. According to the National Hospice Foundation,[13] hospice care involves a team-oriented approach to medical care, pain management, and emotional and spiritual support expressly tailored to the patient's needs and wishes, and extended to the loved ones. Hospice care is based on the belief that everyone has the right to die pain-free and with dignity. The focus is on caring, not curing.

The Health Care Financing Administration (HCFA) has established criteria for eligibility for hospice care for patients with heart failure.[14] A patient is considered to be in the terminal stage of heart disease, and hence eligible for hospice care, if the following characteristics are present.

1) The patient has significant symptoms of heart failure at rest (New York Heart Association class IV). A left ventricular ejection fraction of 20% or less is helpful supplemental objective evidence, but should not be required if not already available.
2) The patient is already optimally treated with diuretics and vasodilators, preferably ACE inhibitors, but continues to experience symptoms.
3) Other factors that may support eligibility for hospice care for patients with optimally treated heart failure include:
   a. treatment-resistant symptomatic arrhythmias;
   b. history of cardiac arrest or resuscitation;
   c. history of unexplained syncope;
   d. brain embolism of cardiac origin;
   e. concomitant HIV disease.

Hospice professionals have become very proficient in caring for people dying of cancer, but are less familiar with the care of people dying of heart failure. Hospice nurses are comfortable with pain management, but may be unfamiliar with treatment for pulmonary edema. Most recent statistics revealed that cancer was the primary diagnosis of 70.6% of patients admitted to hospices in the United States, whereas heart disease was the primary diagnosis of only 6.8%.[15] Given the high prevalence of heart failure – approximately 4.7 million Americans are currently living

with heart failure – the fact that only 6.8% of patients admitted to hospice care have a primary diagnosis of heart disease means that most people are dying elsewhere.

The Regional Study of Care for the Dying was a population-based survey of family members or others who knew about the last year of life of people who died in 1990 in England. Of the 600 people for whom heart disease was the underlying cause of death, the majority (54%) died in a hospital, and 36% were reported to have died alone.[16] In their recent analysis of the experience of patients who underwent continuous outpatient support with inotropes, Hershberger et al reported that 41.7% died in a hospital.[17]

Similarly, Fried et al[18] examined older persons' preferences for site of terminal care. Patients with heart failure made up 47% of their sample (n = 117). Patients were asked where they would prefer to receive treatment if recovery from their illness was unlikely. Of the entire sample (data were not reported by diagnosis), 48% preferred treatment in a hospital, 43% preferred treatment at home, and 9% were not sure. In addition, a small portion of the patients (n = 29) underwent qualitative interviews. When asked the same question, 24% preferred treatment in a hospital, 24% preferred home, 17% nursing home, and 4% hospice. The remainder (31%) would not talk about their preferences. Patients who preferred care in a hospital or nursing home had concerns about burdening their families and the families' ability to care for them. Those who preferred home noted the importance of having family around them.

Our data on patients' experiences living with advanced heart failure indicate that 58% of the patients preferred treatment in a hospital, rather than at home or another facility.[19] We found that patients tended to want access to more aggressive treatment. This is consistent with the observation that the recommended treatment for heart failure, which can be maximized in the hospital setting, should improve symptoms. Although many patients with a poor prognosis related to other terminal conditions refuse medical interventions, patients with advanced heart failure usually prefer to receive maximal medical therapy until death. For example, one woman stated that she would want to be in a major medical center in order to receive the latest and best treatment. Another patient said that he would want the hospital setting because he could receive medications he perceived were not available at home. A preference for receiving curative therapies in the hospital, rather than supportive therapies at home, was a recurring theme in this study.

These four studies support the observation that few patients with advanced heart failure die under hospice care. Perhaps because of the uncertain trajectory of illness and the high incidence of sudden death associated with heart failure, patients, families, and health care providers do not consider the possibility of hospice care. Patients often retain a fairly high level of functioning, and, therefore, may underestimate the severity of their illness. In fact, patients may feel as well at the beginning of the week in which they die as they do in the beginning of any other week. In addition, recent advancements in the treatment of heart failure, such as ventricular resynchronization, may be perceived as offering hope for a cure.

Although patients with heart failure may benefit from hospice care, different models of care may be needed because of the high incidence of sudden death and concern that these patients do not necessarily have a clearly defined terminal phase. Perhaps a modified palliative care model would be appropriate. Hume[20] suggested that a mix of curative and comfort care may be most effective for controlling symptoms and maintaining patients' spirits at the end of life. On the curative side, new technologies would be available to patients as they are developed. These may contribute to better cardiac functioning and symptom control with corresponding improvement in quality of life. On the comfort side, patients would have available to them and their families services that address their psychosocial and spiritual needs. Counseling services, including support groups as well as individual counseling, would offer an outlet for patients to express their worries and concerns. Although hospice care does offer palliative care services for non-cancer patients, the concern is that patients and their caregivers are not offered support soon enough. A program specific to patients with heart failure that would start at the time of diagnosis is needed.

Patients should know that death may come suddenly and if they have important things to 'close', they might want to do so in advance.[7] Most patients have a few episodes of exacerbations of heart failure. These can function as 'rehearsals' for death, and experience with them can be used to help the patient and family make more specific plans and cope better when death occurs. On the other hand, a patient may be 'rescued' from death so many times that when death *actually* occurs, it may be more of a surprise to the family.

Lynn[7] proposes specific clinical strategies for good care at the end of life (see Table 14.1). She points out that listening and open communication, especially regarding

Table 14.1. Clinical strategies for good care at the end of life for patients with heart failure[7]

- Listen
- Honor the search for meaning
- Treat symptoms
- Use time-limited trials
- Set reasonable expectations for prognosis and treatment
- Negotiate stopping treatments
- Ensure continuity
- Plan for the time after death
- Be willing to provide sedation

management of symptoms and attitudes about dying, is one of the most important contributions the clinician can make. The rule is to talk less, listen more, and honor the search for meaning. Lynn advises that beyond pain and dysfunction, people who are dying are often

... absorbed with the annihilation of the self, the impact on loved ones, the terror of the unknown, and the opportunity for transcendence beyond the mortal. Health care professionals must learn how to take an appropriately supportive role in this human drama (p. 1634).[7]

Time-limited trials of aggressive diagnosis and treatment can teach all involved a great deal about the disease, as well as about how the patient's body responds. Key participants agree to reassess the merits of such procedures on a scheduled basis, and to stop the procedures if they are not helping, thereby setting reasonable expectations for prognosis and treatment. Ensuring continuity of clinicians may sometimes be challenging, however, knowing that a trusted clinician will be there to attend to their needs can be profoundly therapeutic for patients and families. Encouraging patients and families to consider what will happen in the time after the patient dies can be difficult, but reassuring for all involved. In addition, explaining that adequate sedation will be available may help alleviate fears of a struggle at the end of life.

Ward[9] proposes another strategy for good care at the end of life. He suggests using 'check lists' to ensure that a reversible etiology or precipitant has not been overlooked and that all reasonable treatment options have been considered.

Resuscitation issues

Although it is common for patients with heart failure not to appreciate the severity or terminal nature of their illness, they do need to plan for the future and complete some form of advanced directive. Because many dying persons will have periods of delirium, somnolence, or inattention and will need someone else to make decisions, it is useful to designate a surrogate with durable power of attorney for health care. Patients and families need to make specific plans for the complications that are likely in their situations. For example, persons with metastatic brain cancer need to prepare for possible seizures, whereas persons with heart failure should expect life-threatening arrhythmias. Clinicians should discuss the patient's desires regarding resuscitation and provide information regarding its effectiveness and possible outcomes. If a patient decides that resuscitation is *not* desired, it is crucial to discuss with family members or caregivers what to do in the event of sudden death. For instance, call a physician, nurse, or hospice worker, rather than 911 (or the equivalent emergency number, e.g. 999 in the UK). If the patient has an implantable defibrillator and has concerns about it prolonging life unnecessarily, he or she should be reassured that it can be turned off in preparation for death.

If deemed appropriate by the health care provider, caregivers could be supplied with an emergency kit to use in a crisis situation.[20] Kits might include such items as emergency phone numbers, nitroglycerin tablets or spray, furosemide tablets, morphine to be administered subcutaneously or by mouth, oxygen, and specific written instructions. Contents of the kit would be established by the health care provider and individualized to the specific patient's needs. The kit would not only provide the patient with more prompt symptom relief, but may also empower the caregiver and lessen feelings of helplessness. An emergency kit could be used both for patients who desire full resuscitative efforts, as well as for those who do not.

Patients' wishes related to resuscitation must be determined early in the course of the illness and reassessed frequently thereafter. Krumholz et al[21] used data obtained as part of SUPPORT to examine resuscitation preferences of patients with severe heart failure. Of the 936 patients in the sample, 69% definitely *did* want to be resuscitated in the case of a cardiac arrest, 23% explicitly stated that they *did not* want to be resuscitated, and 8% were unsure. The physician's perception of the patient's preference was not accurate in 24% of the cases. In response to a follow-up questionnaire 2 months later, 19% of patients had changed their preferences, including 14% of those who initially wanted resuscitation and 40% of those who initially did not. These findings reinforce the need to have frequent conversations regarding preferences for resuscitation.

Table 14.2. *Common symptoms in the Regional Study of Care of the Dying*[21]

Symptom	Occurrence in last year	'Very distressing'
Pain	78%	50%
Dyspnea	61%	43%
Low mood	59%	50%
Sleeplessness	45%	+
Loss of appetite	43%	+
Confusion	*	*
Constipation	37%	43%
Nausea/vomiting	32%	42%
Anxiety	30%	55%
Urinary incontinence	29%	+
Fecal incontinence	16%	64%

+ data not reported

* confusion occurred in 27% of patients < 55 years old and in 42% of patients ≥85. It was very distressing in 43% of patients < 75 years of age and in 33% of patients > 75.

Symptom management at the end of life

Table 14.2 shows the symptoms commonly experienced in the last year of life by people dying of heart disease in the Regional Study of Care for the Dying.[22] The most frequently reported symptoms during the last year of life were pain, dyspnea, low mood, and sleeplessness. These symptoms were said by many to have been 'very distressing'. Similarly, Anderson et al[23] reported that dyspnea, angina, and tiredness were the most troublesome problems for patients in their sample who had heart failure.

Management strategies for these symptoms can include relatively simple interventions. Pain, which is usually related to ischemia, is most effectively treated with nitrates and morphine. Dyspnea can be controlled with diuretics, both long- and short-acting morphine, and oxygen. Although the total daily dose of morphine used for dyspnea is usually less than that used for pain, the following dosing regimen used for pain control can serve as a guide. Initially, 2.5 mg is administered every 4 hours around the clock, with an additional 2.5 mg given between doses as required. After 1–2 days and as necessary thereafter, the every 4-hour dose is recalculated based on the total dose used in the previous 24 hours.[9] Short-term mechanical ventilation and sedation may be used for selected patients while pulmonary edema is being treated. The decision to use a ventilator would need to be revisited over time, as the patient's condition worsens. Mental disturbances (low mood, sleeplessness, anxiety, and confusion) all too commonly obliterate the opportunity for a meaningful closing to life. Each is potentially treatable, or preventable, but is often unrecognized against the background of disease or is accepted as a matter of course. Antidepressants, sleep aids, sedatives, and complementary therapies, such as Reike, may be very beneficial. Gastrointestinal problems (loss of appetite, constipation, nausea/vomiting, and fecal incontinence) can be managed with diet modifications, appetite enhancers, or medications. Urinary incontinence is often related to diuretic use and weakness. It may be alleviated with a change in the timing of diuretic doses, administration of medications to improve bladder function, or managed with a urinary catheter or external device.

Management of fatigue and activity intolerance may require some lifestyle modifications. Energy conservation techniques, such as breathing retraining, spacing activities, meditating, or using assistive devices, may be helpful. A low-level exercise program may have both physical and psychological benefits. Home health aides and homemakers can be very helpful in assisting patients to manage activities of daily living and thus conserve energy. Recently, Hershberger et al[17] in their series of 36 patients, demonstrate that continuous outpatient infusion of an intravenous inotropic agent was useful in decreasing symptoms and increasing quality of life for patients with endstage heart failure.

As patients approach the end of life, symptom management, although challenging, should become a top priority for clinicians. Florence Wald, the founder of the hospice movement in the United States, put this in perspective when she said,

> Managing symptoms of a hospice patient is what I like to call a 'delicate titration.' Keeping a patient awake, pain free, and comfortable enough to interact with the family requires expertise, and those who do this well are as skillful in their own way as a surgeon who repairs a delicate blood vessel (p. 1684).[24]

Conclusions

Although heart failure is associated with a shorter life expectancy than that of many types of cancer, it is not typically considered a terminal illness. Existing end-of-life services, which were originally designed to meet the needs of patients with cancer, may not be appropriate for patients with heart failure. Due to the unpredictable trajectory of illness and the high incidence of sudden death, a model of palliative care that begins at the time of diagnosis and continues through death may be more appropriate. Continued research is needed to evaluate the benefits of such a program for patients with heart failure and their families.

References

1 Stewart S, MacInyre K, Hole DJ, Capewell S, McMurray JJV. More 'malignant' than cancer? Five-year survival following a first admission for heart failure. *Eur J Heart Fail* 2001; **3**: 315–22.

2 Ho KKL, Pinsky JL, Kannel WB, Levy D. The epidemiology of heart failure: the Framingham Study. *J Am Coll Cardiol* 1993; **22:** 6A–13A.

3 Rodeheffer RJ, Jacobsen SJ, Gersh BJ et al. The incidence and prevalence of congestive heart failure in Rochester, Minnesota. *Mayo Clin Proc* 1993; **68:** 1143–50.

4 Narang R, Cleland GF, Erhardt L et al. Mode of death in chronic heart failure: a request and proposition for more accurate classification. *Eur Heart J* 1996; **17:** 1390–403.

5 Kannel WB, Plehn JF, Cupples LA. Cardiac failure and sudden death in the Framingham Study. *Am Heart J* 1988; **115:** 869–75.

6 Cowie MR, Mosterd A, Wood DA et al. The epidemiology of heart failure. *Eur Heart J* 1997; **18:** 208–25.

7 Lynn J. An 88-year-old women facing the end of life. *JAMA* 1997; **277:** 1633–40.

8 Levenson J, McCarthy E, Lynn J, Davis R, Phillips R. The last six months of life for patients with congestive heart failure. *J Am Geriatr Soc* 2000; **48:** S101–S109.

9 Ward C. The need for palliative care in the management of heart failure. *Heart* 2002; **87:** 294–8.

10 Saunders C, Baines M, Dunlop R. *Living with Dying: A Guide to Palliative Care, 3rd edn.* Oxford: Oxford University Press, 1995.

11 World Health Organization, WHO definition of palliative care. www.who.int/dsa/justpub/cpl.htm, retrieved May 31, 2002.

12 Fried TR, Bradley EH, Towle VR, Allore H. Understanding the treatment preferences of seriously ill patients. *N Engl J Med* 2002; **346:** 1061–6.

13 National Hospice and Palliative Care Organization. National Hospice Foundation, what is hospice? www.hospiceinfo.org, retrieved May 31, 2002.

14 National Hospice and Palliative Care Organization, Fax-on-Request. #262 Worksheet for Determining Prognosis – Heart Disease. www.nhpco.org, retrieved April, 22, 2001.

15 National Center for Health Statistics. 1996 National Home and Hospice Care Survey. www.nahc.org, retrieved April 22, 2001.

16 McCarthy M, Addington-Hall J, Ley M. Communication and choice in dying from heart disease. *J R Soc Med* 1997; **90:** 128–31.

17 Hershberger RE, Nauman D, Walker TL, Dutton D, Burgess D. Care processes and clinical outcomes of continuous outpatient support with inotropes (COSI) in patients with refractory endstage heart failure. *J Cardiac Failure* 2003; **9:** 180–7.

18 Fried T, van Doorn C, O'Leary J, Tinetti M, Drickamer M. Older persons' preferences for site of terminal care. *Ann Intern Med* 1999; **131:** 109–12.

19 Hudson KM, Funk M, Sexton DL, Nyström KV, Coviello JS, Tocchi CB. End-of-life issues for patients with heart failure. *Circulation* 2001; **104** (Suppl II): II533.

20 Hume M. Improving care at the end of life. *Quality Letter for Healthcare Leaders* 1998; **10:** 2–10.

21 Krumholz H, Phillips R, Hamel M et al. Resuscitation preferences with severe congestive heart failure: results from the SUPPORT project. *Circulation* 1998; **98:** 648–55.

22 McCarthy M, Lay M, Addington-Hall J. Dying from heart disease. *J R Coll Physns* 1996; **30:** 325–8.

23 Anderson H, Ward C, Eardley A et al. The concerns of patients under palliative care and a heart failure clinic are not being met. *Palliative Med* 2001; **15:** 279–86.

24 Friedrich MJ. Hospice care in the United States: a conversation with Florence S. Wald. *JAMA* 1999; **281:** 1683–5.

15 Psychosocial aspects of heart failure management

Linda S Baas and Ginger Conway

Heart failure, a disorder that diminishes physical energy through impaired cardiac output, can also drain the emotional strength of the person with the diagnosis. The marked reduction in activity tolerance and frequent bouts of fluid overload can lead to negative moods and personality changes as the person adjusts to ever variable symptoms and knowledge of the high mortality rate associated with the diagnosis.[1,2] Depression, anxiety, and anger can be expressions of poor adjustment.[3,4] Some may suffer as they change roles within the family and groups that have been meaningful to them while others struggle with the understanding that they need an ever-increasing support system to manage life with a chronic disorder.[5] The continuous need for increasing supportive resources may lead to feelings of helplessness or hopelessness.[6]

Despite the bleak picture that has been presented, not all persons with heart failure have such severe negative emotional reactions. Many maintain a high level of quality of life. Vigor was a predominant expression in a sample of elderly persons with heart failure.[7,8] In a study of quality of life of those treated medically or with transplant there was no group difference. Most people reported a high degree of well-being.[9]

The purpose of this chapter is to review two theories and the research related to maintaining psychosocial health. Specifically, we will begin with a discussion of the mind–body relationship in heart failure. This will be followed by a description of a conceptual model that describes the shifting perspective of chronic illness.[10] This view defines two different ways that a person with a diagnosis such as heart failure may view life with a chronic health problem. Case studies of patients will be presented to illustrate this model. Next, Modeling and Role-Modeling theory will be discussed as a way to understand how and why perspectives shift and appropriate psychosocial interventions.[11] We will also review research related to a variety of internal and external supportive resources that strengthen the psychosocial energy of the person with a chronic disorder such as heart failure. The case studies will be revisited as we describe theory and research-based interventions appropriate for each person. Throughout the chapter, we will identify ways to be culturally relevant as we provide a framework for providing holistic care of the person with heart failure.

The unique mind–body relationship in heart failure

Those with the diagnosis of heart failure have a more complex relationship between physical and psychosocial aspects of the disorder than persons with many other chronic disorders. An early compensatory mechanism in heart failure is sympathetic nervous system activation to increase cardiac output.[12] In addition, the renin–angiotensin–aldosterone hormonal response is activated. This information is presented in detail in Chapters 3 and 4 of this book. While the initial attempt of these physiologic responses is to compensate for decreased cardiac output, these compensatory mechanisms soon become dangerous and further reduce cardiac function. Thus, the major thrust of management of chronic heart failure is aimed at blunting the neurohormonal responses that further impair cardiac function.[12–14]

The mind is also linked to the neurohormonal responses found in heart failure. When anxious, fearful, or angry, the sympathetic nervous system is activated.[2,15] While these moods do not lead to heart failure in a normal heart, they can exacerbate the problem in someone with the diagnosis of heart failure. Psychosocial interventions that decrease this sympathetic response play an important but often unrecognized role in managing heart failure.[16] Of interest, beta-blockers are medications used to blunt the neurohormonal response in heart failure, but they can result in an increased perception of fatigue and even depression.

The problem with prescribing interventions is that people are holistic and unique individuals with varied needs and resources. Thus, there are multiple interventions that must be individualized to be effective.[11] As heart failure worsens, it can lead to psychosocial problems that may be as challenging as the physiological changes. Not only is the patient with heart failure affected, but family members and friends must also face changes in roles and responsibilities.[17] Holistic care of the patient with heart failure must include the assessment and management of the psychosocial as well as the physical aspects of the disorder. Next, we apply a theory that describes two ways in which people with heart failure may present to health care providers.

The shifting perspectives model of chronic illness: understanding perceptions of illness and wellness in chronic disease

Patterson conducted a metastudy of 292 published, primary qualitative research studies that explored the experience of chronic illness in adults.[10] A rigorous method of data analysis was used to synthesize studies conducted in different countries and by different disciplines. Rather than viewing stages of recovery, the model described two states that people experience and their movement between the conditions. The first state is described as living with illness in the foreground. The alternative is living with wellness in the foreground (see Figure 15.1). Whether illness or wellness is in the foreground, it is the person's perception that is important. Each state will be described in more detail and discussed in terms of how and why people shift between them.

Living with illness in the foreground usually occurs after the diagnosis is made and the person feels overwhelmed by the new burden that must be borne.[10] In this scenario the person focuses on the burden of living with the disease, perception of sickness, and suffering from symptoms or potential loss. In other words, it is a state in which the person responds with a negative and perhaps depressed mood. Focusing on the illness has some protective function, especially for the person who welcomes the 'sick role' as part of a personal identity.[18] Also, a focus on the illness may conserve energy and supportive resources. After the initial diagnosis, the person needs to attend to the illness in order to learn self-care strategies. Effective teaching requires that the person recognizes the presence of the health problem and the need to perform certain behaviors in order to maintain or improve health status. This may mean that a better understanding of the disease and self-care can help move the perspective of illness from the foreground to the background.

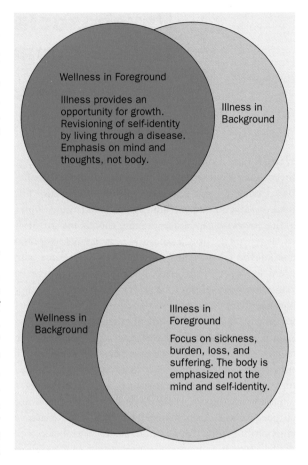

Figure 15.1. *Shifting perspectives model of chronic illness.*

When living with wellness in the foreground, personal identity shifts to the self, not the diseased physical state.[10] Living with the disease is perceived as a challenge and meaningful change. The person feels less a victim of the disease and instead thinks of the body as something that is distant and needs to be fixed. Removing the focus from the disease allows the person to develop the emotional, social, and spiritual context they desire. Often, relationships with family and friends are renewed, providing even more meaning in life.

The shift from illness to wellness in the foreground may be slow and gradual or a sudden awakening.[10] Regardless, the person must recognize that a shift has occurred and express the desire to give up the sick identity by making meaningful changes in behavior. It is not clear what specifically prompts the shift to wellness in the foreground; however, the influence of another with the disease, or a significant family member may support the change. There is limited support from the literature that health care providers influence this shift, but once the change occurs, they can support the individual in the search for ways to maintain healthy living. So, health care providers can facilitate or support a change.

Shifting to illness in the foreground may be the result of an actual or perceived loss of control. When symptoms worsen or new skills are needed, the person may experience hopelessness or helplessness. Furthermore, non-illness-related crises might compound the situation. Regardless of the cause of the shift, the change allows the individual to gain control through self-indulgence. Paradoxically, self-help groups can turn attention to the illness, not the potential for wellness and foster this shift.

Patterson did not discuss cross-cultural implications of this model.[10] However, intuitively there is a recognized strong link between cultural norms and the expression of illness in society. Decades ago, Mechanic described the 'sick role' and the associated social responsibilities.[18] This model described the sick role from the perspective of American culture. Other cultures have prescribed roles for the sick.[19,20] Some cultures are more nourishing for the person who lives with illness in the foreground. In these groups greater attention to the details of one's illness are appropriate and shared with others. However, in other cultures there may be norms that suppress efforts to live with illness in foreground. In such a situation, the person may be compelled to suppress outward signs of living with illness in the foreground whether that is the case or not.

Considering the meaning that the heart has to most individuals, the shifting perspective model may have special implications for the person with heart failure. After all, the heart is believed to be the center of emotions, and to be void in this area is considered to be heartless. The heart is also portrayed in some religions and cultures as the soul or the center of the being. When the heart fails, it may rob the person of their core being and a meaningful existence. The loss of heart function may lead to a focus on illness, while a hopeful heart or a warm heart may focus on wellness. Two patients are presented to illustrate the shifting perspective model.

First case study illustrating the shifting perspectives model

Mrs NB is a 64-year-old Caucasian female diagnosed with cardiomyopathy 7 years ago. She was referred to a cardiac transplant center 5 years ago and was eventually placed on the transplant waiting list due to a left ventricular ejection fraction of 12%, New York Heart Association class III–IV symptoms, and significantly impaired cardiopulmonary exercise capacity. Mrs NB is widowed without any children but has a very close relationship with her sister and brother. Her hobbies include maintaining a small flower garden. Her medication regimen was optimized and her condition remained fairly stable over the past few years. She continued to live her life as fully as possible within the limits imposed by a failing heart. She attended church and called on her 'shut-in' friends.

Mrs NB illustrated the picture of living with health in the foreground until recently when her heart failure worsened requiring a 3-week hospitalization. During that time, her energy was focused on dealing with the acute exacerbation of symptoms. She became despondent and at times withdrawn. She talked of preparing for the end and knowing that she could not live much longer without a heart transplant. She worried that her lungs and kidneys would also fail and that she would then become ineligible for a transplant. She clearly focused most of her attention on the illness during this hospitalization. However, occasionally she expressed a longing to return home and enjoy her life, even if it was limited and she needed to depend upon others for more support.

After discharge Mrs NB returned to her own home with extra support from her brother and sister-in-law. She planned to move to an apartment in her brother's home. During this transition, she refocused her energies from waiting for a new heart to maintaining her health status. She monitored her diet more closely, performed low-level exercise for brief periods daily, and took her medication regularly. After thoughtful consideration of her options, she decided to remove herself from the transplant list. Her medical condition had not improved. The measure of left ventricular ejection fraction had dropped to 8% and she continued to have symptoms with activities such as housework and shopping. While some may describe this behavior as denial, she clearly recognized the extent of her disease. However, she was focused on enjoying her life and was unwilling to undergo the anticipated hospital stay waiting for a transplant. After all, she had been on the waiting list for transplant for the past 5 years. She wanted to focus on the present and not a future that may never come to pass as many die while awaiting a heart transplant. Mrs NB spent more time with her family and moved her gardening attention from outdoor flowers to indoor plants.

When living with wellness in the foreground one cannot ignore the maintenance of one's health and often must pay even closer attention to it. Mrs NB did this by becoming more involved in her self-care by adhering to her diet, medication and activity regimen. However, an individual living with wellness in the foreground may also ignore the progression of their disease, which may contribute negatively to their survival. The important thing for health care providers to remember is that this is the informed decision of the individual. Mrs NB may have given up years but she did so for peace of mind and perhaps for improved quality of life.

Second case study illustrating the shifting perspectives model

Mr DC is a 56-year-old Caucasian male who illustrates several moves in the shifting perspective of illness model. Mr DC is married with two adult children. Mr DC and his wife have attended church regularly. They see their children every few weeks. He worked full-time as a manager in a large corporation. Mr DC first noticed symptoms of heart failure 2 years ago. He was seen by his internist and referred to a cardiologist because he developed the symptoms of dyspnea on minimal exertion, orthopnea, paroxysmal nocturnal dyspnea, and lower extremity edema. His left ventricular ejection fraction was 54% on an echocardiogram. He was referred to a tertiary care center for further evaluation where the diagnosis of diastolic heart failure was made. His medications were adjusted for optimal ventricular relaxation and his condition steadily improved.

Initially he was concerned and had difficulty accepting the fact that he had heart failure despite a 'near normal ejection fraction'. During this time, he seemed to be very focused on his disease but he eventually took responsibility for managing his diet and medications. He began walking daily to increase his functional status so that he could stay connected with friends and enjoy life. Mr DC was very optimistic about his future and although he was not working at the time he planned to eventually return to work, at least part time. His heart failure had been well controlled and he seemed to be improving, with a focus on wellness, until a year ago.

When his symptoms worsened, despite increased therapy, Mr DC was forced to accept permanent disability due to his symptoms of diastolic heart failure. His wife continued to work full time. Recently, she started to go out with her friends in the evening to movies or for dinner. He refused to go out to any social events. Their only time spent together outside the house was occasionally attending church and the monthly heart failure support group. His increase in symptoms continued and he needed frequent adjustments in his diuretic regimen, had two emergency room visits in 1 month and eventually was hospitalized for a week. He denied dietary indiscretion; however, his wife reported he had not stayed on a low sodium diet. He often made sarcastic jokes about his wife's evenings out with her friends and the time she comes home; however, he denied this was of concern to him. He said that he did not have a problem with accepting permanent disability, but he would refer to his present life as useless. He expressed concern frequently by asking 'what is going on or why is this happening'. He consistently focused on his limitations and symptoms.

With this increase in symptoms, Mr DC seemed to slip into a pattern of illness in the foreground. He limited his social circle to those with the same illness. He had many more non-cardiac physical complaints, insisting on many different diagnostic procedures for the variety of aches and pains. No organic basis was found for these reported problems. His affect became flat and he appeared quite depressed but refused antidepressant medications and referrals for counseling. This pattern persisted for more than 6 months. Mr DC clearly demonstrated a shift to 'illness in the foreground'. This shift may have been precipitated by the need to maintain the sick role during an exacerbation of symptoms, by a perceived loss of control, by role changes, or by the loss of employment. Regardless of the cause, he continued to project negativity until he agreed to participate in a cardiac rehabilitation exercise program.

Mr DC had a dramatic turnaround after 8 weeks of cardiac rehabilitation. He began to focus on his 'health' again. He lost 10 pounds and gained physical strength. He became involved in new social circles. His visits to the heart failure center decreased in frequency. Once again, he focused on wellness.

It is not always clear what triggers the shifting perspectives. Regardless of the changes, the health care provider must recognize that changes have occurred and they are the result of perceptions held by the individual. Some external forces, like a negative support group, may trigger a shift to illness, while others like a cardiac rehabilitation program, may shift the person to a wellness perspective. Increased symptoms heralded changes in both case studies presented. One's perception of supportive resources can likewise influence the shift in perspective of illness/wellness. The paradigm, Modeling and Role-Modeling, may add additional understanding to why and how shifting perspectives may appear. Also, Modeling and Role-Modeling provides a framework for examining internal and external supportive resources to regain or maintain psychosocial health despite the physical problems imposed by heart failure.

Modeling and Role-Modeling: a paradigm to guide holistic care of the person with heart failure

Modeling and Role-Modeling is a framework for practice that integrates many non-nursing theories of growth and development, stress, loss and attachment into a collection of middle range theories for practice.[11,21–23] It is easy for many nurses to understand and apply this approach to practice as it builds on the familiar work of Maslow, Erikson, Piaget, Selye, and Engel.[24–28] The authors of the theory, Erickson, Tomlin, and Swain developed the theory based on their clinical, teaching, and research experiences.

The name, Modeling and Role-Modeling, was derived from the overall goals of nursing action.[11] First, the nurse must build a model of the person's world. That is, the nurse must see the uniqueness of the individual and assess the person's myriad needs, strengths, and resources. This emphasis on understanding the beliefs and perceptions of the individual is similar to Patterson's underlying assumption in the Shifting Perspective model of chronic illness. Once the nurse has a model of the person's world, it is time to guide or assist the person in a multitude of ways to regain healthy functioning through an individualized plan of role modeling. Understanding the person is the basis for a therapeutic relationship, but the nurse must also unconditionally accept the person in order to be effective in developing mutual goals and plans for care.

The theorists proposed Modeling and Role-Modeling as a broad paradigm or conceptual model to guide practice and research. Now, several meta-theorists describe it as interrelated middle range theories.[29,30] Four middle range theories (self-care, affiliated individuation, developmental residual, and the adaptive potential assessment model) within the Modeling and Role-Modeling paradigm will be explained here. These theories and the supporting research provide the basis for providing psychosocial care of the person with heart failure.

Self-care theory

The first middle range theory is self-care.[31,32] This theory proposes that the person has self-care knowledge, or the understanding of what is needed to maintain or regain health. Self-care knowledge is more than the factual information about the health problem; it is what the person understands to be the reason that the health care problem happened at this time as well as the personal meaning of the health problem. Based on this knowledge, the person mobilizes internal and external self-care resources to enable self-care actions. Internal supportive resources can include a myriad factors such as hope, control, spirituality, and self-efficacy. External resources can include social support, roles and relationships, financial resources, and health care providers.

In a pilot study of 38 persons with heart failure, the Self-Care Resource Inventory was used to assess needs (self-care knowledge) and resources available in persons with heart failure treated medically or after heart transplantation.[9] This tool measured both internal and external types of needs and resources.[33] There was neither a treatment group difference nor a gender difference in needs or resources available. Furthermore, the two variables predicted 38% of the variance in quality of life, an outcome of self-care actions.[9] Similar results were found in a larger sample of persons with heart failure and in a sample of 81 persons after an acute myocardial infarction.[33] Of interest, self-care needs and resources were better predictors of outcomes such as quality of life than deficits which is the central focus of Orem's theory of self-care.[34]

Affiliated individuation

A second middle range theory within Modeling and Role-Modeling describes affiliated individuation, a coexisting need to be both connected and autonomous. While these may seem to be conflicting needs, they actually exist in a dynamic equilibrium that is situationally based.[11] Which type of relationship is needed at any time depends on the individual's perception, attachments, and needs. Loss of an attachment to a loved one or cherished object can lead to grief. If new attachments are not developed, morbid grief and depression can ensue. Loss of health and functional capacity can be mourned or grieved.

Internal resources are derived from having individuation needs met. Examples may include a hopeful outlook, control, and self-efficacy. External resources are derived from strong affiliation with others and include an adequate social network and support. In a study of caregivers of persons with Alzheimer's disease, a strong sense of both affiliation and individuation provided a buffer against stress related to the burden of caring for a loved one with complex health needs and difficult communication needs.[35]

Developmental residual

Developmental growth progresses through a series of stages defined by Erikson more than 50 years ago.[25] Each stage is described in terms of a challenge. As one meets the challenge, new coping skills are acquired. The new skill provides a resource that helps the person meet additional challenges throughout life. For example, as a child gains trust, autonomy, initiative, and industry through the developmental stages, there are strengths gained from these positive passages that provides strength in adulthood. This developmental residual is particularly relied upon during times of stress or when other resources are insufficient to meet the needs required for growth or adaptation.[11] A health problem, such as an exacerbation of heart failure symptoms, is an example of a stressor that may make the person again face developmental challenges. The person with more developmental residual will resolve the challenge with less difficulty than the person with less developmental residual.

In a study of 138 persons with heart failure, the qualitative analysis of subject goals revealed that all eight of the Eriksonian developmental stages could be identified.[4] Of interest, those under age 45 years had greater negative mood states (depression, anger, and anxiety) than those who were over age 65, but after 6 months, the difference was not statistically significant. It was proposed that the younger person with heart failure faced the adult developmental stages prematurely due to the gravity of their diagnosis. Having a health problem with a high 5-year mortality forces a younger person to meet adult developmental challenges of intimacy, generativity, and integrity before their same-age peers. This leads to depression and anger, but with time, the younger person may be able to meet the developmental challenge. Of interest, those with the highest quality of life had the least anger and depression, regardless of age.[4] Perhaps they had the greatest amount of developmental residual.

Adaptive potential assessment model

The final theory within Modeling and Role-Modeling is the Adaptive Potential Assessment Model, which is deeply rooted in the work of Selye and Engel.[27,28] Selye described the physiological effects of stress and Engel delineated the psychosocial response. During times of

stress, such as one might experience when faced with a new, chronic, and progressively deteriorating illness like heart failure, adaptation depends upon the ability to effectively use the resources that one perceives they have available. Stressors can be either perceived threats or real threats to one's well-being; however, either will elicit the arousal response. This surge in sympathetic nervous system and the related hormonal response is particularly harmful to the person with heart failure who has little reserve. Resources can mitigate the stressor response and the person can return to equilibrium. Impoverishment occurs when resources are depleted. The characteristics of responses in these three states have been validated in adults and adolescents.[36]

Linkages among the modeling and role modeling theories

The perceived availability of both internal and external resources, and the ability to mobilize these resources are the major links among the four middle range theories of Modeling and Role-Modeling. Affiliation is achieved through developing external resources while individuation is derived from strong internal resources. As one moves through developmental stages, resources are accumulated. The greater the accumulation of resources the more strength one has to respond to stressors.[11]

Self-care is a goal for most people with heart failure.[4,9,37] Self-care strategies are the basis for treatment at comprehensive heart failure centers.[38,39] Numerous studies have supported the benefits of treatment at such comprehensive centers demonstrating fewer hospital stays, lower costs, and better management of symptoms.[40–43] Guidelines for the treatment of patients with heart failure further recognize the importance of such programs, which are often nurse-managed centers of care.[12–14]

The self-care model (see Figure 15.2) is depicted in relationship to other components of Modeling and Role-Modeling. Because the potential resources are so important in this model, a review of research related to internal and external resources will be provided next. This will be followed by a discussion of the case studies and nursing interventions in view of both Modeling and Role-Modeling and the theory of shifting perspectives.

Internal resources

Resources that are derived from primarily internal sources include hope, control, self-efficacy, vigor, and spirituality.[11]

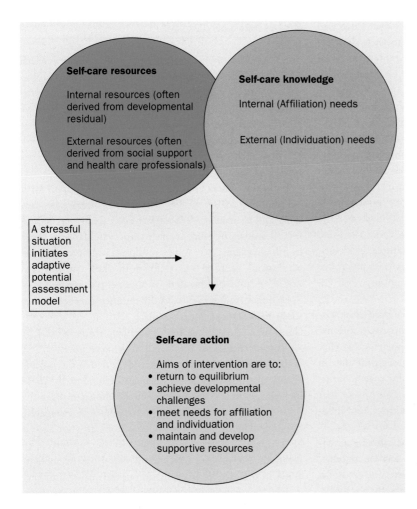

Figure 15.2. *Depiction of how developmental residual, affiliated individuation, and the adaptive potential assessment models are related to self-care ionship among the four constructs of Modeling and Role-Modeling.*

These same factors can be viewed as developmental residual that enables the person to face challenges in life with the determination and confidence that they can make the most of the situation. Internal resources allow one to live in the present and see a future that is possible. Each of these resources will be discussed with research support and clinical application to the care of patients with heart failure.

Hope is a powerful internal resource that is derived from a positive expectation about the future.[44] In several studies, loss of hope with ensuing depression was related to higher mortality in persons with chronic illness.[45–47] Two aspects of hope have been described, generalized hope and particularized hope.[48] Generalized hope is more of a global outlook on life while particularized hope is the desire to see a specific outcome for an identified situation. In a study of community-dwelling elderly, generalized hope was associated with spirituality, trust, and social support.[48]

Particularized hope was related to control. In a study of patients with heart failure, hope was significantly related to morale (r = 0.57) and social (r = 0.50) but not physical (r = 0.15) function.[49]

Control can be actual or perceived.[11,50–52] In a given situation the person may have the actual control to make a change or act in a specific way. In other situations, they may not have full control to do as desired; instead they perceive they have control over some aspect of the decision-making or implementation of a plan of care. Perceived control has been related to lower levels of anxiety, depression, and hostility in the 6 months after an acute myocardial infarction.[51] In qualitative studies of recovery, control was found to be an integral part of the process.[52]

Bandura popularized self-efficacy, the belief that one has both the knowledge and the skills to perform a specified behavior.[53] Self-efficacy is particularly pertinent to the person with heart failure who needs the knowledge and ability to perform self-care behaviors. Many new skills are needed when one first learns of the problem of heart failure. New medication regimens may be complicated. For instance, to prevent hypotension, the schedule for various medications may be staggered by an hour or two. Most need to learn how to monitor fluid status by weighing daily and monitoring edema. Meals should be low in salt and that may require new skills in shopping, cooking, and selecting food when dining out. What may take even more skill is learning to balance periods of activity with rest. As one develops a sense of self-efficacy, positive reinforcement further increases a sense of control over the disease. Self-efficacy has been studied in various chronic illnesses, including heart disease.[54] In a sample of 43 subjects with heart failure, self-efficacy scores were predictive of actual performance on cardiopulmonary exercise testing.[55]

Knowledge has been described as a component of self-efficacy, but it also has broader implications as an internal resource. 'Knowledge is power' is a popular saying that exemplifies how those with heart failure may gain control over their illness. Studies have delineated the specific information that patients request.[56,57] It is not surprising that the areas of information focus on food, activity, and medications; all are important aspects needed for self-care.[56] Knowledge was associated with increased self-care activities.[57] A specific method of teaching focusing on concrete, objective information may provide the most useful method of preparing a person to gain self-care skills. Research has supported this method as one that increases a feeling of control and results in improved outcomes.[58–60] This type of teaching is based on personalization of the experience of living with the disorder and addresses common experiences along with the factual information needed for self-care.

Several additional internal resources have been described in the literature. Vigor is a perception of energy and inner strength that was associated with quality of life but not related to the severity of illness in a sample of elderly with heart failure.[7] Predictors of vigor in a sample of persons with heart failure included general health perceptions, mental health, and energy expended in planned exercise.[8] Spirituality, or a sense of belief in the importance and meaning of life, was found to have a stronger relationship with global and health-related quality of life than participation in religious activities in adults with heart failure.[61]

External resources

Social support, often considered to be the primary external resource, is derived from the actual or perceived helpfulness of others who may be able to assist in some way during an acute or chronic problem.[62] Most of the time we associate social support with improved outcomes, but that is not always the case. Social support is a complex concept that has both positive and negative outcomes that needs further explanation.[63]

Early researchers equated a lack of social support with being unmarried or socially isolated. An increase in mortality and morbidity was found in several large epidemiological studies of persons with cardiovascular and other health problems.[64–66] While results were impressive, the way social support was defined in these studies was not from the perspective of the people studied.[67–69] Subsequent studies examined the number of people in the social network and found positive relationship with outcomes and a greater number of people in the network.[67]

Not all studies of social network were positive.[68] A 'darker side' of social support was identified as the indebtedness that one feels as the recipient of support for those in their network.[70] Reciprocity, or the ability to repay the person for their kindness, could mediate this negative response. The payment need not be monetary, nor need it be proportional to the original gift or support. The meaning behind the repayment was most important. Work in this area led to evaluation of the quality, not necessarily the quantity of support available.

Four major reviews of the literature related to social support in persons with cardiac disease have been published.[5,6,71,72] Results in samples of cardiac patients were similar to what was found in other chronic illnesses. However, when the reviews were conducted, little research had been done in the area of heart failure. Most research in this growing population has been published in the past 7 years. In one study of 50 people with heart failure, those with poorer adjustment had more health problems and lower functional status.[73] They also reported more strained social and family relationships. A group of 359 people waiting for heart transplant reported satisfaction with emotional and tangible support, although neither was a significant predictor of quality of life.[74] In a sample of 65 people, of which one-third were rehospitalized, there were no group differences in social support. However, in a group of 292 older patients with heart failure, those with lower levels of social support had more recurrent cardiac events and higher mortality 1 year after the initial hospitalization.[75] A special concern for the elderly is that the person who is the primary support person is often also older and with chronic health problems of their own.[76]

Support groups provide another example of an external resource. Groups can provide a setting for sharing information and experiences while providing a sense of belonging. The group may provide the opportunity for a person to feel attached to others and remain socially integrated.[77-78] A study of 134 Swedish elderly persons with heart failure who participated in self-help support groups found the experience positive. Group participation resulted in shared information that enhanced confidence in ability to manage their care.[79]

Implications for practice

Based on all of the information about the two theories and much research conducted on various internal and external resources, what should the nurse do to provide competent psychosocial care for the person with heart failure? The theory of Shifting Perspectives describes two profiles that may be recognized in persons with a chronic disease such as heart failure. But this theory does not offer much to help health care providers assist people to move to the state in which illness is in the foreground. It does emphasize that movements can be subtle or sudden and the nurse should be supportive and understanding of the person's perspective of their illness. This is congruent with Modeling and Role-Modeling in that the nurse must unconditionally accept the person. This may also mean that when the person expresses more dependent desires, it is reflecting the greater requirement for affiliation needs. It is better to facilitate obtaining these needs than forcing independence when the person is not able to assume that role yet. Instead of pushing the person into a role of taking responsibility for their own care, ask them when they will be ready to do so, or what can you do to help them be ready for some aspect of self-care.

Based on Modeling and Role-Modeling, there are five aims of intervention. The first is to build trust. This may require much effort but every person needs to accept that you are seeing them as an individual with unique needs and resources. Building a trusting relationship may occur with the initial encounter if the person is living with health in the foreground; however, it may take many interactions to gain trust from the person who is living with

illness in the foreground. The person has a preoccupation of living with the disease and may be mourning lost health and lifestyle. Being consistent, available, and understanding will foster the development of trust.

The second aim of intervention is to provide control. Control is a powerful internal resource that may be the key in shifting one from illness to wellness in the foreground. The loss of control that happens when symptoms worsen may trigger the reverse move to illness in the foreground. Both of the case studies presented earlier in the chapter demonstrated this shift when symptoms worsened. Both individuals exhibited a more positive outlook when control was restored. For Mrs NB, the control was demonstrated by her decision not to undergo a heart transplant, despite no improvement in her cardiac condition. For Mr DC, it came after participating in cardiac rehabilitation and seeing positive physical changes. However, his prior participation in a support group did result in a positive change in outlook.

The third aim of intervention is to promote a positive orientation. Reframing situations to demonstrate a healthier outlook can do this. Seeing the glass as half full instead of half empty is the most familiar example of reframing. Care must be taken when reframing situations so that an unrealistic picture is not painted for the individual. Also, it should be a relevant analogy. In his more depressed mood, Mr DC expressed how his life was worthless. The nurse could point out the many family members and participants in the support group who felt that they benefited from their relationships with him. Specific examples of what was said may reframe the situation. It also would reinforce the strong external supports available. Mrs NB demonstrated reframing her life goals when she stated that she wanted to live for the day instead of the hope for a transplant.

The fourth aim of intervention is to promote strengths. This can be accomplished by pointing out specific examples of behaviors and beliefs that demonstrate the internal resources that the person has exhibited in the past as well as the external resources that may be helpful. When the person is very withdrawn, it may not be possible for him or her to see their strengths. Once the person has developed a sense of trust, and degree of control, this aim of intervention is more feasible. When he was focused on his illness, Mr DC was not able to see that he could increase his exercise capacity. Yet, when he shifted to wellness in the foreground, he could see how his functional status improved and enjoyed telling others of his rehabilitation success.

When Mrs NB moved and no longer had an outdoor garden, she delighted in caring for indoor plants and giving gardening advice to her friends and church members.

The final aim is to set mutual goals. The goals really must be mutually agreed upon. Often, health care providers set goals and later convince the patient to accept them. To be truly mutual, there must be trust and the patient must have control to participate in determining the specific health care outcome and plan. To best accomplish mutual goal setting, the person should be focused on wellness. In addition, there should be adequate resources available. The person can rely on their health care provider to meet affiliation needs while reaching the goals associated with individuation.

The five aims of intervention can provide the basis for psychosocial care of the person with heart failure. Understanding how people view health and illness provides a means of determining which interventions may be most appropriate at a given point in time. Regardless of the specific plan of care, the nurse can do much to promote health and self-care by building a model of the client's world that includes an assessment of affiliation and individuation, developmental residual, adaptive potential, needs, and internal and external resources. Based on this model, the nurse can intervene to promote health. Figure 15.3 relates concepts from Modeling and Role-Modeling with the Shifting Perspective model.

Conclusions

Psychosocial care is a vital component of the treatment plan for a person with heart failure. Theory and research can guide the practitioner to develop the most appropriate and successful plan of care. Recognizing that every individual is different, though influenced by common cultural experiences, will help the nurse to focus on the individual with heart failure, not the heart failure patient.

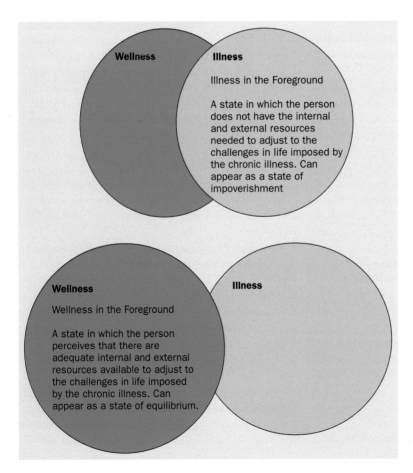

Figure 15.3. *Relationship between the self-care resource model and shifting perspective model of chronic illness.*

References

1 Rowe MA. The impact of internal and external resources on functional outcomes in chronic illness. *Res Nurs Health* 1996; **19:** 485–97.

2 Sotile WM. *Psychosocial interventions for cardiopulmonary patients.* Champaign IL Human Kinetics: 1996.

3 Koening HG. Depression in hospitalized older patients with congestive heart failure. *Gen Hosp Psychiatry* 1998; **20:** 29–43.

4 Baas LS, Beery TA, Fontana JA, Wagoner LE. An exploratory study of development growth in adults with heart failure. *J Holistic Nurs* 1999; **17:** 117–38.

5 Moser D. Social support and cardiac recovery. *J Cardiovasc Nurs* 1994; **9:** 27–36.

6 Yates BC, Skaggs BG, Parker JD. Theoretical perspectives on the nature of social support in cardiovascular illness. *J Cardiovasc Nurs* 1994; **9:** 1–15.

7 Fontana JA. A consideration of vigor as an outcome measure of exercise therapy in chronic illness. *Rehabil Nurs Res* 1995; **4:** 75–81.

8 Fontana JA. The emergence of the person–environment interaction in a descriptive study of vigor in heart failure. *Adv Nurs Sci* 1996; **18:** 75–82.

9 Baas LS, Fontana JA, Bhat G. Relationships between self care resources and the quality of life of persons with heart failure: a comparison of treatment groups. *Prog Cardiovasc Nurs* 1997; **12:** 25–38.

10 Patterson BL. The shifting perspectives model of chronic illness. *J Nurs Scholarship* 2001; **33:** 21–6.

11 Erickson HC, Tomlin E, Swain MA. *Modeling and Role-Modeling: a Theory and Paradigm for Nursing.* Lexington, SC: Pine Press of Lexington; 1988.

12 Grady KL, Dracup K, Kennedy G, Moser DK, Piano M et al. Team management of patients with heart failure: a statement for healthcare professionals from the Cardiovascular Nursing Council of the American Heart Association. *Circulation* 2000; **102:** 2443–56.

13 Hunt SA, Baker DW, Chin MH, Cinquegrani MP, Feldman AM et al. ACC/AHA guidelines for the evaluation and management of chronic heart failure in the adult: a report of the American College of Cardiology/American Heart Association Task Force on Practice Guidelines. 2001; **38:** 2101–13.

14 Heart Failure Society of America (HFSA). HFSA guidelines for management of patients with heart failure caused by left ventricular systolic dysfunction: a pharmacological approach. *J Cardiac Failure* 1999; **5:** 357–82.

15 Dossey BM, Keegan L, Guzzetta CE. *Holistic nursing: a handbook for practice*, 3rd edn. Gaithersburg, MD: Aspen Publication, 2000.

16 Moser D, Dracup K, Woo M, Stevenson L. Voluntary control of vascular tone by using skin-temperature biofeedback-relaxation in patients with advanced heart failure. *Alternative Therapies Health Med* 1997; **3:** 51–9.

17 Friedman MM. Social support sources among older women with heart failure: continuity versus loss over time. *Res Nurs Health* 1997; **20:** 319–27.

18 Mechanic D. *Medical Sociology*, 2nd edn. New York: Free Press, 1968.

19 Spector R. *Cultural diversity in health and illness*, 5th edn. Upper Saddle River, NJ: Prentice Hall, 2000.

20 Campinha-Bacote J. A model and instrument for addressing cultural competence in health care. *J Nurs Education* 1999; **38:** 203–7.

21 Frisch NC, Bowman SS, Erickson HC, Tomlin EM, Swain MAP. In: George J (ed.). *Nursing Theories: the Base for Professional Nursing Practice*, 4th edn. Norwalk, CT: Appleton & Lange, 1995.

22 Kinney CK, Erickson HC. Modeling the client's world: a way to holistic care. *Issues Mental Health Nurs* 1990; **11:** 93–108.

23 Marriner-Tomey A, Allingood MA. *Nursing Theorists and their Works*, 4th edn. St. Louis: Mosby, 1998.

24 Maslow AH. *Toward a Psychology of Being*. New York: Van Nostrand Reinhold; 1968.

25 Erikson E. *Identity, Youth and Crisis*. New York: WW Norton, 1968.

26 Piaget J. *The Psychology of the Child*. New York: Basic Books, 1969.

27 Selye H. *Stress without Distress*. Philadelphia: J.B. Lippincott Co., 1974.

28 Engel GS. *Psychological Development in Health and Disease*. Philadelphia: WB Saunders, 1968.

29 Liehr P, Smith MJ. Middle range theory: spinning research to practice to create knowledge for the new millennium. *Adv Nurs Sci* 1999; **21:** 81–91.

30 Frisch NC, Kelley J. *Healing Life's Crises: a Guide for Nurses*. Albany, NY: Delmar Publishers, 1996.

31 Erickson HC. Self-care knowledge: an exploratory study. In: Erickson HC, Kinney C, eds. *Modeling and Role-Modeling: Theory, Practice and Research*. Austin, TX: The Society for the Advancement of Modeling and Role-Modeling; 1990, 178–202.

32 Erickson HC, Swain MAP. Mobilizing self-care resources: a nursing intervention for hypertension. *Issues Ment Health Nurs* 1990; **11:** 217–35.

33 Baas LS, Curl ED, Hertz JE, Robinson KR. Innovative approaches to theory-based measurement: modeling and role-modeling research. *ANS: Advances in Methods of Inquiry for Nursing*. Gaithersburg, MD: Aspen Publishers; 1994, 147–59.

34 Orem DE. *Nursing: Concepts of Practice*, 6th edn. St. Louis: Mosby, 2001.

35 Acton GJ, Miller EW. Affiliated-individuation in caregivers of adults with dementia. *Issues Ment Health Nurs* 1996; **17:** 245–60.

36 Barnfather J, Swain MA, Erickson H. Construct validity of an aspect of the coping process: potential adaptation to stress. *Issues in Mental Health Nurs* 1989; **10:** 23–40.

37 Baas LS, Trupp RA, Abraham WT. Supportive resources for the patient with heart failure. In: Moser D, Riegel B (eds). *Improving outcomes in heart failure: an interdisciplinary approach*. Gaitherburg, MD: Aspen, 2001, 201–18.

38 Riegel B, Thomason T, Carlson B et al. Implementation of a multidisciplinary disease management program for heart failure patients. *Congest Heart Fail* 1999; **5:** 164–70.

39 Reigel B, Glaser D, Thomas V, Gocka I, Gillespie TA. Development of an instrument to measure cardiac illness dependency. *Heart Lung* 1997; **26:** 448–57.

40 Fonarow GC, Stevenson LW, Walden JA et al. Impact of a comprehensive heart failure management program on hospital readmission and functional status of patients with advanced heart failure. *J Am Coll Cardiol* 1997; **30:** 725–32.

41 Rich MW, Becham V, Wittenberg C, Leven CL, Freedland KE, Carney RM. A multidisciplinary intervention to prevent the readmission of elderly patients with congestive heart failure. *N Engl J Med* 1995; **333:** 1190–5.

42 Roglieri J, Futterman R, McDonough K. Disease management intervention to improve outcomes in congestive heart failure. *Am J Managed Care* 1997; **3:** 1831–9.

43 Hanmanthu S, Butler J, Chomsky D, Davis S, Wilson JR. Effect of a heart failure program on hospitalization frequency and exercise tolerance. *Circulation* 1997; **96:** 2842–8.

44 Farran CJ, Herth KA, Popovich MJ. *Hope and Hopelessness: Critical Clinical Constructs*. Newbury Park, CA: Sage Publications, 1995.

45 Engel GL. A life setting conducive to illness: the giving-up given-in complex. *Ann Intern Med* 1968; **69:** 293–300.

46 Ruberman W, Weinblatt E, Goldberg J, Chardhary B. Psychosocial influences on mortality after myocardial infarction. *N Engl J Med* 1984; **311:** 552–9.

47 O'Malley P, Menke E. Relationship of hope and stress after MI. *Heart Lung* 1988; **17:** 184–90.

48 Curl ED. Hope in the elderly: exploring the relationship between psychosocial developmental residual and hope. *Dissertation Abstracts Int* 1992; **53:** 1782.

49 Rideout E, Montemuro M. Hope, morale and adaptation in patients with chronic heart failure. *J Adv Nurs* 1986; **11:** 429–33.

50 Johnson JL, Morse JM. Regaining control: the process of adjustment after myocardial infarction. *Heart Lung* 1990; **19:** 126–35.

51 Moser DK, Dracup K. Psychosocial recovery from a cardiac event: the influence of perceived control. *Heart Lung* 1995; **24:** 273–80.

52 Baker CA. Recovery: a phenomenon extending beyond discharge. *Schol Inq Nurs Pract Int J* 1989; **3:** 181–97.

53 Bandura A. Self-efficacy mechanism in human agency. *Am Psychol* 1982; **37:** 122–47.

54 Gortner S, Jenkins L. Self-efficacy and activity levels following cardiac surgery. *J Adv Nurs* 1990; **15:** 1132–8.

55 Oka RK, DeMarco T, Haskell WL. Perceptions of physical fitness in patients with heart failure. *Prog Cardiovasc Nurs* **14:** 97–102.

56 Frattini E, Linddsay P, Kerr E, Park YJ. Learning needs of congestive heart failure patients. *Prog Cardiovasc Nurs* 1998; **13:** 11–16, 33.

57 Jaarsma T, Halfeens R, Abu-Saad JJ et al. Effects of education and support on self-care and resource utilization in patients with heart failure. *Eur Heart J* 1999; **20:** 673–82.

58 Johnson JE, Fuller SS, Endress MP, Rice VH. Altering patients' responses to surgery: an extension and replication. *Res Nurs Health* 1978; **1:** 111–21.

59 Suls J, Wan CK. Effects of sensory and procedural information on coping with stressful medical procedures and pain: a meta-analysis. *J Counseling Clin Psychol* 1989; **57:** 372–9.

60 Moore SM. CABG discharge information: addressing women's recovery. *Clin Nurs Res* 1996; **5:** 97–104.

61 Beery TA, Baas LS, Fowler CA. Spirituality in persons with heart failure. *J Holistic Nurs* 2002; **20:** 5–26.

62 Uchino BN, Cacioppo JT, Kiecolt-Glaser JK. The relationship between social support and physiological processes: a review with emphasis on underlying mechanisms and implications for health. *Psychol Bull* 1996; **119:** 488–531.

63 Stewart MJ. *Integrating Social Support in Nursing*. Newbury Park, CA: Sage Publications, 1993.

64 Blazer DG. Social support and mortality in an elderly community population. *Am J Epidemiol* 1982; **115:** 684–9.

65 Berkman LF, Syme SL. Social networks, host resistance and mortality: a year follow-up study of Alameda County residents. *Am J Epidemiol* 1979; **109:** 186–204.

66 House JS, Robbins C, Metsner HL. The association of social relationships and activities with mortality: prospective evidence from the Tecumseh Community Health Study. *Am J Epidemiol* 1982; **116:** 123–40.

67 Norbeck JS. Social support. *Annu Rev Nurs Res* 1998; **6:** 85–105.

68 Stewart MJ. Social support intervention studies: a review and prospectus of nursing contributions. *Int J Nurs Stud* 1989; **26:** 93–114.

69 Bruhn JG, Phillips BU. Measuring social support: a synthesis of current approaches. *J Behav Med* 1994; **7:** 151.

70 Tilden VP, Galen RD. Costs and conflict: the darker side of social support. *West J Nurs Res* 1987; **9:** 9–18.

71 Meagher-Stewart D. The role of social support in recovery from cardiovascular illness. *Can J Cardiovasc Nurs* 1994; **5:** 19–29.

72 McCauley KM. Assessing social support in patients with cardiac disease. *J Cardiovasc Nurs* 1995; **10:** 73–81.

73 Frost MH, Kelly AN, Mangan DB, Zarling KK. An analysis of factors influencing psychosocial adjustment to cardiomyopathy. *Cardiovasc Nurs* 1994; **30:** 1–7.

74 Grady KL, Jalowiec A, White-Williams C et al. Predictors of quality of life in patients with advanced heart failure

awaiting transplantation. *J Heart Lung Transplant* 1995; **14:** 2–10.

75 Bennett SJ, Pressler ML, Hays L, Firestine LS, Huster GA. Psychosocial variables and hospitalization in persons with chronic heart failure. *Prog Cardiovasc Nurs* 1997; **12:** 4–11.

76 Krumholz HM, Butler J, Miller J et al. Prognostic importance of emotional support for elderly patients hospitalized with heart failure. *Circulation* 1998; **97:** 958–64.

77 Karmilovich SE. Burden and stress associated with spousal caregiving for individuals with heart failure. *Prog Cardiovasc Nurs* 1994; **9:** 33–8.

78 Kinney CK, Mannetter R, Carpenter MA. Support groups. In: Bulechek GM, McCloskey JC, eds. *Nursing Interventions: Essential Nursing Treatments*, 2nd edn. Philadelphia: WB Saunders Company, 1992: 326–39.

79 Hildingh C, Fridlund B, Segesten, K. Social support in self-help groups, as experienced by persons having coronary heart disease and their next of kin. *Int J Nurs Stud* 1995; **32:** 224–32.

16 Gender issues in heart failure: meeting the needs of both men and women

Anna Strömberg, Jan Mårtensson and Bengt Fridlund

Introduction

During the last decade, there has been an increasing focus on gender differences in patients who suffer from heart failure. Despite this attention, however, the volume of research involving men with heart failure is still much less compared with that of women. Overall, therefore, we do not yet have a clear picture of the extent and importance of gender differences concerning patients with heart failure. In this chapter we will review and discuss the differences between men and women with heart failure. We will examine the subject with respect to epidemiology, aetiology, diagnostics, prognosis, pharmacological and non-pharmacological treatment, and the impact of heart failure on psychosocial factors and healthcare utilization.

Epidemiology

The incidence of heart failure is higher for men compared with women in all age groups.[1] According to data from the Framingham study, the incidence is one-third lower in women than in men after adjustment for age.[1] Despite this, the overall prevalence rates of heart failure in men and women are quite similar, an approximate 49% vs 51% split.[2–4] There are, however, some important differences related to age. For example, the average age of women hospitalized for heart failure is 7 years greater than that of men.[5–7] Currently, therefore, there is a higher prevalence of men aged less than 80 years with heart failure compared with age-matched women. Conversely, there are many more women aged greater than 80 years with heart failure.[4] Based on current trends and the demographic profile of developed countries, the slight imbalance between the number of men and women with heart failure and the age differential between the two sexes is likely to disappear over the next two decades (i.e. a greater prevalence of older men).[8]

Aetiology

Aetiology and risk factors for heart failure differ between men and women. Ischaemic heart disease is the most common cause of heart failure in men of all ages and in elderly women. Heart failure in younger women is more often due to non-ischaemic heart disease, such as valvular heart disease, hypertension or idiopathic causes.[9] Women are more likely than men to develop heart failure after myocardial infarction[10,11] and coronary artery bypass grafting (CABG).[12] Women with heart failure, but not affected by myocardial infarction, more frequently suffer from diastolic dysfunction than men.[13–15] Among women, the prevalence of diastolic dysfunction increases significantly with age, while no such difference is found between younger and older men.[14] Diabetes[4,13,14] and hypertension[16] appear to be more powerful risk factors in women than in men, which can explain why women suffer more from diastolic dysfunction. Men with heart failure are more likely to have a higher intake of alcohol and smoke[15] and have a higher prevalence of alcoholic cardiomyopathy. On the other hand, alcoholic women are more susceptible when it comes to developing cardiomyopathy secondary to alcohol abuse.[17]

Diagnostics

Gender differences in diagnostic procedures have been evaluated in different settings. A study carried out in the United States showed that women were not as frequently diagnosed by nuclear ventriculogram, Holter monitoring and exercise stress tests compared with men. Alternatively, there were no differences in the use of echocardiography and telemetry monitoring.[18,19] A Swedish study showed that women were less frequently diagnosed with echocardiography.[20] It has been shown that the rate of women with clinical signs consistent with heart failure, but no left ventricular dysfunction when diagnosed with echocardiography, is higher than in men.[21,22]

Both in Europe[23] and in the United States[19] women are more likely to be diagnosed and treated by a general practitioner/primary care physician than a cardiologist and are not referred to hospital to the same extent as men.

Prognosis

Large epidemiological studies[1,3] have reported better survival in women on an age-adjusted basis. In the Framingham study,[1] the 5-year survival was 38% for women compared with 25% for men and median survival after the diagnosis of heart failure was longer for women (3.2 years) than for men (1.7 years). A better long-term survival after 10–15 years has been reported in women across all age groups.[3] In the latest Framingham report, improved survival rates were reported in both men and women.[24] In the SOLVD studies,[25] women were found to have a significantly lower 1-year survival rate of 78% compared with the 83% survival rate for men. The difference between the two large epidemiological studies[1,3] and the SOLVD studies[25] was that all patients in SOLVD had a verified left ventricular dysfunction and that the women had more ischaemic aetiology, which are two causes contributing to a poorer prognosis. In studies of patients with heart failure admitted to clinics or to hospital, women were found to have a lower[9,18,19] or equivalent mortality rate[26] in comparison to men. For example, in a recent UK study of all incident admissions for heart failure, 5-year mortality was 75% in both sexes, despite women being significantly older than their male counterparts.[27]

Overall, these data suggest that women live longer after being diagnosed with heart failure on an age-adjusted basis and this explains why the prevalence of heart failure is equal among men and women, despite a higher incidence of heart failure in men. The reason women survive longer after the onset of heart failure is probably due to the fact that they tend to have better ventricular function and instead more frequently suffer from diastolic dysfunction.[13,14] Other factors that improve their prognosis are that women have less ischaemic heart disease,[1,9] atrial fibrillation[9] and ventricular arrhythmias.[28]

Treatment

Pharmacological treatment

The comprehensive goals of heart failure treatment are to reduce symptoms as well as improve survival, physical activity and quality of life. The choice and combinations of drugs depend on the stage of the disease, the aetiology and type of heart failure. A number of large clinical trials have evaluated a range of drugs to determine their effect on the typical morbidity and mortality associated with chronic heart failure treatment (see Table 16.1).[29–47] These trials have largely evaluated the treatment of patients with systolic dysfunction. There are limited research data and guidelines available for the optimal treatment of diastolic dysfunction, although this is currently being addressed to a greater extent (e.g. the CHARM Study). As described in Chapter 8, the combinations of drugs for basic treatment of systolic dysfunction are angiotensin-converting enzyme (ACE) inhibitors, diuretics and β-blockers.[48–51] The treatment goal is to reduce the increased filling pressure as well as reduce the neurohormonal levels and improve cardiac output. In diastolic dysfunction, the treatment should aim at improving the ventricular relaxation and filling (calcium antagonist, ACE inhibitors and β-blockers) and if there are signs of volume overload, reduce preload (diuretics).[48–51]

According to current guidelines on the treatment of heart failure, men and women should receive the same pharmacological treatment.[48–51] However, this can be questioned with regard to women. The guidelines are based on clinical trials conducted during the last decade. In these trials only 30% or less of the subjects were women (see Table 16.1). Some of the trials have performed subgroup analysis with regard to gender differences, but they were not designed for gender-specific analysis. Other trials have either not included, or completely excluded women and not compared differences in mortality between the sexes.

The V-HeFT trials,[30,31] which investigated the effect of vasodilators in the treatment of heart failure, were performed at Veteran hospitals and did not include women. In the CONSENSUS-1 trial,[29] which evaluated the effect of ACE inhibitors in patients with severe heart failure, subanalyses showed that women had no survival benefit, while men had a 51% reduction in mortality. In the SOLVD studies,[33] women treated with ACE inhibitors showed reduced mortality and morbidity, but to a lesser extent compared with men. However, in a meta-analysis of 30 ACE inhibitor trials, the reduction in mortality and morbidity was similar in both sexes.[52] In the US Carvedilol Heart Failure Study[39] and the MERIT-HF trial,[45] β-blockers reduced mortality similarly in men and women. Other large β-blocker trials did not compare men and women.[38,44] The DIG trial did not initially compare differences in mortality between men and women treated with digoxin,[41] however, a recent post hoc analysis suggested that women but not men treated with digoxin were more likely to die when compared with those assigned to the placebo arm of the study.[53] The Elite trials[40,46] showed

Table 16.1. *Clinical trials evaluating different agents for heart failure treatment. The trials in the table have been important in the guidance of developing treatment strategies*

Trial	Year	Agents tested	Sample (n)	Women (%)	Mean age (years)
CONSENSUS I[29]	1987	Enalapril vs placebo	253	30	71
V-HeFT I[30]	1986	Prazosin vs hydralazine–isosorbide dinitrate	642	0	58
V-HeFT II[31]	1991	Enalapril vs hydralazine–isosorbide dinitrate	804	0	60
PROMISE[32]	1991	Milrinone vs placebo	1088	22	64
SOLVD (symptomatic)[33]	1991	Enalapril vs placebo	2569	20	61
SOLVD (prevention)[34]	1992	Enalapril vs placebo	4228	11	59
SAVE[35]	1992	Captopril vs placebo	2231	17	59
AIRE[36]	1993	Ramipril vs placebo	2006	26	65
MDC[37]	1993	Metoprolol vs placebo	383	27	49
CIBIS[38]	1994	Bisoprolol vs placebo	641	17	60
US Carvedilol[39]	1996	Carvedilol vs placebo	1094	23	58
ELITE[40]	1997	Losartan vs captopril	722	32	73
DIG[41]	1997	Digitalis vs placebo	6800	22	64
RALES[42]	1999	Aldactone vs placebo	1663	27	65
ATLAS[43]	1999	Lisinopril vs placebo	3164	20	64
CIBIS-II[44]	1999	Bisoprolol vs placebo	2647	19	61
MERIT- HF[45]	2000	Metoprolol vs placebo	3991	22	64
ELITE II[46]	2000	Losartan vs captopril	3152	30	71
COPERNICUS[47]	2001	Carvedilol vs placebo	2289	20	63

a similar mortality reduction for men and women treated with an angiotensin II antagonist. There were no difference in mortality between men and women treated with aldactone according to the RALES study.[42]

In evaluations of clinical practice, there are studies showing that women are more seldom treated with ACE inhibitors[54–56] but, in other settings, no differences in treatment[57] or better therapeutic care[19,23,58] have been found. Women have also reported more adverse effects from ACE inhibitors than have men.[59] In a study of younger patients with heart failure men tended to use more diuretics than women.[9] Among elderly patients in the primary care the opposite was observed; 89% of the women were treated with diuretics compared with 80% of the men.[58]

Interventional and surgical treatment

Patients with heart failure caused by ischaemic heart disease or valvular disease can be treated with interven-

tional or surgical interventions. Men more often have invasive cardiac services such as electrophysiological testing, pacemaker implantations, cardiac catheterization, revascularization procedures, cardiac surgery and heart transplantation, compared with women.[18,19] These gender differences were only found between white men and women and seem to be age-related. There were no gender differences between black men and women probably because they are younger when affected by heart disease and no age difference was found between the sexes.[18,19]

Women suffer more from single-vessel disease, they are usually suitable for angioplasty. Women with heart failure are elderly and have more comorbidities, decreased body surface area and smaller coronary arteries, factors that increase the mortality risk during percutaneous transluminal coronary angioplasty and CABG.[60]

Only 20% of the heart transplant recipients are women.[61] This is probably because heart failure develops earlier in men, and women are more likely than men to refuse transplant as a therapeutic option, despite the fact that they would be accepted as candidates.[62] Men have a lower risk of rejection and a higher 1-year survival than women.[61] Women experience a higher level of both symptom frequency and symptom distress related to immunosuppressive therapy, mostly corticosteroid-related, compared to men.[63]

Non-pharmacological treatment

Important complements to the pharmacological regimen are symptom monitoring and lifestyle changes, which include daily weighing, reduced salt intake, fluid restriction, smoking cessation, alcohol restriction/abstinence, infection prophylaxis and exercise.[49,64]

Patients with heart failure suffer from reduced exercise capacity and are limited in their physical activities due to fatigue and dyspnoea. Exercise intolerance is caused by reduced cardiac output, elevated intrapulmonary pressure and skeletal muscle changes, the latter in turn caused by inactivity, malnutrition, underperfusion and increased levels of neurohormones.[65] A number of trials evaluating exercise in heart failure patients have shown that exercise significantly increases quality of life[66–72] and decreases anxiety and depression.[73] However, in most of these trials women have, once again, been in the minority (Table 16.2).[66–76] Women have a weaker body strength and lower aerobic power than men, but healthy women respond to physical exercise in the same way as men.[77] Tyni-Lenné and colleagues conducted two separate studies for men[66] and women[68] showing that exercise tolerance and both physical and psychosocial aspects of health-related quality of life improved both in men and women after 8 weeks of skeletal muscle endurance training. Tyni-Lenné[78] also found that peak exercise performance, skeletal muscle strength and oxidative capacity increased and blood lactate and plasma norepinephrine decreased similarly in both

Table 16.2. Clinical trials evaluating the impact on quality of life of exercise in patients with heart failure

Author	Exercise mode, intensity and length of intervention	Sample (n)	Women (%)	Mean age (years)
Koch et al (1992)[74]	Anaerobic, strength training three times a week during 3 months	25	25	55
Kostis et al (1994)[73]	Aerobic, walking, rowing, cycling, stair climbing, heart rate 40–60% of functional capacity 3–5 times per week during 3 months	20	30	66
Tyni-Lenné et al (1996)[66]	Aerobic, local quadriceps femoris training three times a week during 2 months	21	0	60
Kavanagh et al (1996)[67]	Aerobic, walking, 50–60% of peak O_2 five times a week during 12 months	30	17	62
Tyni-Lenné et al (1997)[68]	Aerobic, local quadriceps femoris training three times a week during 2 months	16	100	62
Wielenga et al (1998)[69]	Aerobic, cycling, walking, ball game, interval training three times a week during 3 months	80	0	64
Willenheimer et al (1998)[70]	Aerobic, cycling, interval training 80% of peak O_2 during 4 months	49	29	64
Belardinelli et al (1999)[71]	Aerobic, cycling 80% of peak O_2 2–3 times per week during 12 months	99	11	59
Quittan et al (1999)[72]	Aerobic, cycling three times per week during 3 months	27	12	55
Gottlied et al (1999)[75]	Aerobic, cycling, treadmill three times per week during 6 months	33	13	66
Owen et al (2000)[76]	Aerobic, circuit with six stations, once a week during 3 months	22	25	81

genders after 8 weeks of training. However, aerobic power measured as peak oxygen uptake increased only in women.[78] Earlier studies have shown that women were less frequently referred to exercise training.[79–81] Since exercise seems to produce similar improvement in women and men, it is important to refer more women to cardiac rehabilitation programmes.

Patient education has become an important component in heart failure management in order to teach the patient self-care,[63,82] and improve compliance,[83] self-efficacy,[84] and quality of life,[85] as well as reduce health care costs.[85,86] Nurses have an important role in the education of patients with heart failure. Written and verbal information is most commonly used and videotapes are sometimes used for additional education.[87] The use of computer-based tools in the education of elderly patients is relatively new and not yet very common.[88] It has been shown that computer-based educational programs improved the patients' knowledge about heart failure more and that the patients retained the knowledge better when compared with traditional teaching methods.[89] The computer seemed to be an especially useful tool for the education of women with heart failure. Education provided by a heart failure nurse did not improve the women's knowledge significantly, but additional computer-based education led to improved and

greater knowledge retention during a follow-up period of 6 months.[90] This gender difference might be explained by the fact that elderly women often have a lower educational level. Patients with low literacy skills benefit more from individualized, interactive education.[91,92] With the computer they can proceed at their own pace, make errors and repeat the material without pressure or embarrassment.[93,94]

In trials evaluating the impact of nurse-led interventions with special emphasis on patient education and intensified follow-up (Tables 16.3[95–102] and 16.4[82,85,86,103–110]), a much higher percentage of the subjects were women compared with the trials evaluating drugs and exercise (Tables 16.1 and 16.2). However, regarding outcomes or clinical and demographical data, no comparisons between men and women were made. Since these trials have a much smaller sample size compared with most drug trials there is a risk that they will lack the statistical power to detect gender differences.

Compliance

Demographic characteristics such as gender, age, race and social class have not been shown to predict compliance.[111] There are almost no studies available addressing differences in adherence to heart failure treatment between the sexes. Monane et al[112] found that women with heart

Table 16.3. *Non-randomized trials evaluating nurse-led or coordinated outpatient heart failure management programmes with special emphasis on patient education and intensified follow-up*

Author	Intervention	Sample (n)	Women (%)	Mean age (years)
Cintron et al (1983)[95]	Outpatient heart failure clinic led by nurse practitioner	15	0	65
Kornowski et al (1995)[96]	Home visits with assessment by internist and nurse	42	43	78
West et al (1997)[97]	Physician supervised, nurse-managed education and telephone follow-up	51	29	66
Hanumanthu et al (1997)[98]	Physician-directed outpatient heart failure clinic with assisting nurse coordinators	187	29	52
Smith et al (1997)[99]	Outpatient heart failure clinic led by cardiologists and nurse practitioner	21	0	61
Fonarow et al (1997)[100]	Outpatient heart failure clinic led by cardiologists and clinical nurse specialists	214	19	52
Shah et al (1998)[101]	Nurse-managed education and monitoring	27	0	62
Heidenreich et al (1999)[102]	Physician-directed, nurse-cordinated home-based education and monitoring	68	59	73

Table 16.4. *Randomized trials evaluating nurse-led or coordinated outpatient heart failure management programmes with special emphasis on patient education and intensified follow-up*

Author	Intervention	Sample (n)	Women (%)	Mean age (years)
Rich et al (1995)[85]	Nurse-directed, multidisciplinary discharge planning, education and follow-up (USA)	282	63	79
Weinberger et al (1996)[103]	Increased access to primary care, close follow-up by nurse and physician (USA)	504	1	63
Cline et al (1998)[104]	Nurse-led education and follow-up at heart failure clinic (SE)	190	47	76
Ekman et al (1998)[105]	Nurse-led education and follow-up at heart failure clinic (SE)	158	42	80
Jaarsma et al (1999)[82]	Nurse-led education, counselling and support (NL)	179	42	73
Stewart et al (1998)[106]	Nurse- and pharmacist-led, home-based education and follow-up (AU)	97	52	75
Stewart et al (1999)[86]	Nurse- and pharmacist-led, home-based education and follow-up (AU)	200	40	76
Naylor et al (1999)[107]	Discharge planning and home-based education led by nurse practitioners (USA)	363	50	75
Blue et al (2001)[108]	Specialist heart failure nurse home-based intervention (UK)	157	41	75
Doughty et al (2002)[109]	Combination of heart failure clinic and increased access to primary care (NZ)	197	39	73
Krumholz et al[110]	Nurse-led education and support combined with telemonitoring	88	43	74

failure had a significantly higher compliance with digoxin therapy. It is not known whether or not there are any gender differences in terms of compliance with non-pharmacological treatment and self-care behaviour. Women with myocardial infarction, who participate in cardiac rehabilitation programmes, drop out more frequently due to comorbidities, family responsibilities and other psychosocial factors.[79–83]

Impact of heart failure

Life situation

The life situation of patients with heart failure is affected by factors such as dyspnoea,[113,114] physical disability,[115,116] anxiety,[117,118] attitude towards heart failure,[119,120] support from health care professionals[58,121] and support from family.[122,123] Some gender differences have been found in the conception of the life situation. Men suffering from heart failure conceived that neither they nor their environment had an influence over their life situation. Their exis-

tence was marked by an acceptance that nothing could be done, except to passively await death.[124] Women with heart failure were more concerned about their present daily lives and did not worry so much about the future. They had accepted their mortality and ascribed more positive meanings to their illness than men.[117,125,126]

The men noted that the physical limitations caused by their heart failure restricted their existence and that they were continually reminded of this in their everyday life. They also experienced social restrictions in their work and leisure activities, hindering them from taking part in activities that previously had been a natural part of their lives.[124] Women with heart failure also described physical and social restrictions due to lack of energy. Difficulties in performing household tasks and supporting those they used to care for in their surroundings were the most difficult to accept.[117,125,126] Women experienced more feelings of being a burden to others compared with men.[117,124] It has been suggested that 'the emotional cost of caring' is responsible for the major part of the distress experienced by these women,[117] i.e. the distress of the women is due to events that occur not to the women themselves but to those around them. The attitude to heart failure also seemed to be important because those who regarded heart failure as a weakness or an enemy were more emotionally burdened than those who were more hopeful and able to ascribe a positive meaning to the illness.[117,124,125] Gender differences have also been shown to be evident in heart failure patients' coping patterns. Men seemed to use coping strategies that were more emotion focused, fatalistic and, at times, evasive.[125] Women, on the other hand, were more hopeful about the future and tended to use more optimistic coping strategies, seeing their illness as a second chance to live.[125]

Quality of life

Quality of life among patients with heart failure is often influenced by limitations in exercise capacity,[66,70] and activities of daily living.[18,127] It is also influenced by reduced sexual activity and satisfaction,[128,129] disruption of work roles and social interactions with family and friends,[130,131] and psychological distress, including depression, hostility and anxiety.[132,133] Women with heart failure reported perceived physical health status, physical symptoms, especially dyspnoea, NYHA class, and life stresses as having the strongest relationship with quality of life.[113,114] As dyspnoea, life stresses, and NYHA class increased, quality of life decreased.[113] The absence of emotional support, such as someone to talk to about one's problems, was found to be associated with a higher risk of fatal and non-fatal cardiovascular events in the year after hospital admission for women, but not for men.[122]

Chin and Goldman[26] found that women with heart failure had lower vitality and physical function than men and that after the 1-year follow-up, the differences were even greater. Cline et al[127] reported that women had more problems with emotions, sleep, energy, pain, mobility, housework and social life than men did. Burns et al[18] found no difference between men and women with heart failure regarding activities of daily living, shortness of breath when walking, and perceived health. The difference between these results can be explained by the fact that Burns[18] used more direct measures of basic functional status, which seems to be of decisive importance for quality of life, whereas Chin and Goldman[26] and Cline et al[127] used more general measures of health-related quality of life. Data from the Framingham study[134] showed that heart failure predicted disability only in women. The dif-

ference between these men and women with heart failure was that men were twice as likely to also have coronary heart disease, which in itself might be so disabling that no additional disability could be detected.[134] Problems with sexual function as a consequence of heart failure are reported as being equally frequent and intense in male and female patients.[128] Functional status has a great impact on quality of life in patients with heart failure. Thus, symptom amelioration, which may improve functional ability, has the greatest potential for increasing quality of life in patients with heart failure. Despite the fact that there are gender differences in the factors that may lead to an impaired quality of life in patients with heart failure (physical symptoms, psychological problems, treatment adverse effects and social limitation),[135] gender has seldom been analysed separately. Previously, study populations have been composed solely or primarily of men, but during the last few years, women have been included to the same extent as men. Gender differences concerning the association between quality of life and outcomes of heart failure need to be explored further. There is no consensus in instrumentation use among the few studies done in this area and it is therefore difficult to make a comparison between them.

Mood disturbances

Patients with cardiac diseases have a higher prevalence of anxiety and depression.[133] There are few available studies of anxiety and depression in heart failure, and the results have been inconsistent. Freedland et al[133] reported that depression was highly prevalent among elderly heart failure patients. On the other hand, Murberg et al[132] did not find that depression was predominant in these patients. Men and women were found to respond differently to the burden of heart failure and women to exhibit more depression and anxiety than men.[132] The gender differences in depression scores are, however, not larger than those typically found among physically healthy samples, with women twice as likely to be diagnosed with depressive symptoms compared with men.[136] Substantial gender differences have been found in the association between scores for physical limitations and depression.[113,132] The differences can be explained by the fact that men are more negatively affected by functional limitations and perceive them as more psychologically invasive than women. Men are more dependent on activities that involve strenuous physical activity for their well-being than women are. Women with heart failure are also older, lead more sedentary lives and therefore accept, more easily than men, the social dependency and passivity associated with advanced heart failure.[113,132,136] Furthermore, younger women with heart failure experience more mood disturbance, specifically anxiety and depression, than older patients, whose expectations may be more consistent with their condition.[113]

Quality of care and healthcare costs

The quality of care for patients with heart failure has been assessed by the thoroughness of history taking, physical examination, as well as recording of functional status, key symptoms and signs.[58] Further, common tests, procedures and standard therapies used have been evaluated, as have access to a cardiologist and follow-up.[20,58] The overall quality of care for heart failure patients has been shown not to differ with gender, but differences have been noted in specific areas.[20,24,58] Physicians were less likely to record findings from the initial physical examination of women,[20,24,58] and women also underwent fewer procedures.[20,137–139] Women were less often managed by cardiologists and more seldom referred to a teaching hospital or transferred to other acute-care hospitals than men.[20,24,58] Compared with women, men had a shorter stay in hospital,[20,137–139] and lower hospital costs.[20] There are inconsistent results regarding gender differences with regard to hospital admission. In the SOLVD studies,[24] women had a higher annual admission rate than men, whereas Opasich and colleagues[55] found no differences between women and men in annual admissions. Readmission rates have been shown to be independent of gender[18,137] or lower in women.[57] Women rated the quality of follow-up and outpatient care lower than men.[26] Women with heart failure are older (see Chapter 13), suffer from more comorbidities[19] and are more likely to be widowed and live alone when the demands due to their illness increase. Children and other relatives cannot fully compensate for the amount of assistance that a spouse can provide in the home.[130] Women with heart failure are therefore more likely to need home health aid after hospitalization,[26] are more often discharged to skilled nursing facilities and receive more home care post discharge.[19,58]

Conclusion

Despite a higher incidence of heart failure in men, the overall prevalence rate is similar in both sexes, due to women surviving longer after the onset of heart failure.

Women tend to be older when diagnosed with heart failure and more often have hypertension and diabetes than men. These factors can explain why a higher proportion of women suffer from diastolic dysfunction compared with men. The research about diastolic dysfunction is still in its infancy and several questions regarding diagnosis, prognosis and treatment need to be resolved.

It is not clear whether or not women should be treated with the same doses and combinations of drugs in order to have the same outcomes as presented in trials dominated by men. The extent of sex differences in treatment, hospital cost and quality of care can partly be explained by age differences. Women affected by heart failure are older, and the elderly in general tend to undergo fewer procedures and are more often treated by general practitioners/primary care physicians than by cardiologists. Considering the fact that women are more likely to live alone, it is natural that they receive more follow-up at home and have longer stays in hospital. The reason women are less willing to undergo heart transplantation needs to be further explored. The life situations for men and women with heart failure are different. Physical and social restrictions affecting daily life activities are experienced as most annoying for men, whereas restrictions affecting the possibility to support family and friends are most difficult to accept for women. Women with heart failure ascribe more positive meanings to their illness. Despite this, women seem to experience a lower overall quality of life than men.

Recommendations for practice and research

Further research is needed in order to examine the importance of and explain differences in aetiology, diagnostics, prognosis, morbidity, mortality, psychosocial factors and health care utilization between men and women suffering from heart failure. It might be the case that men and women need different medical therapy and care. This needs to be investigated further, and the known differences need to be highlighted in guidelines as well as implemented in standard care. Not only do the gender differences need to be highlighted, age and race differences also need to be investigated further. In order to improve the care and treatment and to meet the needs of all patients with heart failure, research trials investigating different aspects of heart failure need to include patients from both sexes as well as all age groups and races.

References

1 Ho KK, Anderson KM, Kannel WB, Groossman W, Levy D. Survival after the onset of congestive cardiac failure in Framingham Heart study subjects. *Circulation* 1993; **88:** 107–15.

2 McDonagh T, Morrison CE, Lawrence A et al. Symptomatic and asymptomatic left ventricular systolic dysfunction in an urban population. *Lancet* 1997; **350:** 829–33.

3 Schocken DD, Arrieta MI, Leaverton PE, Ross EA. Prevalence and mortality rate of congestive heart failure in the United States. *J Am Coll Cardiol* 1992; **20:** 301–6.

4 Ho KK, Pinsky JL, Kannel WB, Levy D. The epidemiology of heart failure: the Framingham study. *J Am Coll Cardiol* 1993; **22:** 6A–13A.

5 Stewart S, MacIntyre K, McCleod ME, Bailey AE, Capewell S, McMurray JJ. Trends in heart failure hospitalisations in Scotland, 1990–1996: an epidemic that has reached its peak? *Eur Heart J* 2001; **22:** 209–17.

6 Mosterd A, Reitsma JB, Grobbee DE. ACE inhibition and hospitalisation rates for heart failure in The Netherlands, 1980–1998. The end of an epidemic? *Heart* 2002; **87:** 75–6.

7 MacIntyre K, Capewell S, Stewart S et al. Evidence of improving prognosis in heart failure: trends in case–fatality in 66,547 patients hospitalised between 1986 and 1995. *Circulation* 2000; **102:** 1126–31.

8 Stewart S, MacIntyre K, Capewell S, McMurray JJV. An ageing population and heart failure: an increasing burden in the 21st century? *Heart* 2002: In press.

9 Adams KF, Dunlap SH, Sueta CA et al. Relation between gender, etiology and survival in patients with symptomatic heart failure. *J Am Coll Cardiol* 1996; **28:** 1781–8.

10 Kannel WB. Epidemiological aspects of heart failure. *Cardiol Clin* 1989; **7:** 1–9.

11 Tofler GH, Stone PH, Muller JE et al. Effects on gender and race on prognosis after myocardial infarction: adverse prognosis for women, particularly black women. *J Am Coll Cardiol* 1987; **9:** 473–82.

12 Hoffman RM, Psaty BM, Kronmal RA. Modifiable risk factors for incident heart failure in the Coronary Artery Surgery Study. *Arch Intern Med* 1994; **154:** 417–23.

13 Samuel RS, Hausdorff JM, Wei JY. Congestive heart failure with preserved systolic function: is it a women's disease? *Women's Health Issues* 1999; **9:** 219–22.

14 Lindenfeld J, Krause-Steinrauf H, Salerno J. Where are all the women with heart failure? *J Am Coll Cardiol* 1997; **30:** 1417–19.

15 Ofili EO, Mayberry R, Alema-Mensah E et al. Gender differences and practice implications of risk factors for frequent hospitalization for heart failure in an urban center serving predominantly African-American patients. *Am J Cardiol* 1999; **83:** 1350–5.

16 Levy D, Larson MG, Vasan RS, Kannel WB, Ho KLK. The progression from hypertension to heart failure. *J Am Coll Cardiol* 1996; **275:** 1557–62.

17 Fernández-Solà J, Estruch R, Nicolás J et al. Comparison of alcoholic cardiomyopathy in women versus men. *Am J Cardiol* 1997; **80:** 481–5.

18 Burns RB, McCarthy EP, Moskowitz MA, Ash A, Kane RL, Finch M. Outcomes for older men and women with congestive heart failure. *J Am Geriatr Soc* 1997; **45:** 276–80.

19 Philbin EF, DiSalvo TG. Influence of race and gender on care process, resource use and outcomes in congestive heart failure. *Am J Cardiol* 1998; **82:** 76–81.

20 Mejhert M, Holmgren J, Wändell P, Persson H, Edner M. Diagnostic tests, treatment and follow-up in heart failure patients – is there a gender bias in the coherence to guidelines? *Eur J Heart Fail* 1999; **1:** 407–10.

21 Remes J, Miettinen H, Reunanen A, Pyörälä K. Validity of clinical diagnosis of heart failure in primary care. *Eur Heart J* 1991; **12:** 315–21.

22 Cowie MR, Struthers AD, Wood DA et al. Value of natriuretic peptides in assessment of patients with possible new heart failure in primary care. *Lancet* 1997; **350:** 1349–53.

23 Clarke KW, Gray D, Hampton JR. Evidence of inadequate investigation and treatment of patients with heart failure. *Br Heart J* 1994; **71:** 584–7.

24 Levy D, Kenchaiah S, Larson MG et al. Long-term trends in the incidence of and survival with heart failure. *N Engl J Med* 2002; **347:** 1397–402.

25 Bourassa MG, Gurne O, Bangdiwala SI et al. Natural history and current practices in heart failure. *J Am Coll Cardiol* 1993; **22(suppl):** 14A–19A.

26 Chin MH, Goldman L. Gender differences in 1-year survival and quality of life among patients admitted with congestive heart failure. *Med Care* 1998; **36:** 1033–46.

27 Stewart S, MacIntyre K, Hole DA, Capewell S, McMurray JJV. More malignant than cancer? Five-year survival following a first admission for heart failure in Scotland? *Eur J Heart Failure* 2001; **3:** 315–22.

28 Aronson D, Burger AJ. The effect of sex on ventricular arrhythmic events in patients with congestive heart failure. *Pacing Clin Electrophysiol* 2002; **25:** 1206–11.

29 CONSENSUS trial study group. Effect of enalapril on mortality in severe congestive heart failure. *N Engl J Med* 1987; **316:** 1429–35.

30 Cohn JN, Archibald DG, Ziesche S et al. Effect of vasodilator therapy on mortality in chronic congestive heart failure. Results of a Veterans Administration Cooperative Study. *N Engl J Med* 1986; **314:** 1547–52.

31 Cohn JN, Johnson G, Ziesche S et al. A comparison of enalapril with hydralazine-isosorbide dinitrate in the

treatment of chronic congestive heart failure. *N Engl J Med* 1991; **325:** 303–10.

32 Packer M, Carver JR, Rodeheffer RJ et al. Effect of oral milrinone on mortality in severe chronic heart failure. The PROMISE Study Research Group. *New Engl J Med* 1991; **325:** 1468–75.

33 The SOLVD investigators. Effect of enalapril on survival in patients with reduced left ventricular ejection fraction and congestive heart failure. *N Engl J Med* 1991; **325:** 293–302.

34 The SOLVD Investigators. Effect of enalapril on mortality and the development of heart failure in asymptomatic patients with reduced left ventricular ejection fractions. *New Engl J Med* 1992; **327:** 685–91.

35 Pfeffer MA, Braunwald E, Moye LA et al. Effect of captopril on mortality and morbidity in patients with left ventricular dysfunction after myocardial infarction. Results of the survival and ventricular enlargement trial. The SAVE Investigators. *N Engl J Med* 1992; **327:** 669–77.

36 The Acute Infarction Ramipril Efficacy (AIRE) Study Investigators. Effect of ramipril on mortality and morbidity of survivors of acute myocardial infarction with clinical evidence of heart failure. *Lancet* 1993; **342:** 821–8.

37 Waagstein F, Bristow MR, Swedberg K et al. Beneficial effects of metoprolol in idiopathic dilated cardiomyopathy. Metoprolol in Dilated Cardiomyopathy (MDC) Trial Study Group. *Lancet* 1993; **342:** 1441–6.

38 CIBIS Investigators. A randomized trial of beta-blockade in heart failure. The Cardiac Insufficiency Bisoprolol Study (CIBIS). *Circulation* 1994; **90:** 1765–73.

39 Packer M, Bristow MR, Cohn JN et al. The effect of carvedilol on morbidity and mortality in patients with chronic heart failure. US Carvedilol Heart Failure Study Group. *N Engl J Med* 1996; **334:** 1349–55.

40 Pitt B, Segal R, Martinez FA et al. Randomised trial of losartan versus captopril in patients over 65 with heart failure. Evaluation of Losartan in the Elderly Study, ELITE. *Lancet* 1997; **349:** 747–52.

41 Digitalis Investigation Group. The effect of digoxin on mortality and morbidity in patients with heart failure. *N Engl J Med* 1997; **336:** 525–33.

42 Pitt B, Zannad F, Remme WJ et al. The effect of spironolactone on morbidity and mortality in patients with severe heart failure. Randomized Aldactone Evaluation Study Investigators. *N Engl J Med* 1999; **341:** 709–17.

43 Packer M, Poole-Wilson PA, Armstrong PW et al. Comparative effects of low and high doses of the angiotensin-converting enzyme inhibitor, lisinopril, on morbidity and mortality in chronic heart failure. ATLAS Study Group. *Circulation* 1999; **100:** 2312–18.

44 CIBIS II Investigators. The Cardiac Insufficiency Bisoprolol Study II (CIBIS-II): a randomised trial. *Lancet* 1999; **353:** 9–13.

45 Hjalmarson A, Goldstein S, Fagerberg B et al. Effects of controlled-release metoprolol on total mortality, hospitalizations, and well-being in patients with heart failure: the Metoprolol CR/XL Randomized Intervention Trial in congestive heart failure (MERIT-HF). *JAMA* 2000; **283:** 1295–302.

46 Pitt B, Poole-Wilson PA, Segal R et al. Effect of losartan compared with captopril on mortality in patients with symptomatic heart failure: randomised trial – the Losartan Heart Failure Survival Study ELITE II. *Lancet* 2000; **355:** 1582–7.

47 Packer M, Coats AJS, Fowler MB et al, for the COPERNICUS Study Group. Effect of carvedilol on survival in severe chronic heart failure. *N Engl J Med* 2001; **344:** 1651–4.

48 The Task Force of the Working Group on Heart Failure of the European Society of Cardiology. Guidelines for the diagnosis and treatment of chronic heart failure. *Eur Heart J* 2001; **22:** 1527–60.

49 Konstam M, Dracup K, Baker D et al. Heart failure: evaluation and care of patients with left-ventricular systolic dysfunction. Clinical practice guideline No. 11. Rockville: AHCPR Publications, 1994.

50 ACC/AHA Task Force Report. Guidelines for evaluation and management of heart failure. *Circulation* 1995; **91:** 580–615.

51 Packer M, Cohn JN. Consensus recommendations for the management of chronic heart failure. *Am J Cardiol* 1999; **83:** 1A–38A.

52 Garg R, Yusuf S, for the Collaborative Group on ACE inhibitors trials. Overview of randomized trials of angiotensin converting enzyme inhibitors on mortality and morbidity in heart failure. *JAMA* 1995; **273:** 1450–6.

53 Rathore SS, Wang Y, Krumholz HM. Sex-based differences in the effect of digoxin for the treatment of heart failure. *N Engl J Med* 2002; **347:** 1403–11.

54 Clinical Quality Improvement Network Investigators. Mortality risk and patterns of practice in 4606 acute care patients with congestive heart failure. *Arch Intern Med* 1996; **156:** 1669–73.

55 Opasich C, Tavazzi L, Lucci D et al. Comparison of one-year outcome in women versus men with chronic congestive heart failure. *Am J Cardiol* 2000; **86:** 353–7.

56 Agvall B, Dahlström U. Patients in primary health care diagnosed and treated as heart failure, with special reference to gender differences. *Scand J Prim Health Care* 2001; **19:** 14–9.

57 Krumholz HM, Parent EM, Tu N et al. Readmission after hospitalisation for congestive heart failure among Medicare beneficiaries. *Arch Intern Med* 1997; **157:** 99–104.

58 Ayanian JZ, Weissman JS, Chasan-Taber S, Epstein AM. Quality of care by race and gender for congestive heart failure and pneumonia. *Med Care* 1999; **37:** 1260–9.

59 The SOLVD investigators. Adverse effects of enalapril in the studies of left ventricular dysfunction. *Am Heart J* 1996; **131:** 350–5.

60 Hussain KM, Kogan A, Estrada AQ, Kostady G, Foschi A, Dadkhah S. Referral pattern and outcome in men and women undergoing coronary artery bypass surgery – a critical review. *Angiology* 1998; **49:** 243–50.

61 Kaye MP. The registry of the international society for heart and lung transplantation: 10th official report. *J Heart Lung Transplant* 1994; **13:** 561–70.

62 Aaronson KD, Schwartz JS, Goin JE, Mancini DM. Sex differences in patient acceptance of cardiac transplant candidacy. *Circulation* 1995; **91:** 2753–61.

63 Moons P, De Geest S, Abraham I, Cleemput JV, Vanhaecke J. Symptom experience associated with maintenance immunosuppression after heart transplantation: Patients' appraisal of side-effects. *Heart Lung* 1998; **27:** 315–25.

64 Dracup K, Baker DW, Dunbar SB, Dacey RA, Brooks NH, Johnsson JC. Management of heart failure. II. Counseling, education and lifestyle modifications. *JAMA* 1994; **272:** 1442–6.

65 Kokkinos PF, Choucair W, Graves P, Papademetriou V, Ellahham S. Chronic heart failure and exercise. *Am Heart J* 2000; **140:** 21–8.

66 Tyni-Lenné R, Gordon A, Sylvén C. Improved quality of life in chronic heart failure patients following local endurance training with leg muscles. *J Cardiac Failure* 1996; **2:** 111–17.

67 Kavanagh T, Myers MG, Baigrie RS, Mertens DJ. Quality of life and cardiorespiratory function in chronic heart failure: effects of 12 months' aerobic training. *Heart* 1996; **76:** 42–9.

68 Tyni-Lenné R, Gordon A, Jansson E, Bermann G, Sylvén C. Skeletal muscle endurance training improves peripheral oxidative capacity, exercise tolerance, and health related quality of life in women with chronic congestive heart failure secondary to either ischemic cardiomyopathy or idiopathic dilated cardiomyopathy. *Am J Cardiol* 1997; **80:** 1025–9.

69 Wielenga RP, Erdman RAM, Huisveld IA et al. Effects of exercise training on quality of life in patients with chronic heart failure. *J Psychosom Res* 1998; **45:** 459–64.

70 Willenheimer R, Erhardt L, Cline C, Rydberg E, Israelsson B. Exercise training in heart failure improves quality of life and exercise capacity. *Eur Heart J* 1998; **19:** 774–81.

71 Belardinelli R, Georgiou D, Gianci G, Purcaro A. Randomized, controlled trial of long-term moderate exercise training in chronic heart failure: effects on functional capacity, quality of life, and clinical outcome. *Circulation* 1999; **99:** 1173–82.

72 Quittan M, Sturm B, Wiesinger GF, Pacher R, Fialka-Moser V. Quality of life in patients with chronic heart failure: a randomized controlled trial of changes induced by a regular exercise program. *Scand J Rehabil Med* 1999; **31:** 223–8.

73 Kostis JB, Rosen RC, Cosgrove NM, Shindler DM, Wilson AC. Nonpharmacologic therapy improves functional and emotional status in congestive heart failure. *Chest* 1994; **106:** 996–1001.

74 Koch M, Douard H, Broustet JP. The benefit of graded physical exercise in chronic heart failure. *Chest* 1992; **101:** 231S–235S.

75 Gottlieb SS, Fisher ML, Freudenberger R et al. Effects of exercise training on peak perfomance and quality of life in congestive heart failure patients. *J Cardiac Failure* 1999; **5:** 188–94.

76 Owen A, Croucher L. Effect of an exercise programme for elderly patients with heart failure. *Eur J Heart fail* 2000; **2:** 65–70.

77 Wilmore JH, Costill DL. *Physiology of sport and exercise.* Champaign: Human Kinetics, 1994.

78 Tyni-Lenné R, Gordon A, Europe E, Jansson E, Sylvén C. Exercise-based rehabilitation improves skeletal muscle capacity, exercise tolerance and quality of life in both women and men with chronic heart failure. *J Cardiac Fail* 1998; **4:** 9–17.

79 Palm M, Penque S, Doll N, Beahrs M. Women and cardiac rehabilitation: referral and compliance patterns. *J Cardiovasc Nurs* 1999; **13:** 83–92.

80 Lieberman L, Meana M, Stewart D. Cardiac rehabilitation: gender differences in factors influencing participation. *J Women's Health* 1998; **7:** 717–23.

81 Fridlund B, Billing E. Cardiac rehabilitation and gender differences. *Nur Sci Res Nord Count* 2002; **22:** 48–51.

82 Jaarsma T, Halfens R, Huijer Abu-Saad H et al. Effect of education and support on self-care and resource utilization. *Eur Heart J* 1999; **20:** 673–82.

83 Rich MW, Baldus D, Beckham V, Wittenberg C, Luther P. Effect of a multidisciplinary intervention on medication compliance in elderly patients with congestive heart failure. *Am J Med* 1996; **101:** 270–6.

84 Ni H, Nauman D, Burgess D, Wise K, Crispell K, Hershberger RE. Factors influencing knowledge of and adherence to self-care among patients with heart failure. *Arch Intern Med* 1999; **159:** 1613–19.

85 Rich MW, Beckham V, Wittenberg C et al. A multidisciplinary intervention to prevent the readmission of elderly patients with congestive heart failure. *N Engl J Med* 1995; **333:** 1190–5.

86 Stewart S, Marley JE, Horowitz JD. Effects of a multidisciplinary, home-based intervention on unplanned readmissions and survival among patients with chronic congestive heart failure. *Lancet* 1999; **354:** 1077–83.

87 Strömberg A, Mårtensson J, Fridlund B, Dahlström U. Nurse-led heart failure clinics in Sweden. *Eur J Heart Fail* 2001; **3:** 139–44.

88 Lewis D. Computer-based approaches to patient education: a review of the literature. *J Am Med Inform Assoc* 1999; **6:** 272–82.

89 Strömberg A, Fridlund B, Dahlström U. Effects of an interactive, computer-based education on knowledge, compliance and quality of life in patients with heart

failure. A randomized, controlled, multicentre trial. *Eur Heart J* 2000: P1250.

90 Strömberg A, Dahlström U, Fridlund B. Computer-based education for patients with chronic heart failure. A randomized, controlled, multicentre study of the effects on knowledge, compliance and quality of life. *J Adv Nurs*; in press.

91 Pernotto D, Bairnsfather L, Sodeman W. 'Informed consent' interactive videodisc for patients having a colonoscopy, a polypectomy and an endoscopy. *Medinfo* 1995; **8:** 1699.

92 Liao L, Jollis J, Delong E, Peterson E, Morris K, Mark D. Impact of an interactive video on decision making of patients with ischemic heart disease. *J Gen Intern Med* 1996; **11:** 373–6.

93 Wetstone SL, Sheehan TJ, Votaw RG, Peterson MG, Rothfield N. Evaluation of a computer based education lesson for patients with rheumatoid arthritis. *J Rheumatol* 1985; **12:** 907–12.

94 Strömberg A, Ahlén H, Fridlund B, Dahlström U. Interactive education on CD-ROM – a new tool in education of heart failure patients. *Patient Educ Couns* 2002; **46:** 75–81.

95 Cintron G, Bigas C, Linares E, Aranda J, Hernades E. Nurse practitioner's role in chronic heart failure clinic: in-hospital time, costs, and patient satisfaction. *Heart Lung* 1983; **12:** 237–40.

96 Kornowski R, Zeeli D, Averbuch M et al. Intensive home-care surveillance prevents hospitalization and improves morbidity rates among elderly patients with severe congestive heart failure. *Am Heart J* 1995; **129:** 762–6.

97 West JA, Miller NH, Parker KM et al. A comprehensive management system for heart failure improves clinical outcomes and reduces medical resource utilization. *Am Heart J* 1997; **79:** 58–63.

98 Hanumanthu S, Butler J, Chomsky D, Davis S, Wilson JR. Effect of a heart failure program on hospitalization frequency and exercise tolerance. *Circulation* 1997; **96:** 2842–8.

99 Smith LE, Fabri SA, Pai R, Ferry D, Heywood T. Symptomatic improvement and reduced hospitalization for patients attending a cardiomyopathy clinic. *Clin Cardiol* 1997; **20:** 949–54.

100 Fonarow G, Stevenson L, Walden J. Impact of a comprehensive heart failure management program on hospital readmission and functional status of patients with advanced heart failure. *J Am Coll Cardiol* 1997; **30:** 725–32.

101 Shah NB, Der E, Ruggerio C, Heidenreich P, Massie B. Prevention of hospitalizations for heart failure with an interactive home monitoring program. *Am Heart J* 1998; **135:** 373–8.

102 Heidenreich PA, Ruggerio CM, Massie BM. Effect of a home monitoring system on hospitalization and resource use for patients with heart failure. *Am Heart J* 1999; **138:** 633–40.

103 Weinberger M, Oddone EZ, Henderson WG. Does increased access to primary care reduce hospital

readmissions? Veterans Affairs Cooperative Study Group on Primary Care and Hospital Readmission. *N Engl J Med* 1996; **334:** 1441–7.

104 Cline C, Israelsson B, Willenheimer R, Broms K, Erhardt L. Cost-effective management programme for heart failure reduces hospitalisation. *Heart* 1998; **80:** 442–6.

105 Ekman I, Andersson B, Ehnfors M, Matejka G, Persson B, Fagerberg B. Feasibility of a nurse-monitored, outpatient-care programme for elderly patients with moderate-to-severe chronic heart failure. *Eur Heart J* 1998; **19:** 1254–60.

106 Stewart S, Pearson S, Horowitz J. Effects of a home-based intervention among patients with congestive heart failure discharged from acute hospital care. *Arch Intern Med* 1998; **158:** 1067–72.

107 Naylor MD, Brooten D, Campbell R et al. Comprehensive discharge planning and home follow-up intervention of elders hospitalized with common medical and surgical cardiac conditions. *JAMA* 1999; **281:** 613–20.

108 Blue L, Strong E, Murdoch DR et al. Improving long-term outcome with specialist nurse intervention in heart failure: a randomized trial. *BMJ* 2001; **323:** 715–18.

109 Doughty RN, Wright SP, Walsh HJ et al. Randomized, controlled trial of integrated heart failure management: the Auckland Heart Failure Management Study. *Eur Heart J* 2002; **23:** 139–46.

110 Krumholz HM, Amatruda J, Smith GL et al. Randomized trial of an education and support intervention to prevent readmission of patients with heart failure. *J Am Coll Cardiol* 2002; **39:** 83–9.

111 De Geest S, von Renteln-Kruse W, Steeman E, Degraeve S, Abraham IL. Compliance issues with the geriatric population, complexity with aging. *Nurs Clin North Am* 1998; **33:** 467–81.

112 Monane M, Bohn RL, Gurwitz JH, Glynn RJ, Avorn J. Noncompliance with congestive heart failure therapy in the elderly. *Arch Intern Med* 1994; **154:** 433–7.

113 Riedinger MS, Dracup KA, Brecht M-L. Predictors of quality of life in women with heart failure. *J Heart Lung Transplant* 2000; **19:** 598–608.

114 Friedman MM. Older adults' symptoms and their duration before hospitalization for heart failure. *Heart Lung* 1997; **26:** 169–76.

115 Bennett SJ, Baker SL, Huster GA. Quality of life in women with heart failure. *Health Care Women Int* 1998; **19:** 217–29.

116 Friedman MM, King KB. Correlates of fatigue in older women with heart failure. *Heart Lung* 1995; **24:** 512–18.

117 Mårtensson J, Karlsson J-E, Fridlund B. Female patients with congestive heart failure: how they conceive their life situation. *J Adv Nurs* 1998; **28:** 1216–24.

118 Freedland KE, Carney RM. Psychosocial considerations in elderly patients with heart failure. *Clin Geriatr Med* 2000; **16:** 649–61.

119 Rideout E. Hope, morale and adaptation in patients with cronic heart failure. *J Adv Nurs* 1986; **11:** 429–38.

120 Stull DE, Starling R, Haas G, Young JB. Becoming a patient with heart failure. *Heart Lung* 1999; **28:** 284–92.

121 Krumholz HM, Baker DW, Ashton CM et al. Evaluating quality of care for patients with heart failure. *Circulation* 2000; **101:** E122–40.

122 Krumholz HM, Butler J, Miller J et al. Prognostic importance of emotional support for elderly patients hospitalized with heart failure. *Circulation* 1998; **97:** 958–64.

123 Murberg TA, Bru E, Aarsland T, Svebak S. Social support, social disability and their role as predictors of depression among patients with congestive heart failure. *Scand J Soc Med* 1998; **26:** 87–95.

124 Mårtensson J, Karlsson J-E, Fridlund B. Male patients with congestive heart failure and their conceptions of the life situation. *J Adv Nurs* 1997; **2:** 579–86.

125 Evangelista LS, Kawaga-Singer M, Dracup K. Gender differences in health perceptions and meaning in persons living with heart failure. *Heart Lung* 2001; **30:** 294–301.

126 Friedman MM. Stressors and perceived stress in older women with heart disease. *Cardiovascular Nursing* 1993; **29:** 25–9.

127 Cline CMJ, Willenheimer RB, Erhardt LR, Wiklund I, Israelsson BYA. Health-related quality of life in elderly patients with heart failure. *Scand Cardiovasc J* 1999; **33:** 278–85.

128 Jaarsma T, Dracup K, Walden J, Warner L. Sexual function in patients with advanced heart failure. *Heart Lung* 1996; **25:** 262–70.

129 Westlake C, Dracup K, Walden JA, Fonarow G. Sexuality of patients with advanced heart failure and their spouses or partners. *J Heart Lung Transplant* 1999; **18:** 1133–8.

130 Friedman MM. Social support sources and psychological well-being in older women with heart disease. *Res Nurs Health* 1993; **16:** 405–13.

131 Walden JA, Stevenson LW, Dracup K et al. Extended comparison of quality of life between stable heart failure patients and heart transplant recipients. *J Heart Lung Transplant* 1994; **13:** 1109–18.

132 Murberg TA, Bru E, Aarsland T, Svebak S. Functional status and depression among men and women with congestive heart failure. *Int J Psychiatry Med* 1998; **28:** 273–91.

133 Freedland KE, Carney RM, Rich MW et al. Depression in elderly patients with congestive heart failure. *Int J Geriatr Psych* 1991; **24:** 59–71.

134 Pinsky J, Jette A, Branch L, Kannel W, Feinleib M. The Framingham disability study: relationship of various coronary heart disease manifestations to disability in older persons living in the community. *Am J Pub Health* 1990; **80:** 1363–7.

135 Berry C, McMurray J. A review of quality-of-life evaluations in patients with congestive heart failure. *Pharmacoeconomics* 1999; **16:** 247–71.

136 Nolan-Hoeksema S. Sex differences in unipolar depression: evidence and theory. *Psychol Bull* 1987; **101:** 259–82.

137 McMurray J, McDonagh T, Morrison CE, Dargie HJ. Trends in hospitalization for heart failure in Scotland 1980–1990. *Eur Heart J* 1993; **14:** 1158–62.

138 Doughty R, Yee T, Sharpe N, MacMahon S. Hospital admissions and deaths due to congestive heart failure in New Zealand. *N Z Med J* 1995; **108:** 474–5.

139 Reitsma JB, Mosterd A, de Craen AJM et al. Increase in hospital admission rates for heart failure in the Netherlands, 1980–1993. *Heart* 1996; **76:** 388–92.

17 Approaches for patient education

Sandra B Dunbar, Rosemary Gee and Patricia C Clark

Introduction

The high incidence and prevalence of congestive heart failure (CHF) and its resulting high medical resource consumption require comprehensive strategies to improve clinical and fiscal outcomes of care. Many of the costs associated with heart failure care emanate from multiple hospital readmission events due to decompensation with readmission rates reported to be as high as 25–47%.[1–3] Approximately one-third to one-half of CHF hospital readmissions are considered preventable. Factors contributing to preventable hospitalization include inadequate patient and caregiver education; inadequate symptom self-assessment, interpretation and management; inadequate social support, poor discharge planning and follow-up; and failure to adhere to diet, medication and activity regimens.[4–8] In addition to adequate knowledge about heart failure and care, social support and motivation to learn and manage health behaviors are critical for successful adherence to complex self-care heart failure regimens. Thus patient education and counseling are important cornerstones for quality heart failure care.

A variety of heart failure inpatient and outpatient management programs have been developed over the past decade. These include approaches such as multidisciplinary inpatient care guided by evidence-based guidelines and pathways, and outpatient approaches such as disease management, specialty heart failure clinics, nurse practitioner managed clinics, primary care–cardiologist specialist partnerships, and combination approaches.[9] Regardless of the way care is organized or the specific health care personnel involved, provision of clear and organized patient education regarding key aspects of heart failure is the foundation for successful outpatient patient self-management and, ultimately, improved patient outcomes.

Patient education is essential but not entirely sufficient to result in adequate skills for behavioral change and self-care. In spite of teaching, patients may not make choices recommended to them by their health providers. For many persons with heart failure, self-care requires attention to and motivation to change long-standing routines and lifestyles. These changes may influence other family members and require integration into the family's daily routines. Additionally, characteristics of persons with heart failure are important considerations in designing educational strategies. Because there is greater incidence of heart failure with increased age, learning approaches successful with elders need to be incorporated. In addition, female and African-American patients may experience worse patient outcomes, suggesting a need to emphasize specific aspects of the educational program.[10,11] Literacy is another important factor associated with patients' ability to comprehend the large amount of information imparted in heart failure educational programs. For these reasons, this chapter will emphasize topics and approaches for heart failure patient education as well as examine the needs of special populations, and suggest approaches that integrate behavioral strategies (see also Chapter 9).

State of the science in heart failure patient education

Patient learning needs

Current education for patients with CHF is aimed at improving self-care, minimizing symptoms and hospital admissions, and improving the CHF patient's quality of life.[12–14] Patients report that they value the education received during hospitalization for CHF, as do patients diagnosed with other types of cardiac diseases, indicating a desire for increased knowledge to manage their disease.[15–17] As patients improve their self-care abilities and play an active role in reducing distressing symptoms, they begin to experience greater perceived control of their daily life.

Traditionally, educational programs have centered on educational needs as identified by health care providers. Results from several studies suggest that CHF patients and health care providers may differ on what is important to learn indicating a need to develop educational programs that are more in congruence with the perceived learning priorities of CHF patients. Hagenhoff et al[15] developed the Congestive Heart Failure Patient Learning Needs Inventory (CHFPLNI), and this tool has been used in two published studies to address the perceived learning needs of CHF patients. These studies indicated that patients place a high priority on learning about medication, risk factors and anatomy and physiology. In a study comparing patient and nurse rankings of the importance of learning needs, the top categories reported by American patients (medications, anatomy and physiology, risk factors) were slightly different than the top four categories reported by nurses (medication, risk factors, dietary information and activity).[15] Interestingly, patients ranked activity as least important. In a later study of a Canadian population, Frattini et al[12] found that psychological issues in addition to medications, risk factors, and anatomy and physiology were in the top categories of perceived importance to patients whereas once again, nurses ranked medications, diet, risk factors, and activity as the most important information for patients to know. Although both studies were composed of small sample sizes, the data suggest important implications for designing CHF patient education programs and provide guidance for prioritizing learning activities to address patient concerns.

For example, the CHF patients may have rated the need for anatomy and physiology information high in that a better understanding of the relationship of fluid (through diet) and mechanisms of heart failure is required for patients to clearly make the connections between 'extra fluid' and the effect on the heart and symptoms such as shortness of breath, peripheral edema, and interpreting daily weights. Dietary control of sodium and fluid, and engaging in daily activity/exercise, are vital behaviors for CHF self-care, yet patients consistently ranked dietary information and physical activity as low on the priority list of learning needs. There are several explanations for this finding which underscore the difficulty of these two behaviors for CHF patients. Dietary sodium restriction is frequently perceived as unpalatable and difficult to maintain in a family meal context and other social situations. Maintaining activity levels is confusing as patients try to conserve energy associated with activities of daily living and initiate increased exercise in the context of distressing symptoms of shortness of breath. Both activity and diet patterns are developed habitually over time and require motivational strategies in addition to knowledge for change. The implication for patient education programs is to emphasize the role of these behaviors as part of managing risk factors and preventing aggravation of symptoms. Family implications are paramount and are discussed later.

Suggested approaches and innovations

Use of adult education principles

Adult education theory provides some direction for how to approach CHF patient and family education. Because adults want to know what is essential vs what is nice to know and prefer immediate applicable material,[18] it is essential that an assessment of individual CHF learning

Table 17.1. *Topics for heart failure education and counseling*

- General topics
  - Explanation of heart failure
  - Physiological responses
  - Psychological responses
  - Prognosis
  - Advanced directives
- Symptom assessment and management
  - Expected symptoms vs symptoms of worsening heart failure
  - Self-monitoring with daily weights
  - Action plan in case of increased symptoms
  - Dealing with psychological symptoms
  - Smoking cessation
- Dietary recommendations
  - Sodium restriction
  - Fluid restriction
  - Alcohol restriction
  - Compliance strategies
- Activity, exercise, and rest
  - Work and leisure activities
  - Exercise program
  - Sexual activity
  - Energy-conserving suggestions
  - Adherence strategies
- Medications
  - Nature of each drug, dosing, and side-effects
  - Coping with a complicated regimen, refills
  - Adherence strategies
  - Cost issues

Adapted from Konstam et al[28] and Grady et al[51]

needs, usual patterns of behavior, perceived benefits and barriers to behavior change, available family support and resources occur prior to initiating educational activities. Assessment of individual CHF knowledge and needs can occur through formalized assessment tools that are used in either written or interview formats depending on the literacy level of the patient and the time demands or the provider. The assessment should be guided by the topics traditionally included in CHF education (see Table 17.1). Examples of published assessment tools that have been used in heart failure include 'Perceived Benefits and Barriers of Medication and Dietary Compliance', and 'Self-management in Heart Failure'.[19,20] Some institutions use a clinical assessment tool to examine knowledge of areas of self-care and symptom management strategies such as that used by the heart failure disease management program of the Cleveland Clinic Foundation.[21] The information obtained by knowledge and self-care assessment logically leads to the design of individualized learning goals and strategies.

Adult learners are characterized by several additional, important factors including a self-concept that moves from dependency to self-direction, capability of making decisions, accumulation of life experiences, a learning orientation congruent with development tasks and social roles,

and the need for immediate application.[18] One approach might be to provide opportunities for practice of self-care behaviors in the acute care setting, for example the nurse could encourage and assist patients to perform, record and interpret their daily weight, and to select appropriate foods in collaboration with the dietician. This collaborative or empowerment approach is important for adults who also view themselves as producers, and derive self-esteem from contributions (see Table 17.2). A more informal and friendly approach that values CHF patients as individuals and makes the learning fun is important. Anecdotal evidence suggests that CHF patients and families have responded well to games (e.g. CHF jeopardy, role playing), and humor incorporated into CHF education.

Reinforcement of learning

Planning for repeat education sessions is critical to ongoing outpatient management of chronic CHF. Because patient and family situations change, comorbidities evolve or heart failure worsens, those involved with patient education must repeatedly assess the learning needs of the CHF patient and their family members, and provide appropriate reinforcement, new information, or additional counseling. A successful patient education session does not assume retention and application of self-care knowledge.

Table 17.2. Empowerment components of patient education with a person with heart failure

Empowerment component	Application to heart failure patient education
Sufficient knowledge to make rational informed decisions	Nurse provides patient with all the information to make informed decisions about management of heart failure including pharmacologic (medications, importance, and side-effects) and non-pharmacologic (diet, exercise, daily weights, symptoms) aspects. Patient is informed of complications of heart failure and the role of self-care, and is encouraged to read more about heart failure, to talk to friends and relatives about self-care regimen.
Sufficient control and resources to implement decisions	Nurse provides additional written materials and self-care records to assist patient in decisions. Options for dietary management, exercise approaches and treatment, for example, are reviewed; patient is encouraged to set own goals for heart failure outcomes.
Sufficient experience to evaluate the effectiveness of their decisions	Nurse continues to monitor patient's response to treatment by telephone assessment of symptoms; serves as a coach to help interpret symptoms, suggest alternative foods or activities, medications, and continues to support patient goals without pressure or judgment.

Adapted from Rankin and Stallings (p. 82)[45] and Funnell et al[58]

Table 17.3. *Suggestions for written heart failure patient education and self-management materials*

- Understanding heart failure
  - Definitions, causes, understandable anatomy and physiology
  - Treatment approaches, and prognosis
  - Simple diagrams of normal hearts and hearts with congestive heart failure
  - Sample advanced directive appropriate for region or state
- Understanding how to assess and manage symptoms
  - Dyspnea
  - Orthopnea and sleep difficulties
  - Fatigue
  - Weight gain
  - Swelling
  - Irregular or fast heart beat
  - Nausea and appetite changes
  - Confusion, mental changes
  - Dizziness, fainting
- Medications – why are they important?
  - Information about specific medications
  - Flexible diuretic regimen explanations
  - Tips for remembering to take medications
  - Medication administration chart
  - Suggestions for resources (pill boxes, timers, etc.)
- Importance of a low sodium diet
  - Role of sodium and fluid in symptoms and management
  - How to calculate sodium intake from food charts, reading product labels
  - Examples of high sodium foods to avoid
  - Importance of potassium: sources of potassium-rich food sources
  - Seasoning alternatives
  - Sample menus and recipes
  - Tips for dining in restaurants
  - Food and fluid diary
- How to handle fluid restriction
  - Calculating fluid intake
  - Hidden sources of fluid
  - Tips for managing the symptom of thirst
- Avoiding alcohol and smoking
  - Effects of alcohol on the heart
  - Effects of smoking on the heart
  - How to stop smoking
  - Helpful resources
- Measuring daily weight successfully
  - Focus is on fluid, not total weight management
  - Guidelines for weighing daily
  - Weight record

Table 17.3. *Continued*

- Exercise
  - Exercise guidelines
  - Activity logs
  - Tips for energy-conserving routines
  - Information on sexual activity
- Stress management
  - Instructions for relaxation exercises
  - Taking care of your emotional health
  - Maintaining a positive outlook
  - Seeking support from family and friends
- Additional resources
  - Internet sites
  - Clinic contacts (nutritionist, social workers, nurse practitioners, pharmacists, exercise specialist, physician, etc.)
  - Organizations
  - Support groups

Persons with heart failure may have depression, congestion and poor oxygen delivery, and subtle cognitive impairment that interfere with concentration during an educational session and subsequently, they fail to recall the seriousness of the need for self-care or the specific instructions.[22,23] Several studies of patient knowledge and self-care behavior after discharge from the hospital have documented inadequate knowledge of medications, purpose and effects of treatment, and how and why to perform self-care behaviors such as daily weights[7,24] Planning for individualized repeat education can occur with adequate discharge planning, during outpatient clinic or office visits, telephone follow-up or home visits.

Comprehensive discharge planning for CHF patients has demonstrated improved patient outcomes of fewer rehospitalizations, lengthened time between discharge and readmission, and decreased the cost of providing care.[25] Various models of discharge planning exist, and effective elements include home follow-up by advanced practice nurses, problem-solving, provision of long-term education and counseling and referral to other resources. Stewart et al[26] report that a one-time, home care visit by a nurse/pharmacist team for the purpose of optimizing medication management, identifying clinical deterioration and improving caregiver vigilance led to reduced hospitalizations for CHF. While the details of the educational interventions are not made explicit, these studies provide evidence for the benefit of some type of ongoing assessment and education.

Provision of written materials that reinforce one-on-one or group discussions is also essential. Written materials can be used during individual teaching sessions, and patients and their families can refer to them at home. Suggestions for reinforcing written information and self-management records (to track diet, exercise, medications, and weight) are listed in Table 17.3. Several commercially available booklets can be used or the development of materials with an institution's imprimatur may be preferred. One example of a commercially available booklet is 'A Stronger Pump' (Atlanta, GA: Prichett & Hull, Inc.). Once again, follow-up contact by the health care provider with suggestions of how to use the written materials and review of the self-management records reinforces earlier teaching. Serial mailings of educational materials have been noted to reduce total admissions and costs and to improve self-care of weighing behaviors and following dietary sodium advice.[27] Videotapes may also be used for reinforcement, and although little research is available on this technique in heart failure, audiotapes have been successful in promoting recovery in other cardiac populations.

Family-focused approaches

Heart failure education has implications for including the patient's family and/or support system due to the complex home management regimen required, and evidence that inadequate social support contributes to readmissions.[3,7] The importance of including families in CHF education is advocated,[28,29] although the role of the family caregiver in heart failure remains poorly defined. Considerable research has demonstrated that cardiovascular disease has a powerful impact on the family, and the family influences the course of heart disease through adaptation, social support, coping mechanisms and adherence.[30] Although research on the responses of CHF family members and the role they play in patient self-management is sparse, the literature on other chronic diseases provides some support that family involvement may result in better patient outcomes. Morisky et al,[31] for example, compared three different psychoeducational interventions (brief individual counseling, spouse counseling, and patient support groups) in hypertension patients. Their results demonstrated that spouse counseling improved overall compliance to appointment-keeping and medications, and contributed significantly to lowering blood pressure and mortality. A descriptive study of patients with diabetes found that family support explained 17% of the variance in self-care behavior.[32] Information, positive affect or/and actual assistance diminished the impact of the illness in family members of cancer patients, and both social support and education provided resources to interpret and obtain assistance with the illness.[33] Thus, family members can play an important role, but they need both the knowledge and guidance of how to be supportive of self-care in heart failure. Family members may also need counseling to encourage appropriate activity levels in CHF patients and to overcome their tendency to do everything for the CHF patient who is experiencing distressing symptoms.

One approach to family education for heart failure may be found in the literature on self-determination. Self-determination theory suggests that lasting behavior change is not simply complying with demands for change but rather accepting the regulation for changes as one's own.[34] Autonomous behaviors are ones for which the regulation is experienced as chosen and emanating from self vs controlled behaviors which are viewed as pressured or coerced by another. According to the theory, successful accomplishment of CHF behaviors would occur when the patient viewed that change, e.g. limiting sodium in the diet or increasing physical activity, was important for their health benefits, not because one's spouse or health care provider insisted on the change. Self-determination theory suggests that autonomy supportive contexts – ones in which the significant others offer choice, provide alternatives, minimize pressure, and acknowledge the individual's feelings and perspectives – will facilitate more autonomous regulatory processes and thus promote effective behavior change.[34,35]

Caregivers of CHF patients may feel a responsibility to help persons with CHF adhere closely to dietary and fluid restrictions and other treatment recommendations. Monitoring another person's behavior may lead to negative family interactions if the person with CHF is not making choices consistent with treatment recommendations. Autonomy support influences individuals by increasing their individual autonomy and by increasing individual feelings of competence in a situation. Specifically in health care situations, the use of autonomy supportive environments has resulted in positive outcomes in educational, work and health care situations. These studies have demonstrated increased adherence in long-term medication adherence,[36] weight loss and maintenance,[37] and alcoholism treatment participation.[38]

The autonomy supportive approach involves listening fully, providing choice, offering a clear rationale, and encouraging self-initiation of behaviors, whereas a controlling context refers to pressuring one to think, feel or behave in specific ways.[35] Building a partnership between the CHF patient and their family members for disease management facilitates the autonomy approach. Autonomy support is currently being tested in a study of the effect of a family partner intervention on self-management behaviors in heart failure.[39] In addition to the usual heart failure topics, family members are taught concrete, specific ways to support the patient making lifestyle changes. It is hypothesized that the family partner intervention may enable the caregiver to use a different approach to be supportive, directly and indirectly, of the person with CHF trying to adhere to recommended treatments.[40]

It is important to note that interventions that prepare families to perform illness-related behaviors may in fact increase anxiety and caregiver burden if these are not addressed as demonstrated by Dracup et al[41] who tested the effect of teaching CPR to family members of high-risk patients. A study of 41 (75% female) spouses of CHF patients revealed that caregiving was burdensome and stressful.[42] These data indicate the serious effect of the disease on the family as well as the individual, and findings of caregiver stress are consistent with research from other chronic illness populations which demonstrate that caregivers are psychologically and physically vulnerable.[43,44] As family-focused educational strategies are developed, addressing family self-care must also receive attention. On the other hand, changing the social context in which the illness is experienced by providing education and support may promote greater perceived autonomy for both the patient and family.[35]

While educational principles and common sense suggest that patients and families should hear and learn the same material, separate patient and family teaching sessions may be preferred in certain cases. These include (a) when it is difficult to assess learning needs; (b) when there are marked differences between the patient and family member in literacy and comprehension; and (c) when family members coopt the teaching session and make the patient feel guilty about past non-compliance or risk behavior.[45]

Incorporating behavioral strategies into education

Because adequate self-care requires not only learning about the needs, but also becoming motivated to change behavior, identifying resources needed to support making and sustaining the change, and actually making and sustaining the change, behavioral strategies are essential to incorporate into the patient educational process.[46] Several behavioral theories and strategies may be relevant to the heart failure patient, and although a detailed discussion is beyond the scope of this chapter, a few approaches are discussed briefly below and in Table 17.4.

The stage of change model developed by Prochaska et al characterizes behavior as a series of stages responsive to different and specific interventions.[47] The stages are *precontemplation* (person does not see the need to change behavior), *contemplation* (person declares change may be needed but has not initiated the change), *planning* (person is preparing to make a change), *action* (change is enacted), and *maintenance* (change is sustained, and relapses into old patterns are avoided). The health care provider and patient can decide upon the specific stage and set learning needs appropriately to move to the next stage.

Self-efficacy and outcome expectations theory gives another direction to the health provider for how to structure the physical and social environment in which learning occurs.[48] Self-efficacy refers to the patient's confidence in their ability to perform the behavior and achieve its intended outcomes and is achieved through personal mastery, verbal persuasion, vicarious experiences and physiological cues that the appropriate behavior has taken

Table 17.4. *Using behavioral strategies to enhance congestive heart failure patient education*

Behavioral theory or strategy	Application to CHF education
Stage of change[47]	Consider whether patient is at precontemplation, contemplation, preparation, action or maintenance phase for CHF self-care behaviors of sodium and fluid management, exercise, medication administration, and daily weighing; tailor educational messages to the stage.
Self-efficacy and outcome expectations[48]	Provide opportunity to master behavior; provide verbal encouragement and positive reinforcement, promote interactions with other CHF patients for vicarious learning; emphasize relationship between successful self-care behavior and physiological change (i.e. reduced symptoms, increased exercise tolerance).
Health belief model[50,59]	Review potential barriers and costs associated with dietary sodium compliance, medication acquisition, and exercise performance.
Health promotion model[51]	Emphasize the preventive role of self-care behaviors; reframe dietary restrictions into dietary recommendations
Motivational interviewing[46]	Solicit patient beliefs about diet, medications, exercise, symptom assessment and management; identify benefits of self-care behaviors; encourage confidence; emphasize that it is the patient's decision to change; actively listen to patient's point of view; support and encourage.
Social support[35,49]	Create family or caregiver partnerships; goals are developed and shared by family/caregiver.

place. Some have combined stage of change theory and self-efficacy concepts to set up dynamic behavioral interventions. Social support is another behavioral construct that is hypothesized to mediate the stress associated with behavior change and reinforce mastery.[49]

Originally developed to examine compliance, the Health Belief Model has been recently reviewed,[50] and research findings suggest that it is most useful for identifying the barriers and costs that prevent participation in health behaviors. For heart failure patients, this may be most salient in examining perceived difficulties and fiscal implications of dietary recommendations and medications. Pender's Health Promotion Model may be most useful for reframing and translating the avoidance and restricting CHF self-care behaviors into a health protection viewpoint.[51] Motivational interviewing is a technique used to establish patient perceptions about need, rationale and commitment to behavior change. Motivational interviewing has been an effective intervention with persons trying to change smoking behaviors or recover from alcohol and food addictions.[46] Using one or a combination of these behavioral approaches will significantly strengthen the effectiveness of CHF patient education to achieve the desired patient outcomes.

Special populations
Elders

Tailoring patient education for elders involves consideration of factors they are much more likely to have than younger patients. These include coexisting problems related to comorbidities, polypharmacy, financial concerns, sensory impairments, physical and cognitive limitations, social isolation, and depression. Older adults are a heterogeneous group, and the person planning the education session needs to carefully assess for individual needs. Health care providers need to be aware of the 'myths' of aging, have a strong understanding of normal aging changes, and keep an open mind about the types of changes that older adults are willing to make. In general, there are some issues that affect the learning process that the educator will want to consider when teaching older adults. Vision changes such as presbyopia or macular degeneration may require some modification of teaching materials including the use of enlarged print or other low vision aids such as 'talking watches' for timing of medication. Strong contrasts between text and print will facilitate visual teaching aids. Instructions on medication bottles are typically written in very small print, and larger print labels or magnification can be used. In addition, when teaching

older adults, one may need to plan for extra time so the session will not be rushed allowing for adequate time to think and formulate questions. Older adults may have a sensorineural hearing loss, presbyacusis, which typically causes difficulty with conversational speech. An effective technique is to ask patients to repeat critical information, such as medication dosages, to verify that they heard the instructions correctly.

Because of the changes of aging and cormobidities, it may be more difficult for the older adult to identify important symptoms that may require action or communication with their health care provider. An interesting resource is a publication entitled, 'Talking with your Doctor: A Guide for Older People',[52] which can be obtained at no cost from the National Institute of Aging. This booklet was designed to help older adults develop effective interactions with their health care providers. Because older adults may be on numerous medications, providing a printed form of all their medications, dosages, and schedules is useful for them to have for health care visits and emergencies. This list needs to be carried with them at all times, updated when medications are changed, and a family member needs to be aware of where to find the list in an emergency.

Since family members often play a substantial support role for older adults, prior to teaching, the provider should ask the older adult if they desire family participation in the teaching session. Often family members help with the shopping and/or preparation of meals, administering medications and observing for changes in symptoms. As discussed earlier, family members have an important role in encouraging adherence to self-management activities. With older adults, it is particularly important for them to address the topic of advance directives and durable health care power of attorney (in states where applicable) with their families. They may need specific guidance in how to approach this topic

Women

Women have not been included in the same numbers as men in large CHF clinical trials; however, existing information does suggest that there may be gender differences in response to both CHF as an illness and its treatment. Women with CHF may have different outcomes in areas of overall physical functioning and exercise tolerance.[11] These differences have been hypothesized to be related to trends that women with CHF tend to be older and may have greater prevalence of underlying hypertension and diastolic dysfunction. Even when controlling for age, left ventricular ejection fraction and New York Heart Association class, women tend to have worse quality of life ratings on intermediate activities of daily living and social activities than men.[53] These emerging data about women have implications for patient teaching and underscore the importance of assessing and addressing topics for individuals such as exercise and activity tolerance, and comorbidities (i.e. hypertension) in the self-care plan.

Low literacy

CHF patients with low literacy or functional illiteracy present special challenges for patient and family education and require use of modified teaching approaches and materials. While some suggest the use of videotapes, these are not quick answers in that the inability to read may be accompanied by an inability to process and assimilate information.[54] Teaching strategies for lower literate

patients include focusing on the *core* knowledge and skills necessary to learn, teaching the smallest amount possible, making points vivid, using pictures and illustrations, and asking patients to restate or demonstrate the knowledge.[45] To accomplish successful learning with the low literacy patient with heart failure, the educator and patient together must prioritize what is most important for the individual patient to know based on the degree to which the patient and/or caregiver assumes responsibilities. Initially, the goal may be on the stabilization of fluid and symptom status through medications, daily weights and sodium restriction, with delay of teaching content on activity and psychological issues until a later time. Emphasize activities that the patient should *do* and reframe what they should *not do* to avoid confusion.[45,55]

Suggestions for adapting CHF teaching materials for lower literacy are listed in Table 17.5. For example, a low

Table 17.5. *Adapting congestive heart failure patient education for low literacy*

Topic	Adaptation for low literacy
Understanding heart failure	• Illustrations of hearts with normal and low cardiac output • Illustration of consequences of fluid retained in CHF
How to assess and manage symptoms	• Diagram of person with anatomical locations of symptoms highlighted • Pictures of self-care activity to alleviate symptoms
Heart failure medications	• Place color-coded dots on medication bottle; develop a chart with coordinating explanatory information (e.g. yellow dot for 'water pill') • Provide a medication-specific administration time chart vs teaching 'take three times a day' • Provide resources such as pill boxes using color codes
Diet and fluid	• Pictures of potassium-rich food sources • Pictures of seasoning alternatives to sodium • Pictures of salt shaker, sodium rich foods, and alcohol stamped with large X • If fluid restriction, provide timetable with amount of fluid distributed throughout the day
Exercise	• Pictures of recommended exercise behaviors • Pictures of how to conserve energy during daily routines
Stress management	• Pictures of groups of family and friends in social settings • Pictures of activities used for relaxation
Other resources	• Important phone numbers • Appropriate low literacy internet sites • Provide appropriate videotape or audiotape

literacy 'to do' teaching guide might include a chart of self-care activities organized around the time of day. The chart would include illustrations of a person doing the following: getting out of bed in the morning, performing daily weight activity, recording the weight on a chart, phoning the physician's or nurse's office if weight gain increased by a specified amount, taking medications (color-coded with matching color-coded dots on the actual medication bottle) at certain times, sitting down to the table for meals with no salt shaker on the table, etc. Additional illustrations can be provided for symptoms for which the health care provider should be called. The patient can be asked to review the chart and explain to the provider what the self-care pictures mean and how they will adapt this to their own daily routine. Care should be exercised so that the low literacy patient is not made to feel embarrassed or ashamed of their level of reading ability.

Creative adaptation of patient teaching materials for special populations, cultures or low literacy requires a multidisciplinary approach and additional time and resources. The emergence of multimedia technology that combines computer graphics, sound and patient inter-action may be important adjuncts to heart failure education in the future.[56]

Conclusion

This chapter has provided an overview of the learning needs of CHF patients and their families, suggested approaches to education and advocated incorporation of behavioral strategies. Although patient education is vital to quality heart failure care, there is little research to guide practice. Research is needed to develop evidenced-based care and to guide decisions about teaching activities as a selection of strategies, group vs individual approaches, and essential vs nice to know content. The dose of education and cost-effective follow-up approaches that achieve the best outcomes also need to be developed and tested. Clearly, studies of various approaches that incorporate behavioral strategies should be conducted. When patient education is considered to be the cornerstone for achieving optimal self-care and patient outcomes, the health care provider is well-positioned to greatly improve quality of life for heart failure patients and their families.

References

1 Brass-Mynderase N. Disease management for chronic congestive heart failure. *J Cardiovasc Nurs* 1996; **11:** 54–62.

2 Lasater M. The effect of a nurse-managed CHF clinic on patient readmission and length of stay. *Home Healthcare Nurse* 1996; **14:** 352–6.

3 Vinson J, Rich MW, Sperry JC et al. Early readmission of elderly patients with congestive heart failure. *J Am Geriatr Soc* 1990; **38:** 1290–5.

4 Ghali JK, Kadakia S, Cooper R et al. Precipitating factors leading to decompensation of heart failure. Traits among urban blacks. *Arch Intern Med* 1988; **148:** 2013–16.

5 Conn VS, Taylor SG, Kelley S. Medication regimen complexity and adherence among older adults. *J Nurs Scholar* 1991; **23:** 231–5.

6 Monane M, Bohn RL, Gurwitz JH et al. Noncompliance with congestive heart failure therapy in the elderly. *Arch Intern Med* 1994; **154:** 433–7.

7 Happ M, Naylor M, Roe-Prior P. Factors contributing to rehospitalization of elderly patients with heart failure. *J Cardiovasc Nurs* 1997; **11:** 75–84.

8 Bennett S, Huster GA, Baker SL et al. Characterization of the precipitants of hospitalization for heart failure decompensation. *Am J Crit Care* 1998; **7:** 168–74.

9 Moser DK. Heart failure management: optimal health care delivery programs. *Ann Rev Nurs Res* 2000; **18:** 91–126.

10 Yancy CW. Heart failure in African-Americans: a cardiovascular engima. *J Cardiac Fail* 2000; **6:** 183–6.

11 Richardson LG, Rocks M. Women and heart failure. *Heart Lung* 2001; **30:** 87–97.

12 Frattini E, Lindsay P, Kerr E et al. Learning needs of congestive heart failure patients. *Progr Cardiovasc Nurs* 1998; **13:** 11–6,33.

13 Jaarsma T, Haltens R, Tan F et al. Self-care and quality of life in patients with advanced heart failure: the effect of a supportive educational intervention. *Heart Lung* 2000; **29:** 319–30.

14 Knox D, Mischke L, Williams R. Heart failure patient and family education. In: *Improving Outcomes in Heart Failure*, Moser DK, Riegel B eds. Gaithersburg, MD: Aspen Publishers, Inc. 2001; 178–198.

15 Hagenhoff B, Feutz C, Conn VS et al. Patient education needs as reported by congestive heart failure patients and their nurses. *J Adv Nurs* 1994; **19:** 685–90.

16 Karlik BA, Yarcheski A. Learning needs of cardiac patients: a partial replication study. *Heart Lung* 1987; **16:** 544–51.

17 Karlik BA, Yarcheski A, Braun J et al. Learning needs of patients with angina: an extension study. *J Cardiovasc Nurs* 1990; **4:** 70–82.

18 Knowles M. *Adult Learner: the Definitive Classic in Adult Education and Human Resource Development*. Houston: Gult Publishing Company, 1998.

19 Bennett SJ, Milgrom LB, Champion V et al. Beliefs about medication and dietary compliance in people with heart failure: an instrument development study. *Heart Lung* 1997; **26:** 273–9.

20 Riegel B, Carlson B, Glaser D. Development and testing of a clinical tool measuring self-management of heart failure. *Heart Lung* 2000; **29:** 4–15.

21 Albert N. *Your Guide to Managing Heart Failure*. Cleveland, OH, Cleveland Clinic Foundation, 2001.

22 Cacciatore F, Abete P, Ferrava N et al. Congestive heart failure and cognitive impairment in an older population. Osservatorio Geriatrico Campano Study Group. *J Am Geriatr Soc* 1998; **46:** 1343–8.

23 Moser DK, Worster PL. Effect of psychosocial factors on physiologic outcomes in patients with heart failure. *J Cardiovasc Nurs* 2000; **14:** 106–15.

24 Stewart S, Pearson S, Horowitz JD. Effects of a home-based intervention among patients with congestive heart failure discharged from acute hospital care. *Arch Intern Med* 1998; **158:** 1067–72.

25 Naylor MD, Brooten D, Campbell R et al. Comprehensive discharge planning and home follow-up of hospitalized elders: a randomized clinical trial. *JAMA* 1999; **281:** 613–20.

26 Stewart S, Marley JE, Horowitz JD. Effects of a multidisciplinary, home-based intervention on unplanned readmissions and survival among patients with chronic congestive heart failure: a randomised controlled study. *Lancet* 1999; **354:** 1077–83.

27 Serxner S, Miyaji M, Jeffords J. Congestive heart failure disease management: a patient education intervention. *Congest Heart Fail* 1998; **4:** 23–8.

28 Konstam M, Dracup K, Baker DW et al. Heart failure: management of patients with left ventricular systolic dysfunction. Clinical Practice Guidelines for Clinicians No. 11. Rockville, MD: Agency for Health Care Policy and Research, Public Health Service, US Department of Health and Human Services, 1994.

29 Dunbar SB, Dracup K. Agency for health care policy and research. Clinical practice guidelines for heart failure. *J Cardiovasc Nurs* 1996; **10:** 85–8.

30 Campbell T, Patterson J. The effectiveness of family interventions in the treatment of physical illness. *J Marital Family Therapy* 1995; **21:** 545–83.

31 Morisky D, Levine DM, Green LW et al. Five year blood pressure control and mortality following health education for hypertensive patients. *Am Pub Health* 1983; **73:** 153–62.

32 Wang C, Fenske M. Self care of adults with non insulin dependent diabetes mellitus: influence of family and friends. *Diabetes Educ* 1996; **22:** 465–70.

33 Lewis F, Woods NF, Hough EE et al. The family's functioning with chronic illness in the mother: the spouse's perspective. *Soc Sci Med* 1989; **29:** 1261–9.

34 Deci E, Ryan R. *Intrinsic Motivation and Self Determination in Human Behavior*. New York: Plenum, 1985.

35 Williams G, Deci E, Ryan R. Building health-care partnerships by supporting autonomy: promoting maintained behavior change and positive health outcomes. In: Suchman A, Hinton-Walker P, Botelho R, eds. *Partnerships in Healthcare: Transforming Relational Process*. Rochester: University of Rochester Press 1998.

36 Williams G, Rodin G, Ryan R et al. Autonomous regulation and long-term medication adherence in adult outpatients. *Health Psychol* 1998; **17:** 269–76.

37 Williams G, Grow V, Freedman A. Motivational predictors of weight loss and weight loss maintenance. *J Personality Soc Psychol* 1996; **70:** 115–26.

38 Ryan R, Plant R, O'Malley S. Initial motivations for alcohol treatment: relations with patient characterisitics, treatment involvement and dropout. *Addictive Behav* 1995; **20:** 279–97.

39 Dunbar SB, Clark PC, Deaton C et al. *The effect of a family focused intervention on self management behaviors in congestive heart failure*. Atlanta, GA: Emory University: 1999.

40 Dunbar SB, Clark PC, Deaton CD, Smith A, De A. A family focused intervention improves dietary sodium consumption. *J Cardiac Failure* 2002; **8:** 5.

41 Dracup K, Moser DK, Taylor SE et al. The psychological consequences of cardiopulmonary resuscitation training for family members of patients at risk for sudden death. *Am J Pub Health* 1997; **87:** 1434–9.

42 Karmilovich S. Burden and stress associated with spousal caregiving for individuals with heart failure. *Progr Cardiovasc Nurs* 1994; **9:** 33–8.

43 Schulz R, Visintainer P, Williamson G. Psychiatric and physical morbidity effects of caregiving. *J Gerontol* 1990; **45:** P181–91.

44 Kiecolt-Glaser JK, Glaser R, Shuttleworth EC et al. Chronic stress and immunity in family caregivers of Alzheimer's disease victims. *Psychosomatic Med* 1987; **49:** 523–35.

45 Rankin SH, Stallings KD. *Patient Education: Principles and Practice*. Philadelphia: Lippincott, 2001.

46 Saarmann L, Daugherty J, Riegel B. Patient teaching to promote behavioral change. *Nurs Outlook* 2000; **48:** 281–7.

47 Prochaska JO, Redding CA, Harlow LL et al. The transtheoretical model of change and HIV prevention: a review. *Health Ed Q* 1994; **21:** 471–86.

48 Bandura A. *Self Efficacy: the Exercise of Control*. New York: WH Freeman, 1977.

49 Pearlin LI, Skaff MM, Stress and the life course: a paradigmatic alliance. *Gerontol* 1996; **36:** 239–47.

50 Janz NK, Becker MH. The health belief model: a decade later. *Health Ed Q* 1984; **11:** 1–47.

51 Pender NJ. *Health Promotion in Nursing Practice.* Stamford: Appleton and Lange, 1996.

52 NIA. *Talking with Your Doctor: a Guide for Older People.* Vol. NIH Publication No. 94–3452. Washington, DC: US Department of Health and Human Services, Public Health Services, National Institutes of Health, National Institute of Aging, 2000.

53 Riedinger MS, Dracup K, Brecht ML et al. Quality of life in patients with heart failure: do gender differences exist? *Heart Lung* 2001; **30:** 105–16.

54 Williams MV, Parker RM, Baker DW et al. Inadequate functional health literacy among patients at two public hospitals. *JAMA* 1995; **274:** 1677–82.

55 Baker DW, Parker RM, William MV et al. The health care experience of patients with low literacy. *Arch Family Med* 1996; **5:** 329–34.

56 Bennett SJ, Hays LM, Embree JL et al. Heart Messages: a tailored message intervention for improving heart failure outcomes. *J Cardiovasc Nurs*, 2000; **14:** 94–105.

57 Grady KL, Dracup K, Kennedy G et al. Team management of patients with heart failure: a statement for healthcare professionals from the Cardiovascular Nursing Council of the American Heart Association. *Circulation* (Online) 2000; **102:** 2443–56.

58 Funnell MM, Anderson RM, Arnold MS et al. Empowerment: an idea whose time has come in diabetes education. *Diabetes Educator* 1991; **17:** 37–41.

59 Janz NK. The health belief model in understanding cardiovascular risk factor reduction behaviors. *Cardiovasc Nurs*, 1988; **24:** 39–41.

18 Challenges in heart failure care for the 21st century

Susan J Bennett and Milton L Pressler

The 20th century was witness to many advances in health care – the virtual eradication of polio and smallpox, the development of effective therapies for hypertension and diabetes mellitus, development of anesthetic and surgical techniques permitting complex corrective surgeries in the tiniest newborns. Health care delivery has changed radically in the past 20 years – spurred by a desire to contain costs and reduce society's obligations to the elderly and disabled. Care has become more depersonalized, less hospital-based, but also more interdisciplinary – changes imposed by economics but with the hope of not compromising outcomes and quality of life. People are living longer but not always better; increasingly death occurs not from acute illness but after prolonged, progressive, chronic diseases associated with aging.

Heart failure is the disabled child of the new millennium – a legacy from advances made in the 20th century in coronary care, hypertension management, and treatment of acute infectious diseases. Heart failure is becoming increasingly prevalent as more people survive acute myocardial infarction[1] and live into the seventh and eighth decades of life.[2–4] Overall, 1–2% of the adult population suffers from heart failure but prevalence increases 10-fold in those over 75 years of age (Figure 18.1).[5] Identifying heart failure in the elderly is often difficult because symptoms may be unusual and comorbid conditions may obscure the diagnosis.[3] Similarly, optimal treatment in the elderly is often difficult because of the high degree of confounding medical, psychosocial, and economic factors. How we manage heart failure in the 21st century will benchmark the chronic care of the elderly and our ability to surmount the vexing issues of compliance and quality management.

Current heart failure management

Implementation of proper treatment for heart failure depends upon several interconnected elements:

- accuracy of diagnosis;
- knowledge of medications and non-pharmacologic interventions (e.g. exercise training; sodium restriction) that improve symptoms and lengthen life;
- avoidance of detrimental factors; and
- compliance with the prescribed health care plan.

On all aspects, current therapies for the management of heart failure are unsatisfactory – a case study crying out for wholesale improvement. Documentation of heart

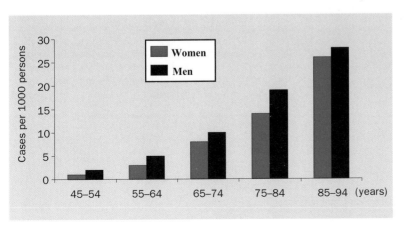

Figure 18.1. Age-related incidence of heart failure. Reprinted with permission from Kannel.[5]

failure is lacking in almost one-third of all admissions for same[6] and approximately one-half of primary care for heart failure is given to patients not meriting the diagnosis.[7,8] Medications proven to increase survival (e.g. angiotensin-converting enzyme (ACE) inhibitors, beta-blockers) are prescribed for a fraction of those diagnosed with heart failure. Dietary counsel on salt avoidance – an elementary intervention known for decades – can be documented in only 54% of patients admitted for heart failure decompensation.[6] Compliance is likewise poor for prescribed medications and lifestyle changes (e.g. smoking cessation; salt avoidance; abstinence from alcohol) – sometimes blamed on cost but often related to lack of patient education and understanding. Without improvement in systems of care delivery, heart failure will remain the number one cause for hospitalization in those over age 65.

Diagnosis for heart failure is complicated by the lack of ironclad, simple parameters to validate the clinical assessment. Signs and symptoms, e.g. fatigue, lack of energy, dyspnea on exertion, cough, weight gain, swollen legs or ankles, may be attributed to other conditions (e.g. obesity, lung disease, infirmities of aging) or conversely, those with other conditions may be falsely diagnosed with heart failure. Clinical signs, e.g. diastolic gallop (S3), cardiomegaly, jugular venous distension, end-inspiratory crackles, pleural effusion, hepatomegaly, dependent edema, may be difficult to discern or be overlooked by time-pressed practitioners. Diagnostic measures (chest X-ray, echocardiography, radionuclide ventriculography, magnetic resonance imaging) are most often inpatient- or specialty care-based and open to interpretation. Taking as an example ventricular function, left ventricular ejection fraction can range from normal to very depressed yet still be consistent with the diagnosis of heart failure. The latter condition, so-called diastolic dysfunction (Figure 18.2), accounts for perhaps one-third of patients with heart failure, is more prevalent in the elderly and those treated

in a primary care setting, and has a more favorable outlook for survival than heart failure with impaired left ventricular systolic function (ejection fraction < 45%).[9] Heart failure remains an inexact diagnosis based on the composite of relevant symptoms and signs complemented by documentation of abnormal ventricular function (either systolic, diastolic or both) or accompanying heart failure signs on chest X-ray (e.g. cardiomegaly, pleural effusion, redistribution of vascularity, interstitial infiltrates). New York Heart Association (NYHA) classes have been a rough guide to functional status and prognosis.[10]

Current pharmacologic therapies

Guidelines for the use of heart failure medications have been published and should be consulted for details of approach to dosing and follow-up care.[11–13] The discussion below gives a brief overview of prescriptive approaches for management of outpatients with chronic heart failure. Current pharmacologic therapies are directed partly at symptom relief and partly to improve survival. Market surveys have shown that symptom relief often takes precedence over length of life for many patients.[14] The first drug prescribed for many patients is a diuretic. The urgency to induce diuresis, and hence dose and route of administration, is dictated by the severity of pulmonary congestion, respiratory distress, and magnitude of peripheral edema. Once respiratory distress is relieved, excretion of accumulated salt and water should be accomplished gradually aiming at 0.5–1.5 kg weight loss/day. The target weight is based upon physical assessment of peripheral edema and the extent of prerenal azotemia. Although practice varies, the authors aim for 'trace' pretibial edema mitigated by no more than 20-fold ratio of blood urea nitrogen (BUN) to creatinine. Occasionally patients require diuresis resulting in more marked prerenal azotemia (40–50-fold ratio of BUN/creatinine) in order to resolve pulmonary congestion and respiratory distress, but

- Accounts for one-third of all heart failure
- Greater prevalence: elderly, primary care
- Lower annual mortality
  - 19% deaths/year (systolic and other heart failure)
  - 8% deaths/year (diastolic heart failure)
- Criteria for diagnosis
  - signs/symptoms of chronic heart failure
  - ~ normal systolic function (left ventricular ejection fraction > 45%)
  - abnormal left ventricular relaxation, filling, or diastolic stiffness

Figure 18.2. *Diastolic heart failure: characteristics. From the European Study Group on Diastolic Heart Failure.[9]*

this approach ought to be reserved for settings that allow for close patient monitoring and follow-up by specialists.

Another mainstay of pharmacotherapy is the initiation and titration of an ACE inhibitor, a drug class with compelling evidence for symptom relief and improvement in survival.[11–13,15] Keys to successful ACE inhibitor management include the following:

> • low initial dose (e.g. for creatinine clearance ≥ 30 ml/min, 6.25 mg tid captopril, or once daily 2.5 mg enalapril, 5 mg lisinopril, or 5 mg quinapril) to lessen the likelihood of first-dose hypotension;
> • gradual uptitration with several week (up to 2 months) intervals between dose adjustments;
> • readjustment of diuretic dose (often reduction) as edema resolves and/or systolic blood pressure lessens.

Many patients with heart failure are never given an adequate period of treatment with an ACE inhibitor. Practitioners should be wary not to automatically discontinue ACE inhibition if a patient with heart failure complains of cough but rather should search for signs of underlying pulmonary congestion (that may precipitate cough) and the need for additional diuretic. Older age (above 75 years), borderline hyperkalemia (up to 5.5 mmol/l) and significant impairment of renal function (up to creatinine of 3.0 mg/dl) should not deter implementation of ACE inhibition. However, these patients may be more sensitive – hence the initial dose and maximum tolerated dose is often less and one must be vigilant for further changes in renal function and serum potassium.

Two other drug classes with long-term survival benefit in heart failure are the beta-blockers (carvedilol, metoprolol, succinate, bisoprolol) and aldosterone antagonists (spironolactone, eplerenone). Figure 18.3 demonstrates the reproducible improvement in survival with the beta-blocker carvedilol compared with placebo plus usual care.[16] Similar to ACE inhibitors, β-blockers need to be initiated at a low dose (3.125 mg carvedilol twice daily) and uptitrated at 2-week or greater intervals to the maximum dose tolerated (depending on body weight, up to 25–50 mg carvedilol twice daily). Some patients develop worsening heart failure during initiation and uptitration of β-blocker therapy but many improve after the episode is surmounted. As with ACE inhibitors, dosages of concomitant diuretics may need readjustment (often increased) depending on congestive symptoms. Careful attention should be paid to heart rate and A–V conduction (e.g. PR interval; A–V conduction block) since β-blockade may lead to bradycardia or A–V conduction delay. Spironolactone demonstrated survival benefits among patients with severe (NYHA class IV) heart failure in the RALES trial.[17] Importantly, these patients experienced improvement in symptoms, as evidenced by a reduction in NYHA class.

Lastly, one of the older drugs used for heart failure, digoxin, may be indicated in those with more severe symptoms (NYHA class III–IV) and/or those with concomitant chronic atrial fibrillation. The DIG trial[18] demonstrated no added survival benefit in over 7000 NYHA class II–III patients but similar to two earlier trials (PROVED; RADIANCE), admission to hospital for worsening heart failure was reduced by 28% in those treated with digoxin.[19,20] Elderly patients treated with digoxin should be started on a low initial dose (0.125 mg daily) and an even lower dose employed for those with renal failure (0.125 mg every

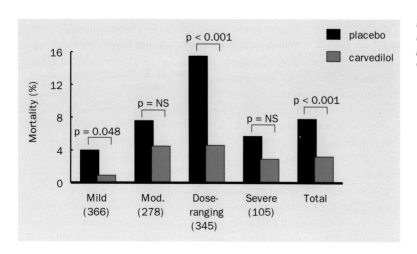

Figure 18.3. *Effect of carvedilol on mortality: US Carvedilol heart failure program (n = 1094). From Packer et al.*[16]

other day). Monitoring of serum potassium is particularly important for those patients treated with digoxin because hypokalemia can lower the threshold for digitalis toxicity. Periodic sampling of trough plasma digoxin levels can aid in dose adjustment of frail, elderly, or other higher risk patients (e.g. renal insufficiency, multisystem disorders). As with β-blockers, bradycardia or A–V conduction delay may be signs of excessive dosage of digoxin.

Non-pharmacologic management

Most non-pharmacologic interventions to manage heart failure are not as well-studied as pharmacologic interventions, but are integral to achieving improved quality of life and optimizing symptom relief when used in conjunction with appropriate medications. Patient education and behavioral change interventions are required for effective self-management in the areas of medication compliance, physical activity, nutrition, and self-monitoring of weight and edema. Psychosocial and counseling interventions are necessary in order to promote psychosocial adjustment and enhance the quality of life for patients and families.

Education and behavior change

Intensive and comprehensive education is required for patients and their caregivers to implement the required complex medical regimens and self-manage their heart failure.[21] This education should provide content about:

- complying with a complex medication regimen;
- following a low sodium and nutritionally adequate diet;
- monitoring and evaluating symptoms that indicate decompensation or worsening heart failure; and
- reducing cardiovascular risk factors through lifestyle modification.[21]

In Chapter 17, Dunbar et al present detailed descriptions of the education necessary for patients with heart failure as well as approaches to providing effective education. Many of these strategies need to be tested for effectiveness among patients with heart failure. Special learning needs of groups of patients, such as the elderly and/or patients with low literacy skills, are discussed with interventions that can be used with these groups to enhance learning.

Restrictions of sodium and fluid, particularly diets limited to 2 or 3 grams of sodium daily, have been a cornerstone of heart failure therapy, although studies have not documented the effectiveness of low sodium diets among patients with heart failure. Deficiencies of other elec-

trolytes, e.g. potassium and magnesium, often arise from diuretics employed to remedy sodium retention. Better adherence to low sodium diets might obviate some of the need for diuretics and replacement of urinary losses of potassium and magnesium. Understanding the consequences of chronic diuretic use, e.g. deficiencies of trace elements, forced swings in body volume, etc., await the development of better means of management of sodium retention above and beyond current pharmacologic and non-pharmacologic therapies. Strategies for helping patients to follow a low sodium diet are offered in Chapter 9 by Moser et al.

Moser et al offer a broader view of nutrition beyond sodium restrictions. The malnutrition that occurs in heart failure patients, i.e. cardiac cachexia, is an independent predictor of mortality.[22] Although existing data are not available about the effects of early and ongoing assessment of heart failure patients' nutritional status, one could hypothesize that close clinical assessment of nutritional status might lead to prevention or early detection of malnutrition. Interventions to assist patients in maintaining adequate caloric and protein intake as well as sodium restrictions might be associated with improved outcomes, especially if implemented early in the disease process before significant wasting occurs. Appetite enhancements – beyond aperitifs – need more study in the heart failure population. The challenge is significant because the added intake must be accomplished without further myocardial depression (as alcohol imparts) and without further compromising fluid balance.[23]

Other dietary factors (i.e. obesity, hypercholesteremia) are important components of nutrition that require intervention in some patients. Obesity can contribute to increased myocardial workload and hypertension, both of which aggravate existing failure. However, recent data suggest that obesity may confer a survival benefit in heart failure. More research is needed to clarify this issue. Recent studies[24] support links between insulin resistance, the development of diabetes mellitus, and heart failure, although more needs to be learned before guidelines can be established for clinical practice. Hypercholesteremia is now treatable with diet and medications yet studies show that this condition remains a major unsolved health care problem. Among heart failure patients, no prospective studies have been done that examined the outcomes of reducing serum cholesterol in patients with chronic heart failure. Confounding the issue is underlying coronary artery disease – for which statins have already been proven beneficial in primary and secondary prevention of ischemic events. It remains to be shown whether independent benefit for heart failure outcomes can be derived from cholesterol reduction above and beyond that related to coronary disease. Effects of new therapies directed at cholesterol transport, e.g. high-density lipoprotein elevation; reduction in oxidized low-density lipoprotein, etc., awaits the development of specific inhibitors. More basic knowledge is needed before specific interventions can be recommended as guidelines for care. Providing nutritional care by dietitians is likely to be indicated for many heart failure patients, but the cost of providing this care remains a challenge.

In Chapter 10, Adams discussed the many benefits of exercise for patients with heart failure. Despite these benefits, specific protocols are incomplete for recommending exercise and physical activity programs for patients with varying degrees of heart failure severity. Those who might need physical reconditioning the most, i.e. those with muscle atrophy, are often those with more severe heart failure and/or afflicted with other infirmities (e.g. advanced age, osteoarthritis, osteoporosis). Cardiac rehabilitation programs are available for some patients, but are not available for all patients due to barriers such as lack of financial reimbursement and lack of accessible programs in some areas. Patients with heart failure who are not candidates for cardiac rehabilitation and/or high-intensity training may still benefit from physical activity programs. Currently, we are lacking knowledge about (1) what specific physical activity recommendations to make for patients, (2) the effectiveness of low-intensity exercise or increased activities of daily living programs, and (3) the feasibility of implementing physical activity programs in busy cardiology and primary care practices.

We need attainable interventions that will help clinicians make evidence-based recommendations about physical activity and exercise programs for all patients with heart failure. These interventions could be targeted to different groups of heart failure patients depending upon their physical status and recommendations of their physician. For example, patients who are eligible for enrolment in cardiac rehabilitation based on their physical status, insurance status, and physician evaluation could be assigned to a formal program. Patients who are not eligible for cardiac rehabilitation could be enrolled in a group or home-based program tailored to their exercise needs. For some patients the exercise program might involve a walking program that advances to a specific walking distance. For patients with severe functional limitations, such a program might only involve working to maintain the patient's current functional status or increasing functional

status in minimal amounts. If these interventions were effective in improving outcomes, particularly functional status and health-related quality of life, they could be implemented in primary care settings and acute care settings with minimal cost, time, or personnel. These programs could be delivered into patients' homes by computerized methods.

Psychosocial care

Improving the psychosocial care of patients with heart failure is a priority for clinicians and researchers. A steadily expanding body of research is documenting the problems of depression and poor quality of life among heart failure patients that require specific psychosocial interventions.[24–29] Given the high mortality rates among patients with heart failure, palliative care is essential to alleviate the suffering of both patients and family caregivers.

Even though we have known for some time that patients with heart failure experience poor quality of life, the psychosocial care of these patients appears to have received less emphasis than the compliance and self-management components. This may not be true; it may be that the emphasis of research studies with multidisciplinary interventions has obscured the psychosocial care being provided to patients. It is likely that the awareness of the costly hospitalizations for patients with heart failure spurred the interest in finding strategies to decrease costs, including hospitalizations. One could argue that reducing hospitalizations improves the patient's quality of life, but until recently, there were limited data to support this view since most multidisciplinary interventions that reduced hospitalizations did not demonstrate corresponding changes in quality of life.[30,31] Recently, multidisciplinary and community-based interventions have been effective in not only reducing hospitalizations but also in improving quality of life.[32–34] Implementing these types of interventions into a variety of practice settings is now a major challenge of heart failure care.

Patients with heart failure experience higher levels of depression than healthy individuals.[27–29] The point prevalence estimates of depression among heart failure patients ranges from 17% to 37% in the literature.[27–29] Undertreatment of depression appears to be a problem that will provide challenges for clinicians to treat adequately.

In past studies, perceived social support was satisfactory among patients with heart failure.[35,36] However, there is a critical gap in our knowledge about the family caregivers of patients with heart failure. The burden imposed by other chronic disorders such as stroke leads to poor health and depression among family caregivers.[37] Given the burden associated with heart failure, it seems likely to expect that family caregivers may be experiencing problems that impede their ability to provide care and lead to poor health among the caregiver.

Even though treatment of heart failure has improved a great deal in the past two decades, we can still anticipate many deaths due to the epidemic proportions of this problem. Funk and Hudson discuss palliative care of patients and families in Chapter 14. Symptom management is a priority of palliative care; strategies are available to keep patients with endstage heart failure comfortable. Systematic methods for assessing preferences for care (for example, resuscitation, mechanical ventilation) at regular intervals are needed because patients' preferences change over time.[38] Because it is difficult to predict when death will occur in heart failure patients, and palliative care programs such as hospice care are based on prediction of time of death, Funk and Hudson advocate a new model of palliative care for patients with heart failure. Research directed toward identifying and validating such models is urgently needed.

Challenges and future advances in heart failure management

Advances in diagnosis and pharmacotherapy

For the management of heart failure patients to make a significant leap forward in the 21st century, simpler means need to be developed to identify and diagnose persons afflicted with the problem. Ventricular imaging (e.g. by echocardiography or radionuclide scans) to detect systolic or diastolic dysfunction requires special facilities and diagnostic acumen not widely available to primary care practitioners. Physical signs (diastolic gallop, inspiratory crackles) and symptoms (fatigue, exercise intolerance) of heart failure may be subtle and easily misinterpreted. Fortunately, elevation of a plasma neurohormone (brain natriuretic peptide, BNP) has been found to correlate with other measures diagnostic of heart failure.[39] Measurement of natriuretic peptides, particularly BNP, may permit easy identification of heart failure in minimally symptomatic patients.[40]

Historically, it has taken nearly a decade for significant new pharmacotherapies to emerge for the treatment of patients with heart failure. The challenge has been to prove incremental benefit in symptoms and/or length of life in the backdrop of multiple concomitant medications (e.g. ACE inhibitors, β-blockers, digoxin, diuretics,

spironolactone) and in an elderly population with multiple comorbidities. The most recent strategy for drug development has involved more specific and/or comprehensive inhibition of the renin–angiotensin–aldosterone system (e.g. angiotensin-receptor blockers ± an ACE inhibitor, ± a selective aldosterone antagonist) but also safer inotropic drugs loom on the horizon. In addition, more effective and safer treatments for comorbid conditions, e.g. arrhythmias, pulmonary hypertension, hypercholesteremia, are likely to be a topic of investigation over the next 5–10 years. In the more distant future, perhaps a decade or more away, gene transfer methods offer the hope of achieving myocardial tissue repair or regeneration and/or upregulation of the diminished contractile force of myocardial cells. Cytokines, transducers coupled to adrenergic receptors, subcellular transducers of force generation, and pathways connected with calcium release/reuptake have all been proposed as potential molecular targets needing remediation in heart failure. Many good ideas will surely fall by the wayside but one or two may provide a breakthrough that can bring patient function to a new level. While awaiting such a breakthrough, some patients may qualify for surgical alternatives (e.g. cardiac transplant, left ventricular assist devices), or benefit from ventricular pacing to achieve resynchronization.[41] Availability of viable, matched organs and high cost (> $50 000) constrain the widespread implementation of such therapies. The ultimate challenge for drug developers and practitioners alike is achieving a 'remission' in heart failure, i.e. halting the inexorable progression of symptoms and disability. In the short term, more optimum use of existing medications – understanding the best combinations, dosages, and when to initiate them – could offer tangible benefits for quality and length of life for many. An easier and more accessible diagnostic tool, e.g. plasma BNP, may enable primary caregivers to make earlier and more accurate diagnosis and thereby implement treatment before the patient has deconditioned and/or required hospitalization for decompensation. Quality of life might be easier to maintain when it has not degraded to the point of significant disability.

Advances in technology interventions

Today's rapidly expanding technology offers exciting new roles for health care professionals to design educational and behavioral change interventions that have documented efficacy and effectiveness. The internet allows people access to health care information that was previously only available to providers. People can be educated consumers of health information and true partners in care.

Three specific areas of opportunity for patient education that we can begin to address immediately are: (1) testing educational and behavioral change interventions that are targeted and/or tailored to patients' needs; (2) developing educational materials as resources for clinicians and patients to use in practice; and (3) expanding the use of technology to deliver patient care.

New strategies offer hope for delivering individualized educational interventions to large groups of patients cost-effectively. Computers now allow for the use of targeted and tailored interventions for education and behavior change. Numerous studies have documented the effectiveness of these types of communications in other groups.[42–44] Targeted interventions (designed for a specific segment of the population who share similar characteristics) and tailored interventions (based on individualized assessment of each person) have been tested in computerized formats among patients with heart failure to improve compliance with medication and dietary restrictions, reduce hospitalizations, and enhance quality of life.[45–47] Sociocultural aspects of individuals are integrated into the interventions through pictures and language to make the content more salient to the viewer.

A second challenge for the future is the urgent need for high quality educational materials designed by health care professionals that can be used with patients in multiple settings. The lack of accurate, relevant, and tested patient education materials is a major barrier to educating patients with heart failure. Individual clinicians have developed their own materials, but this is a costly process in terms of time and money and may not result in the best outcomes. The ideal would be to have materials demonstrated through research to be effective in changing behavior and improving outcomes. In addition to education materials, methods for disseminating the education cost-effectively need to be available in health care settings (hospital units, physicians' offices, clinics), including televisions with videocassette players and computer stations with internet access and color printers.

The third challenge yet to be addressed in any detail in the heart failure population is extending the delivery of care through telehealth. As technology becomes increasingly available in homes, virtual office visits can be made allowing providers to assess and treat patients while patients remain in the comfort of their homes. The Committee on Quality of Health Care in America, part of the Institute of Medicine, is recommending that 24-hour access to providers be implemented in health care systems by computerization.[48] Education can be delivered systematically and at regularly scheduled intervals with monitoring of compliance. Managing patients' symptoms might be particularly amenable to telehealth interventions. Groups of patients could be organized for a virtual support group or exercise interventions. These strategies could alleviate some of the burden of patients and caregivers traveling to clinics and offices.

In summary, we have made significant advances in heart failure care during the past century. These advances include pharmacological agents such as angiotensin-converting enzyme inhibitors, beta-adrenergic antagonists, and aldosterone antagonists (eplerenone,[49] spironolactone). The benefits of caring for these patients by multidisciplinary teams and specialized providers are now known. Challenges remain in bringing these new therapies to the practice settings where much of heart failure care is delivered. Importantly, the numbers of people with heart failure continue to climb and mortality, morbidity, and quality of life impairments remain unacceptably high. In the 21st century, the challenges are to continue to extend and improve the quality of life of these patients until heart failure can be put into complete remission.

References

1 Kannel WB, Sorlie P, McNamara PM. Prognosis after initial myocardial infarction: the Framingham study. *Am J Cardiol* 1979; **44**: 53–9.

2 Mosterd A, Hoes AW, de Bruyne MC, Deckers JW, Linker DT et al. Prevalence of heart failure and left ventricular dysfunction in the general population; the Rotterdam Study. *Eur Heart J* 1999; **20**: 447–55.

3 Rich MW. Heart failure. *Cardiol Clin* 1999; **17**: 123–35.

4 Morgan S, Smith H, Simpson I, Liddiard GS, Raphael H et al. Prevalence and clinical characteristics of left ventricular dysfunction among elderly patients in general practice settings: cross-sectional survey. *BMJ* 1999; **318**: 368–72.

5 Kannel WB. Vital epidemiologic clues in heart failure. *J Clin Epidemiol* 2000; **53**: 229–35.

6 Bennett SJ, Huster GA, Baker SL, Milgrom LB, Kirchgassner A et al. Characterization of precipitants of

hospitalization for heart failure decompensation. *Am J Crit Care* 1998; **7:** 168–74.

7   Remes J, Miettinen H, Reunanen A, Pyorala K. Validity of clinical diagnosis of heart failure in primary health care. *Eur Heart J* 1991; **12:** 315–21.

8   Cowie MR, Wood DA, Coats AJS et al. Incidence and aetiology of heart failure. A population-based study. *Eur Heart J* 1999; **20:** 421–8.

9   Working Group Report. How to diagnose diastolic heart failure. European Study Group on Diastolic Heart Failure. *Eur Heart J* 1998; **19:** 990–1003.

10 Braunwald E. *Heart Disease: A Textbook of Cardiovascular Medicine*, 4th edn. Philadelphia, PA: W.B. Saunders, 1992: 452.

11 Adams KF, Baughman KL, Dec WG, Elkayam U, Forker A et al. HFSA guidelines for the management of patients with heart failure caused by left ventricular systolic dysfunction. Pharmacological approaches (A report of the Guidelines Committee and the Executive Council of the HFSA). *J Card Fail* 1999; **5:** 357–82.

12 Hunt SA, Baker DW, Cin MH, Cinquegrani MP, Feldman AM et al. ACC/AHA guidelines for the evaluation and management of chronic heart failure in the adult: a report of the American College of Cardiology/American Heart Association Task Force on Practice Guidelines (Committee to Revise the 1995 Guidelines for the Evaluation and Management of Heart Failure). 2001. American College of Cardiology Web site. Available at: http://www.acc.org/clinical/guidelines/failure/hf_index.htm, accessed January 17, 2002.

13 The Task Force of the Working Group on Heart Failure of the European Society of Cardiology. The treatment of heart failure. *Eur Heart J* 1997; **18:** 736–53.

14 Oates MB, Stanek EJ, DeNofrio D et al. Analysis of congestive heart failure patient preferences for treatment outcomes: symptoms vs. survival. *J Am Coll Cardiol* 1999; **33:** 181a.

15 Swedberg K, Kjekshus J, Snapinn S, for the CONSENSUS investigators. Long-term survival in severe heart failure in patients treated with Enalapril. Ten year follow-up of CONSENSUS I. *Eur Heart J* 1999; **20:** 136–9.

16 Packer M, Bristow MR, Cohn JN et al, for the US Carvedilol Heart Failure Study Group. The effect of carvedilol on morbidity and mortality in patients with chronic heart failure. *N Engl J Med* 1996; **334:** 1349–55.

17 Pitt B, Zannad F, Remme WJ, Cody R, Castaigne A et al. The effect of spironolactone on morbidity and mortality in patients with severe heart failure. *N Engl J Med* 1999; **341:** 709–17.

18 DIG trial, The Digitalis Investigation Group. The effect of digoxin on mortality and morbidity in patients with heart failure. *N Engl J Med* 1997; **336:** 525–33.

19 Uretsky BF, Young JB, Shahidi FE et al. Randomized study assessing the effect of digoxin withdrawal in patients with mild to moderate chronic congestive heart failure: results of the PROVED trial. *J Am Coll Cardiol* 1993; **22:** 955–62.

20 Packer M, Gheorghiade M, Young JB et al. Withdrawal of digoxin from patients with chronic heart failure treated with angiotensin-converting enzyme inhibitors. *N Engl J Med* 1993; **329:** 1–7.

21 Grady KL, Dracup K, Kennedy G, Moser DK, Piano M et al. Team management of patients with heart failure: a statement for healthcare professionals from The Cardiovascular Nursing Council of the American Heart Association. *Circulation* 2000; **102:** 2443–56.

22 Anker SD, Ponikowski P, Varney S et al. Wasting as independent risk factor for mortality in chronic heart failure. *Lancet* 1997; **349:** 1050–3.

23 Goldberg IJ, Mosca L, Piano MR, Fisher EA. Nutrition Committee, Council on Epidemiology and Prevention, and Council on Cardiovascular Nursing of the American Heart Association. AHA Science Advisory: Wine and your heart: a science advisory for healthcare professionals from the Nutrition Committee, Council on Epidemiology and Prevention, and Council on Cardiovascular Nursing of the American Heart Association. *Circulation* 2001; **103:** 472–5.

24 Swan JW, Anker SD, Walton C, Godsland IF, Clark AL et al. Insulin resistance in chronic heart failure: relation to severity and etiology of heart failure. *JACC* 1997; **30:** 527–32.

25 Dracup K, Walden JA, Stevenson LLW, Brecht M. Quality of life in patients with advanced heart failure. *J Heart Lung Transplant* 1992; **11:** 273–9.

26 Konstam V, Salem D, Pouleur H et al. Baseline quality of life as a predictor of mortality and hospitalization in 5,025 patients with congestive heart failure. *Am J Cardiol* 1996; **78:** 890–5.

27 Freedland KE, Carney RM, Rich MW, Caracciolo A, Krotenberg JA et al. Depression in elderly patients with congestive heart failure. *J Psychiatric Gerontol* 1991; **24:** 59–71.

28 Freedland KE, Carney RM. Psychosocial considerations in elderly patients with heart failure. *Clin Geriatr Med* 2000; **16:** 649–61.

29 Koenig HG. Depression in hospitalized older patients with congestive heart failure. *General Hospital Psychiatry* 1998; **20:** 29–43.

30 Rich MW. Heart failure disease management: a critical review. *J Card Fail* 1999; **5:** 64–75.

31 McAlister FA, Lawson FME, Teo KK, Armstrong PW. A systematic review of randomized trials of disease management programs in heart failure. *Am J Med* 2001; **110:** 378–84.

32 Moser DK, Moser DK, Mack MJ, Worster P. Community case management decreases rehospitalization rates and costs, improves quality of life in heart failure patients with preserved and non-preserved left ventricular function: a randomized controlled trial. *Circulation*, 2000; **102:** II740.

33 Naylor MD, Brooten D, Campbell R et al. Comprehensive discharge planning and home follow-up of hospitalized elders: a randomized clinical trial. *JAMA* 1999; **281:** 613–20.

34 Riegel B, Carlson B, Kopp Z, LePetri B, Unger A, Glaser D. Effect of a standardized nurse case management telephone intervention on resource use in chronic heart failure patients. *Arch Internal Med* 2002; **162:** 705–12.

35 Friedman M, King KB. The relationship of emotional and tangible support to psychological well-being among older women with heart failure. *Res Nurs Health* 1994; **17:** 433–40.

36 Bennett SJ, Perkins SM, Lane KA, Deer M, Brater DC, Murray MD. Social support and health-related quality of life in chronic heart failure patients. *Quality Life Res* 2001; **10:** 671–82.

37 Bakas T, Burgener S. Prediction of emotional distress, general health, and caregiving outcomes in family caregivers of stroke survivors. *Topics Stroke Rehab* 2002; **9:** 34–45.

38 Krumholz HM, Phillips RS, Hamel MB et al. Resuscitation preferences among patients with severe congestive heart failure: results from the SUPPORT project. *Circulation* 1997; **126:** 97–106.

39 Maisel A. B-type natriuretic peptide levels: a potential novel 'white count' for congestive heart failure. *J Cardiac Failure* 2001; **7:** 183–93.

40 McDonagh TA. Asymptomatic left ventricular dysfunction in the community. *Curr Cardiol Rep* 2000; **2:** 470–4.

41 Abraham WT, Fisher WG, Smith AL et al. Multicenter InSync Randomized Clinical Evaluation (MIRACLE): results of a randomized, double-blind, controlled trial to assess cardiac resynchronization therapy in heart failure patients. *Circulation* 2001; **104:** 2921a.

42 Skinner CS, Campbell MK, Rimer BK, Curry S, Procheska JO. How effective is tailored print communication? *Ann Behav Med* 1999; **21:** 290–8.

43 De Vries H, Brug J. Computer-tailored interventions motivating people to adopt health promoting behaviours: introduction to a new approach. *Patient Educ Couns* 1999; **36:** 99–105.

44 Krueter M, Farrell D, Olevitch L, Brennan L. *Tailoring health messages*. Mahwah, NJ: Lawrence Erlbaum Associates, 2000.

45 Bennett SJ, Hays LM, Embree J, Arnould M. Heart messages: a tailored message intervention for improving heart failure outcomes. *J Cardiovasc Nurs* 2000; **14:** 94–105.

46 Riegel B, Carlson B, Glaser D, Kopp Z, Romero T. Standardized telephonic case management in a Hispanic heart failure population. An effective intervention *Dis Manage Health Outcomes* 2002; **10:** 421–9.

47 Linne AB, Liedholm H, Israelsson B. Effects of systematic education on heart failure patients' knowledge after 6 months. A randomized, controlled trial. *Eur Heart J* 1999; **1:** 219–27.

48 Committee on Quality Health Care in America, Institute of Medicine. Crossing the quality chasm: a new health system for the 21st century. Washington, DC: National Academy Press, 2001.

49 Pitt B, Remme W, Zannad F et al. Eplerenone, a selective aldosterone blocker, in patients with left ventricular dysfunction after myocardial infarction. *NEJM* 2003; **348:** 1309–21.

Index